phenomenology and treatment of
ALCOHOLISM

phenomenology and treatment of ALCOHOLISM

Edited by

William E. Fann, M.D.,
Ismet Karacan, M.D., (Med) D.Sc.,
Alex D. Pokorny, M.D.
and
Robert L. Williams, M.D.
all of the Department of Psychiatry,
Baylor College of Medicine,
Houston, Texas

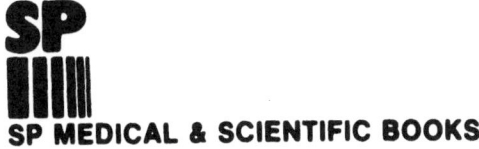

SP MEDICAL & SCIENTIFIC BOOKS

New York • London

SPECTRUM PUBLICATIONS, INC.
175-20 Wexford Terrace, Jamaica, N.Y. 11432

Library of Congress Cataloging in Publication Data

Main entry under title:

Phenomenology and treatment of alcoholism.

   Includes index.
   1. Alcoholism—Addresses, essays, lectures.   I. Fann, William E.
RC565.P45   616.8′61   79-23224

ISBN-13: 978-94-011-7711-5   e-ISBN-13: 978-94-011-7709-2
DOI: 10.1007/978-94-011-7709-2

Acknowledgments

The following pharmaceutical manufacturers provided partial financial support of the symposium from which this volume was developed:

Boehringer-Ingelheim Ltd.
Endo Laboratories
McNeil Laboratories
Merrell National Laboratories
Pfizer Laboratories
Sandoz Pharmaceuticals
Schering Corporation
Smith Kline & French Laboratories

The editors and conference participants are most grateful to these organizations for their valuable assistance and for their dedication to the continuing education of physicians and other health care professionals.

Additional thanks are due Dr. David Mumford, Mrs. Margaret Klug and the staff of Baylor College of Medicine's Office of Continuing Education; Nancy L. Berry, who prepared the manuscript; and Bruce W. Richman, M.A., Assistant Professor of Scientific Communication in Baylor's Department of Psychiatry, who has served as managing editor of all the volumes in the Baylor Psychiatry Series.

Contributors

HAROLD ALTSHULER, Ph.D.
Associate Professor
Dept. of Pharmacology
Baylor College of Medicine
Chief, Neuropsychopharmacology
Texas Research Institute of Mental Sciences
Houston, Texas

STANLEY APPEL, M.D.
Professor & Chairman
Dept. of Neurology
Baylor College of Medicine
Houston, Texas

LAUREN BOEHME, B.A.
Psychosomatic Research Laboratory
Veterans Administration Hospital
Houston, Texas

G. LaVONNE BROWN, M.D.
Biological Psychiatry Branch
National Institute of Mental Health
Bethesda, Maryland

NANCY E. DAWSON, B.S.
Psychosomatic Research Laboratory
Veterans Administration Hospital
Houston, Texas

DONALD I. DAVIS, M.D.
Assistant Professor
Dept. of Psychiatry and Behavioral Science
Director, Family Therapy Program
George Washington University Medical
  Center
Washington, D.C.

SABRIT DERMAN, M.D., Ph.D.
Assistant Professor
Department of Psychiatry
Baylor College of Medicine
Houston, Texas

MICHAEL H. EBERT, M.D.
Laboratory of Clinical Science
National Institute of Mental Health
Bethesda, Maryland

JOHN A. EWING, M.D.
Professor of Psychiatry
Director, UNC Center for Alcohol Studies
University of North Carolina School of
  Medicine
Chapel Hill, North Carolina

WILLIAM E. FANN, M.D.
Department of Psychiatry
Baylor College of Medicine
Chief, Psychiatry Service
Veterans Administration Medical Center
Houston, Texas

DONALD GOODWIN, M.D.
Professor & Chairman
Department of Psychiatry
University of Kansas Medical Center
Kansas City, Kansas

PETER HARTOCOLLIS, M.D., Ph.D.
Medical Director
C.F. Menninger Memorial Hospital
Associate Clinical Professor of Psychiatry
University of Kansas School of Medicine
Topeka Institute of Psychoanalysis
Menninger School of Psychiatry
Topeka, Kansas

PITSA C. HARTOCOLLIS, Ph.D.
Menninger School of Psychiatry
Topeka, Kansas

ROBERT G. M. JOHNSTON,
  M.B., B.Ch., M.P.H.
Medical Director, Day Hospital
Veterans Administration Hospital
Assistant Professor
Department of Psychiatry
Brown University School of Medicine
Providence, Rhode Island

THOMAS E. KANAS, MSW
Research Assistant Professor of Social Work
Dept. of Psychiatry
Baylor College of Medicine
Psychiatric Social Worker
Veterans Administration Hospital
Houston, Texas

HOWARD KAPLAN, Ph.D.
Professor of Sociology
Dept. of Psychiatry
Baylor College of Medicine
Houston, Texas

ISMET KARACAN, M.D. (Med) D.Sc.
Professor of Psychiatry
Baylor College of Medicine
Associate Chief of Staff for Research
Veterans Administration Hospital
Houston, Texas

DAVID C. KAY, M.D.
NIDA Addiction Research Center
Lexington, Kentucky

MARTIN KEELER, M.D.
Professor of Psychiatry
Baylor College of Medicine
Director of Alcoholism Treatment
Veterans Administration Hospital
Houston, Texas

DAVID W. KRUEGER, M.D.
Assistant Professor
Department of Psychiatry
Baylor College of Medicine
Houston, Texas

C. RAYMOND LAKE, Ph.D., M.D.
Assistant Professor of Psychiatry
Uniformed Services Medical School
Bethesda, Maryland

JOHN M. LENNON, B.A., B.S.
Psychosomatic Research Laboratory
Veterans Administration Hospital
Houston, Texas

F. LESLIE MAJOR, M.D.
Clinical Neuropharmacology Branch
National Institute of Mental Health
Bethesda, Maryland

DEMMIE MAYFIELD, M.D.
Professor of Psychiatry
University of Kansas Medical Center
Chief, Psychiatry Service
Veterans Administration Hospital
Kansas City, Missouri

ROY B. MEFFERD, Ph.D.
Professor of Physiology
Departments of Psychiatry and Physiology
Baylor College of Medicine
Director, Psychosomatic Research
   Laboratory
Veterans Administration Hospital
Houston, Texas

E. MANSELL PATTISON, M.D.
Professor & Chairman
Departments of Psychiatry and
   Health Behavior
Medical College of Georgia
Augusta, Georgia

ALEX D. POKORNY, M.D.
Professor and Vice Chairman
Department of Psychiatry
Baylor College of Medicine
Houston, Texas

HENRY ROSETT, M.D.
Associate Professor
Department of Psychiatry
Boston University School of Medicine
Director, Prenatal Clinic
Maternal Health and Child Development
   Program
Boston City Hospital
Boston, Massachusetts

PATRICIA J. SALIS, M.S.
Research Assistant Professor
Dept. of Psychiatry
Baylor College of Medicine
Houston, Texas

MARC A. SCHUCKIT, M.D.
Professor of Psychiatry
University of California at San Diego
School of Medicine
Director, Alcoholism Research
Veterans Administration Hospital
San Diego, California

REGINALD SMART, Ph.D.
Addiction Research Foundation
Toronto, Ontario
Canada

SCOTT SNYDER, M.D.
Research Fellow
Department of Psychiatry
Baylor College of Medicine
Houston, Texas

LYNN WEINER
Dept. of Psychiatry
Boston University School of Medicine
Boston, Massachusetts

CHARLES L. WHITFIELD, M.D.
Associate Professor of Medicine
Assistant Professor of Psychiatry
Director, Alcohol and Drug Abuse
   Education
NIH Career Teacher in Drug Abuse
University of Maryland School of Medicine
Baltimore, Maryland

ROBERT L. WILLIAMS, M.D.
D.C. and Irene Professor and Chairman
Department of Psychiatry
Baylor College of Medicine
Houston, Texas

MICHAEL G. ZIEGLER, M.D.
Assistant Professor
Department of Pharmacology
University of Texas Medical Branch
Galveston, Texas

Foreword

Phenomenology and Treatment of Alcoholism is the fourth in a series of texts on the major psychiatric disorders developed by the Department of Psychiatry at Baylor College of Medicine in Houston. Like the previous three volumes on depression, schizophrenia, and anxiety, this text represents the proceedings of a two day symposium conducted by Baylor. Psychiatrists and other physicians and scientists who have made major contributions to the field of study were invited to discuss important aspects of their work with a large group of other medical professionals. Questions of definition, diagnosis, and clinical management were addressed with a degree of specificity and detail not normally found in general psychiatric texts nor in books presenting an individual outlook or treatment approach.

More than most other psychiatric ailments, alcoholism generates considerable interest among the general medical profession. Psychosis and affective disorders are clearly and specifically within the province of the psychiatrist. Neurotic disorders are often treated by the primary care practitioner in their more moderate manifestations, but by psychiatrists when they reach their most malignant stages. Alcoholism, on the other hand, is confronted by virtually every medical practitioner, whether generalist or specialist.

Alcoholism is among the most prevalent and difficult disorders afflicting human beings. It may exist discretely, as a precipitant, or as a complication of other major diseases, intruding upon virtually every physiological and psychological symptom complex. The family or general practitioner will often be the first medical professional to perceive and attempt intervention in a "drinking problem." Psychiatrists will often see alcohol abuse or dependency in the context of underlying affective, psychotic, or characterological disorders. The internist will usually be responsible for managing medical detoxification of the advanced alcoholic, and for treating organ systems impaired by alcohol. Neurologists are asked to deal with the physiological effects of alcohol on the brain and nervous system tissues. Even surgeons and anesthesiologists must confront problems of alcoholism when their clinical options are limited or complicated by the disease.

Although this volume treats issues in alcoholism primarily as psychiatric concerns, we have valuable contributions from neurologists such as Dr. Appel, internists such as Dr. Whitfield, and social scientists such as Drs. Kaplan and Smart, as well as Dr. Altshuler, a basic scientist, Dr. Mefferd, a physiologist, and Dr. Lake and his group of pharmacologists. Among the contributing psychiatrists, the subspecialties of psychoanalysis, psychopharmacology, gerontology, family therapy, epidemiology, clinical science, and hospital practice are represented here. We compiled the work of leading thinkers and clinicians in so many disciplines in order to approach the medical aspects of alcoholism from as many fronts as are necessary to demonstrate the complexity of the ailment and to solve the problems of definition and treatment which are resistant to individual modalities. As Drs. Ewing, Mayfield, and Pattison attest in their chapters, alcoholism is a disease system with biological, psychological, and social implications, and the proper understanding and intervention must account for them all.

William E. Fann, M.D.
Ismet Karacan, M.D., D.Sc.
Alex D. Pokorny, M.D.
Robert L. Williams, M.D.

Contents

CHAPTER 1

Biopsychosocial Approaches
to Drinking and Alcoholism

JOHN A. EWING

INTRODUCTION

All physical disease and malfunctioning have psychological aspects as well as social and biomedical components. Thus, only a viewpoint that is truly "biopsychosocial" can provide an adequate position from which to take a holistic view of illness. Therefore, I invite you to look at all drinking and alcoholism from a biopsychosocial viewpoint. Indeed, we must see alcoholism as a biopsychosocial disease.

FOUR FACTORS

There are four major groups of factors that can be identified as important in any approach to alcoholism. These are illustrated in Figure 1. As the central part of the figure indicates, alcoholism is the final outcome of problems with beverage alcohol and I will say no more about that since Dr. Pokorny will review stages in the development of alcoholism. The four factors illustrated must not be thought of as independent. For example, social factors affect availability since a society that wishes easy access to alcohol will eventually get it. Similarly, the psychological make-up of individuals contributes to aspects of society and social forces provide major components in the development of the personality of each

1

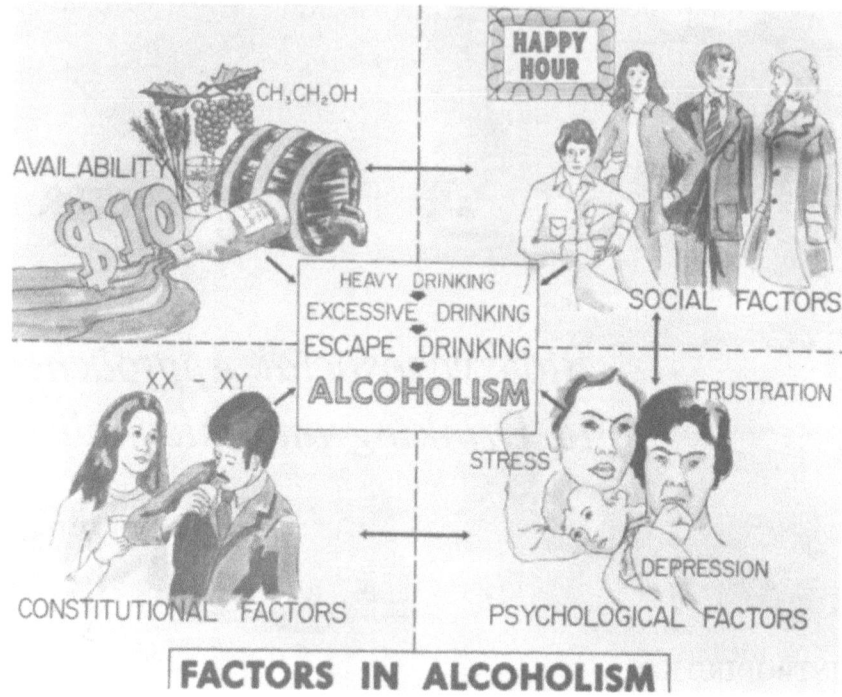

Figure 1.

individual. Constitutional and psychological factors are also interdependent with the personality, reflecting, to a considerable extent, the constitutional endowment inherited by the individual. Each of these four factors must be seen as contributing, more or less, toward the drinking habits of any individual and toward the development of alcoholism in any instance. Indeed, it is my objective to demonstrate how these factors can provide both predisposing and protecting forces.

AVAILABILITY

In most societies today alcohol is relatively freely available but government controls, representing the wishes of the people, vary from country to country. In addition to determining who may manufacture and who may sell alcoholic beverages, governments control who may purchase and who may consume. The almost universal appeal of alcoholic beverages (for instance, about 72% of adults in the U.S.A. consume alcoholic beverages at least once a year) leads governments to see beverage

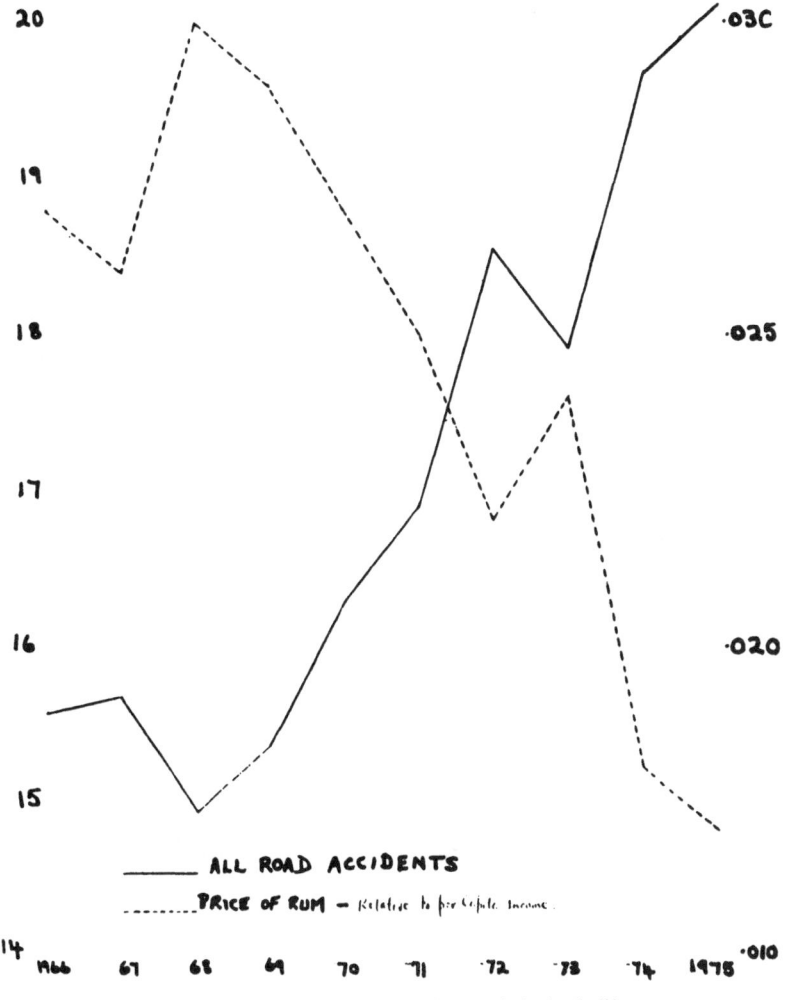

ALL ROAD ACCIDENTS
PRICE OF RUM — Relative to per Capita Income.

FROM: Beaubrun, M.H., "Epidemiological Research in the Caribbean
Context Road Accidents and the Price of Rum in Trinidad & Tobago 1966-1975."
Paper presented at Addiction Research Foundation Seminar on International
Collaboration, Toronto, 1977.

Figure 2.

taxes as an important source of revenue. However, there is always the
danger that crippling levels of taxation will increase motivation for the
illegal manufacture and distribution of alcoholic beverages.[1]

I am indebted to Professor Michael Beaubrun of Trinidad for the next
illustration which demonstrates traffic accidents on the Island of Trinidad
relative to the price of rum, the preferred drink there.

In 1968 tax increases raised the price of rum between 5 and 10%. A

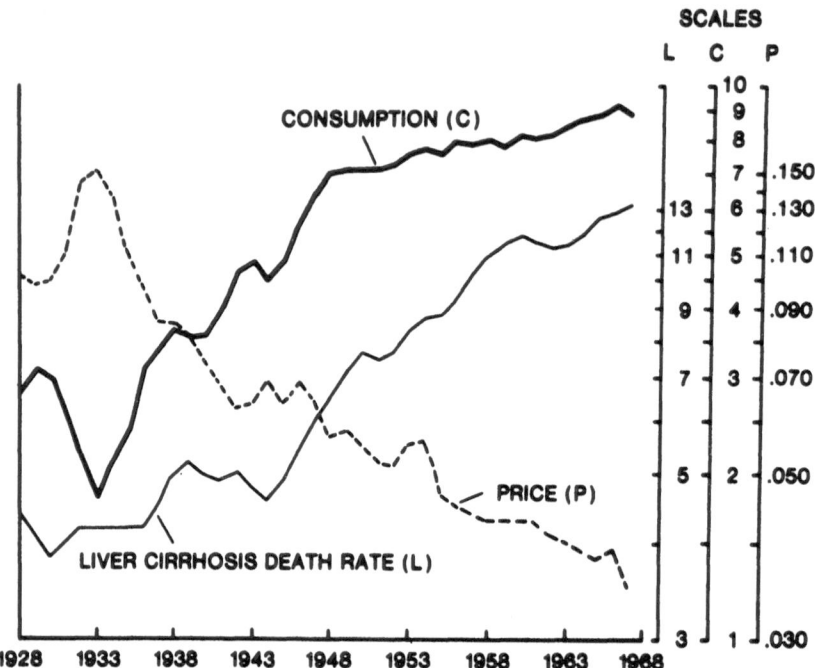

Figure 14-1. Alcohol price and consumption and liver cirrhosis death rates, Ontario, 1928-1967.

Ewing, J.A. & Rouse, B.A. <u>Drinking, Alcohol in American Society-Issues and Current Research.</u> Nelson-Hall Publishers, Chicago, IL 1978.

Figure 3.

similar increase occurred in 1972 with a 10 to 20% rise. The 1974 increase was due to the price being raised by the distillers. However, because of inflation the relative price of rum has been going down fairly steadily in spite of these recorded increases. Professor Beaubrun has used the relative price of rum to predict the number of highway accidents. For example, he told his fellow members of the Trinidad Senate that highway accidents would reach 20,500 in 1975. In fact, they went to 20,550!

The significance of price is also demonstrated in Figure 3 showing that as price diminishes relative to spendable income, consumption and cases of liver cirrhosis rise. In the chapter of our recently published book, *Drinking,* our colleagues from the Addiction Research Foundation of

Ontario make a case for trying to stabilize the cost of alcoholic beverages relative to disposable income and the price of other commodities.[2]

Current statistics indicate that about one out of every twelve drinkers becomes an alcoholic. Researchers should concern themselves about the eleven of twelve drinkers who do *not* develop alcoholism. What are the forces that protect such people? Undoubtedly they involve all four factors.

SOCIOCULTURAL FACTORS

Now, let us take a look at some of the social and cultural influences that impinge upon us. Advertisements frequently carry the theme that it is "smart," "cultured," "sexy" and "attractive" to drink. In addition magazines, radio, television and films carry overt as well as subtle messages about drinking. A recent study showed that many of the soap operas watched by millions of American housewives portray a great deal of drinking.[3]

The makers of alcoholic beverages claim that the advertising campaigns they sponsor merely change the preference of the consumer from one brand to another. I have never seen any proof of this and we are entitled to wonder if the preference is being changed from nonalcoholic to alcoholic beverages, but whether or not this is correct remains to be demonstrated. The impact of advertising and similar social pressures relative to alcohol need to be studied in some depth.

TABLE 1.

SOCIAL CLASS AND AMOUNT OF DRINKING

SOCIAL CLASS*	ABSTAINERS AND LIGHT	MODERATE	MEDIUM-HEAVY	HEAVY
UPPER (1 AND 2)	38%	52%	66%	74%
MIDDLE (3)	31%	33%	30%	17%
LOWER (4 AND 5)	31%	15%	4%	9%

$$\chi^2 = 16.64 \qquad p < 0.02$$

*HOLLINGSHEAD'S 2 FACTOR INDEX

Table 1 demonstrates drinking practices among male undergraduate students at an American university.[4] As can be seen, there is a correlation between social class and drinking with the heaviest drinking occurring in those of upper social class. This appears to represent not just a social class factor but also an economic one in that the students from the upper income homes have more money to spend. Spare funds tend to be spent on recreational activities including drinking of alcoholic beverages. Students at the university have the choice of living in university dormitories or lodging in private homes or in a fraternity. Most fraternities have a reputation for giving parties at which alcoholic beverages flow freely and, indeed, an abstainer who joined a fraternity would be under much pressure to learn to drink. Thus, those who enter fraternities must be presumed to be intending to drink alcoholic beverages.

As Table 2 shows we could find no total abstainers, and very few light drinkers, who belonged to fraternities.[4]

TABLE 2.

PLACE OF RESIDENCE AND AMOUNT OF DRINKING

RESIDENCE	ABSTAINERS	LIGHT	MODERATE	MEDIUM-HEAVY	HEAVY
DORMITORY	80%	64%	55%	48%	28%
FRATERNITY	--	4%	24%	26%	39%
PRIVATE	20%	32%	21%	26%	33%

In the same study we asked people their reasons for drinking. As can be seen from Table 3 the more people drink the more reasons they give for drinking. The reasons themselves are either personal (to relax; to feel good) or social (to celebrate; because others are drinking).

TABLE 3.

REASONS FOR DRINKING BY QUANTITY GROUPS

MAIN REASONS GIVEN	PERCENTAGE OF GROUP MAKING STATEMENT:			
	LIGHT	MODERATE	MEDIUM-HEAVY	HEAVY
TO CELEBRATE	77%	94%	100%	100%
TO RELAX	64%	67%	70%	85%
BECAUSE OTHERS ARE DRINKING	55%	73%	63%	72%
BECAUSE I LIKE THE TASTE	55%	85%	96%	83%
TO FEEL GOOD	45%	85%	78%	89%

PSYCHOLOGICAL FACTORS

Now, let us go to psychological factors. Very many psychological studies of alcoholism have been carried out, although to date there has been no clear demonstration of a "pre-alcoholic personality." Three examples will suffice here.

David McClelland, a Harvard professor of psychology, has studied drinking in social drinkers as well as alcoholics. His methods are detailed in his book and there is no way that I can adequately present them at this time.[5] However, one finding is worthy of note.

Socialized power as represented in Figure 4 refers to feelings of well-being and well-wishing toward one's fellowmen. On the other hand,

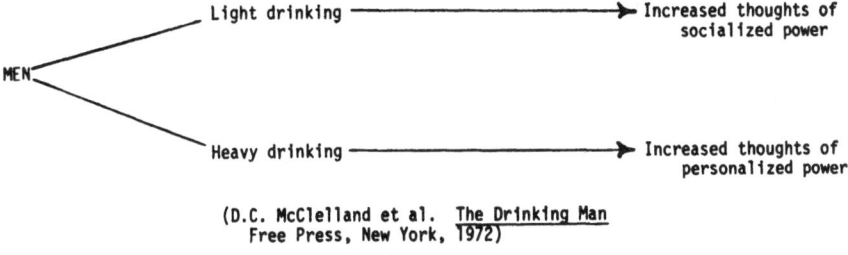

Light drinking ⟶ Increased thoughts of socialized power

MEN

Heavy drinking ⟶ Increased thoughts of personalized power

(D.C. McClelland et al. The Drinking Man
Free Press, New York, 1972)

Figure 4.

personalized power refers to competitiveness and how the individual can do things to benefit himself. Heavy drinking appears to promote these feelings which may provide an escape from inner conflict, particularly in males who have doubts about themselves as masculine figures.

Sharon Wilsnack was a student who worked with McClelland and in her studies (summarized in Fig. 5) she has demonstrated a similar resolution of conflicts in females, with drinking helping them to feel "more feminine" should there be doubts and conflicts about this role hidden within their personality.[6] A substance that can resolve inner conflicts in this way is a powerful drug indeed, and we can begin to understand why there will be psychological needs to experience this conflict resolution again and again.

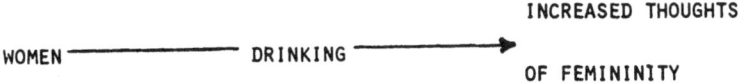

INCREASED THOUGHTS

WOMEN ⟶ DRINKING ⟶

OF FEMININITY

(S.C. WILSNACK, PSYCHOLOGY TODAY
APRIL, 1973)

Figure 5.

As another example Marlatt and his colleagues have explored the role of frustration of aggression and drinking.[7] Again, their methodology is too complex to be detailed at this time but their results are important.

Experimental subjects who received an insult were compared with those who received no insult and others who were insulted but had an opportunity to retaliate within the experimental design. In this study the subjects clearly differentiated themselves when it came to drinking after these experimental manipulations had occurred. The insulted subjects drank more than the controls, whereas those who had an opportunity to deal with their emotions drank less.

The implication of this work is summarized in Figure 6 which suggests that, in states of frustrated aggression, individuals, whether social drinkers

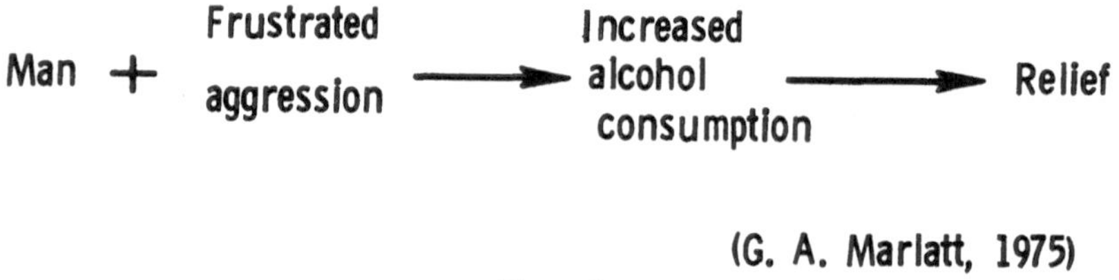

Man + Frustrated aggression ⟶ Increased alcohol consumption ⟶ Relief

(G. A. Marlatt, 1975)

Figure 6.

or alcoholics, may be more likely to turn to alcohol. Indeed, this has therapeutic implications for alcoholism since patients who are trying to remain totally abstinent may need to find other ways of dealing with pent-up emotions. In this area, assertiveness training can be helpful.

BIOLOGICAL FACTORS

During this decade a series of studies has indicated a high probability that there is some inheritable quality that increases the risk for alcoholism.

Twin studies have suggested a case for nature over nurture as have half-sibling researches. Now, a series of adoption studies beginning with that performed by Goodwin et al. provides strong positive evidence for a biological factor.[8]

Goodwin and colleagues studied 55 adoptees who had been born to an alcoholic parent and compared them with 78 who were also adopted but did not have an alcoholic parent.[8] They themselves, their adoptive families and the psychiatrist who interviewed them were not aware of the history of alcoholism or absence of alcoholism in the biological parent.

The results of that study showed a significantly greater probability of complications of heavy drinking and alcoholism appearing in those who had a biological parent with alcoholism even though that parent had no

TABLE 4.

CHILDHOOD DIFFERENCES

	ALCOHOLICS N=14	NON-ALCOHOLICS N=119
BELOW AVERAGE SCHOOL PERFORMANCE	43	15
HYPERACTIVE	50	15
OFTEN TRUANT OR ANTISOCIAL	21	2
COMBINATION OF ABOVE	57	15
SHY, SENSITIVE, INSECURE	64	20
AGGRESSIVE, IMPULSIVE, HOT TEMPERED	50	18
OFTEN DISOBEDIENT	29	4

participation in the rearing of the child. Since this study was published some other family studies have appeared with equally significant positive results.[9-11]

In addition, from Sweden comes a study indicating a greater probability for alcoholism developing, at least after the age of 35, in men whose grandfathers were alcoholics.[12]

Table 4 reminds us that personality and behavior are a reflection, in part, of inherited characteristics. It represents the childhood characteristics as defined by school teachers of those men in the Danish study who later became alcoholics compared with those who did not.[13] All of the characteristics, listed by incidence percentage, differentiated the two groups with statistical significance. They represent the pre-alcoholic child as being restless, concentrating poorly, showing impulsive and even aggressive behavior while at the same time having significant interpersonal problems. Indeed, the list is reminiscent of the features seen in children who are diagnosed as suffering from hyperactivity or the hyperkinesia syndrome. Is it possible that such children have inherited some physiologic characteristics, probably within the central nervous system, that make them more liable to have problems with alcohol if they drink? Some corroborative and affirmative information comes from a recent study by Tarter and his colleagues who divided a clinical population of alcoholics into those with "primary alcoholism" as opposed to those perceived as "secondary."[14]

TABLE 5.

Criteria for Classification as Primary Alcoholics

A. No known precipitating cause for excessive drinking plus at least 6 of the
   following:
B. 1. Increased alcohol tolerance
   2. Withdrawal symptoms
   3. Euphoria after first drinking experience
   4. Euphoria with first drink following
      period of abstinence
   5. No history of social drinking
   6. Abnormal drinking before age 40
   7. Problems from alcohol before age 40
   8. Loss of control

From: Tarter et al., Arch. Gen. Psychiatry,
      34:761-768, 1977.

The primary alcoholics had no known precipitating cause for the onset
of the excessive drinking plus at least six of these eight listed
characteristics in Table 5. Secondary alcoholics, on the other hand, tended
to have developed alcoholism later in life. Their history did not meet the
listed criteria.

When Tarter and colleagues looked at the childhood characteristics of
the primary alcoholics they found no fewer than twelve items that
significantly differentiated these alcoholics from the secondary alcoholics
as well as from control groups of psychiatric patients and nonpatients as
shown in Table 6. The features listed here are remarkably similar to those
identified as childhood characteristics of the Danish adoptee alcoholics.
Cadoret and Gath also noted an association between "childhood socialized
conduct disorder" and adult alcoholism in their adoption study.[11] Of
course, we are a long way from understanding what biological mechanism
might lie behind this, but the evidence strongly suggests that a biological
predisposition does exist.

In some of our studies we have taken healthy normal drinkers and
explored the possible role of the sympathetic nervous system in terms of

TABLE 6.

12 Items in Childhood History Significantly Differentiating Primary Alcoholics from Secondary Alcoholics, Psychiatric Patients and Healthy Controls

Childhood Characteristic

1. Daydreaming	7. Can't accept correction
2. Feeling left out	8. Poor handwriting
3. Impulsivity	9. Short attention span
4. Working below ability	10. Fidgeting
5. Easily frustrated	11. Doesn't complete projects
6. Can't sit still	12. Overactive

From: Tarter et al., Arch. Gen. Psychiatry
34:761-768, 1977.

alcohol euphoria or stimulation.[15] Before our subjects have done any drinking we have taken a blood sample for later determination of the level of dopamine beta-hydroxylase (DBH), the enzyme responsible for the production of noradrenaline from dopamine. In one series of three separate studies we obtained the same results.

Subjects falling into the lower quartile (in terms of DBH levels) had a different kind of response compared with those from the upper quartile after both groups had taken identical quantities of alcohol. In brief, the lower group felt more drunk and sick whereas the upper group felt more stimulated or euphoric (see Table 7). In another study where free drinking was allowed over a period of several hours, subjects differentiated themselves by the amount they chose to drink and, therefore, by the blood levels of alcohol achieved.[16]

Again, these results were in the same direction, with the subjects whose DBH levels fell above the mean choosing to drink more, presumably because they got more enjoyment from drinking (see Table 8).

We are continuing to study this aspect of man's use of alcohol, but in yet another study we had our results significantly confounded by a social factor, as far as we can determine. Briefly, we invited subjects to come with

TABLE 7.

UPPER AND LOWER QUARTILES IN TERMS OF DBH ACTIVITY AND CORRESPONDING BLOOD ALCOHOL AND MOOD LEVELS

	LOW DBH GROUP (N=9) (6♂ 3♀)	HIGH DBH GROUP (N=9) (6♂ 3♀)
RANGE OF DBH VALUES	0-7.51	20.7-31.8
BLOOD ALCOHOL CONCENTRATION	66±39mg%	62±46mg%
FINAL MOOD SCORE (MEANS)		
BEST EVER FELT	62.4	74.2***
MOST DRUNK	66.1	52.0**
MOST SICK	34.0	20.1*

*** $P < .025$

** $P < .10$

* $P < .05$

a spouse or a friend and found that under these conditions the social factors appeared to overshadow the biological ones.[16]

ANIMAL RESEARCH

Some supporting evidence for the role of the noradrenergic system in the mediation of ethanol response is provided in animal studies that have been recently reported. Experimental rats treated with drugs to inhibit the activity of DBH have been shown, under these conditions, to reduce their voluntary intake of ethanol significantly.[17]

Other important animal studies also point to the presence of a significant biological factor behind alcohol use. Two examples will suffice.

Figure 7 represents my interpretation of work done by Ahtee and Eriksson at the Research Laboratories of the State Alcohol Monopoly of Finland.[18] By outbreeding rats they have produced those that drink alcohol readily in preference to other fluids, and others that avoid alcohol. Significant differences in brain levels of serotonin and dopamine were demonstrated. Here, then, we have a biological difference that reflects behavior relative to the drinking of alcohol.

TABLE 8.

BLOOD ALCOHOL LEVELS AND DRINKS CONSUMED BY 14 SUBJECTS WHO REMAINED TO DRINK BEYOND 2 HOURS, IN TERMS OF LEVEL OF DBH ACTIVITY

	LOW DBH GROUP (N=7) (3♂ 4♀)	HIGH DBH GROUP (N=7) (6♂ 1♀)
RANGE OF DBH VALUES	5.3-28.8	38.1-92.9
FINAL BLOOD ALCOHOL CONCENTRATION (MEAN)	66MG%	131MG%**
AVERAGE NUMBER OF DRINKS	5.43	9.58*

**$P < .025$

* $P < .05$

Early in this decade it was suggested that alkaloids found in plants (such as the opium poppy) might be elaborated within the human body by a mechanism involving the combination of naturally occurring substances with the first metabolic breakdown product of alcohol, acetaldehyde.[19,20] Since then, animal studies have shown that such substances can be identified as occurring within the living brain under certain conditions.[21,22] Now, in a recent series of animal studies Myers and his colleagues have shown that the injection of incredibly small amounts of these substances into the brains of animals can significantly alter their alcohol intake.[23,24]

Injected animals voluntarily select amounts of alcohol sufficient to cause the development of tolerance and a withdrawal reaction on cessation of drinking. Equally important, such animals, after prolonged abstinence from alcohol, have been shown to return to that drinking pattern once the opportunity is provided without further injections. The implication is that some permanent change has occurred within the brain of these animals that influences their behavior relative to alcohol. Such experiments lead us to speculate that there may be humans who accumulate these chemicals within the brain on ingesting alcohol, thereafter experiencing a craving to drink more alcohol. The persistence of the effect in the experimental rat is reminiscent of the popular concept, "Once an alcoholic always an

From Ahtee and Eriksson 1975*

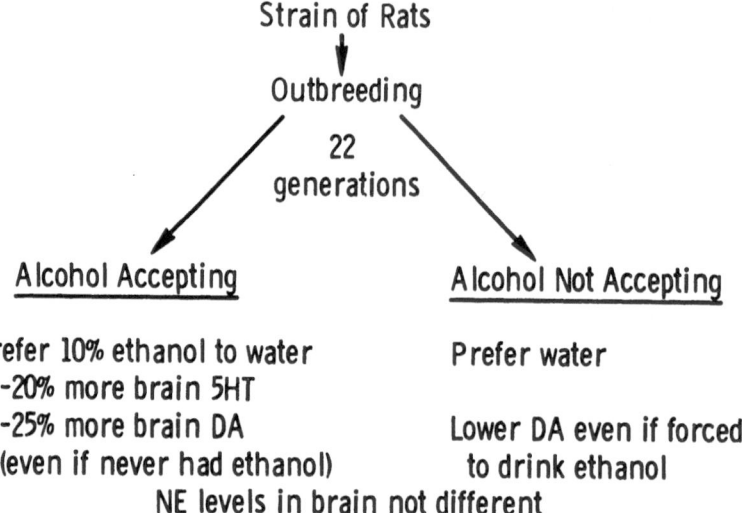

Strain of Rats

Outbreeding

22
generations

Alcohol Accepting   Alcohol Not Accepting

Prefer 10% ethanol to water   Prefer water
15-20% more brain 5HT
15-25% more brain DA   Lower DA even if forced
(even if never had ethanol)   to drink ethanol
NE levels in brain not different

* Acta Physiol. Scand. 93:563-565.

Figure 7.

alcoholic." The work being done by Myers has exciting implications for the biomedical aspect of alcoholism and invites research workers to elucidate this mechanism in detail as well as to look for possible antidotes.

RACIAL DIFFERENCES

One possible protecting factor with a biological basis is the hypersensitivity or flushing reaction to alcohol that is found among a majority of

SCHEME FOR OXIDATION OF ETHANOL IN THE LIVER

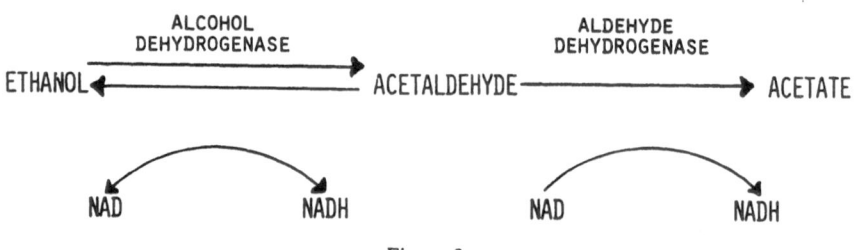

Figure 8.

Oriental subjects that have been studied so far. This is interesting since there is evidence that alcoholism prevalence rates in the Orient fall below the rates found in most parts of the world.[25,26] Even a small quantity of alcohol can be sufficient to produce a reaction within 15 minutes after swallowing it. The face often becomes flushed and the individual feels a sense of intoxication.

Our studies have demonstrated significantly greater heart rate increases in Orientals who have swallowed alcohol compared with people of European descent. In addition, subjective feelings of these groups differ. Pounding in the head is reported only by Orientals whereas the sensations of feeling relaxed, confident and happy are significantly more reported by the non-Orientals.

Figure 8 shows that when alcohol is metabolized the very reactive chemical acetaldehyde is produced as an intermediate metabolite.

In one study we looked at levels of acetaldehyde in the blood of our subjects. There are methodological and technical problems in measuring blood levels and, although the Orientals had somewhat higher levels of acetaldehyde, these did not reach statistical significance.[27] However, more

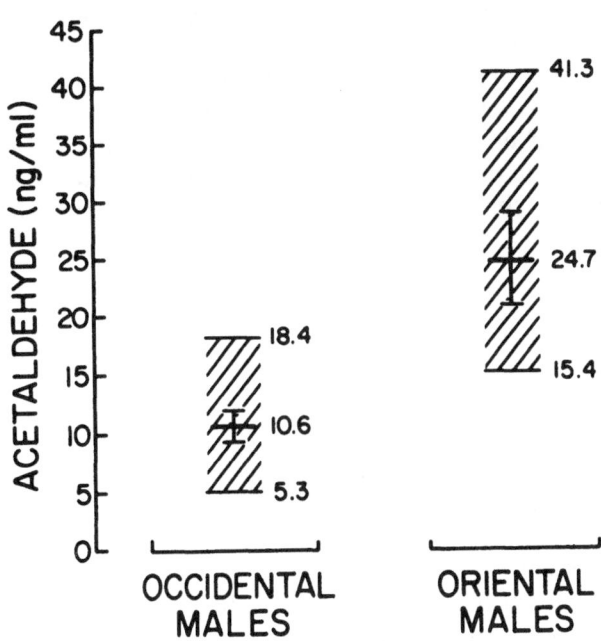

BREATH ACETALDEHYDE RANGES, MEANS
AND STANDARD ERRORS IN 2 RACIAL GROUPS

Figure 9.

recently I have been giving alcohol intravenously to subjects of various races and, with the use of a portable gas chromatograph have been able to analyze the breath of the subjects for acetaldehyde.

Alveolar breath is analyzed immediately, and, as shown in Figure 9 we have evidence that the levels found in our Oriental subjects are significantly higher than in non-Orientals.[28] Thus, although further details of this phenomenon must be elucidated, it is reasonable to say at the present time that the Oriental sensitivity to alcohol appears to involve acetaldehyde toxicity. About three quarters of all Oriental subjects studied so far have a different type of the liver enzyme that is involved in the breakdown of alcohol. This "atypical" liver alcohol dehydrogenase was first identified by von Wartburg[29] who has more recently suggested that it should be called the "Oriental" enzyme.[30] It seems likely that this very active enzyme, when present in an Oriental subject who receives alcohol, leads to the rapid release of acetaldehyde in the circulation and produces the sensitivity response. Since the response is not perceived as a desirable or pleasant one by most subjects and, indeed, some feel quite ill with it, it becomes understandable that such individuals are less liable to drink alcohol to excess. It would be possible to provide other examples of predisposing and protecting factors under the headings of availability, sociocultural, psychological and biomedical areas. However, space does not permit this and it is also evident that future studies in a variety of disciplines will begin to provide more and more examples. All workers in alcoholism whether themselves biologically, psychologically, or socially oriented should keep each of the other factors in mind. Another important point is that each of us in whatever discipline should strive to look for factors pushing people toward, as well as away from alcohol use and abuse. In other words, the concept of identifying predisposing and protecting forces is essential.

SUMMARY AND CONCLUSIONS

Table 9 summarizes my paper by giving examples of predisposing and protecting components under each of the four factor areas. Under availability we have the issues of access and price. Under sociocultural factors we have the attitudes within the society and the drinking practices of peers. Psychological factors of a predisposing nature include problems with frustration and power and sexual roles. However, some individuals are protected by an inner need to feel in control of themselves and of course a relative freedom from conflicts can also be beneficial. Under biomedical factors the first issue is whether alcohol produces discomfort or a relief of

TABLE 9.

Predisposing and Protecting Factors in Alcohol Use and Abuse

FACTOR	PREDISPOSING EXAMPLES	PROTECTING EXAMPLES
AVAILABILTY of beverage alcohol	Easy access; Cheap price	Controlled access; High price
SOCIO-CULTURAL factors	Attitudes encouraging heavy drinking; Heavy drinking by peers	Attitudes discouraging heavy drinking; Light drinking by peers
PSYCHOLOGICAL factors	Problems with feelings of aggression and frustration; Conflicts over power and sexual roles	Inner need to feel in control of self; Relative freedom from conflicts
BIOMEDICAL factors	Relief of discomfort by alcohol; Tendency for alcohol to be stimulating and produce euphoria	Discomfort produced by alcohol; Tendency for alcohol to be depressing and produce dysphoria

discomfort. In addition, as I have already demonstrated, there is the question of whether alcohol produces what the individual perceives as "desirable" feelings or "undesirable" ones.

I hope that this paper has convincingly demonstrated why only a holistic biopsychosocial approach can provide an adequate understanding of alcohol use and abuse.

ACKNOWLEDGMENTS

I am grateful to numerous colleagues for collaboration. Their names appear as coauthors in the reference list. Essential services have also been provided by various technicians and secretaries Elva DeBoy and Elaine Woody.

REFERENCES

1. Ewing, J.A., and Rouse, B.A. *Drinking: Alcohol in American Society—Issues and Current Research.* Chicago: Nelson-Hall, 1978.
2. Popham, R. Schmidt, W., and de Lint, J. Government control measures to prevent hazardous drinking, Chapter 14 in Ewing, J.A. and Rouse, B.A. (eds.), *Drinking: Alcohol in American Society—Issues and Current Research.* Chicago: Nelson-Hall, 1978.
3. Garlington, W.K. Drinking on television; a preliminary study with emphasis on method. *J. Stud. on Alcohol* 38:2199-2205, 1977.
4. Ewing, J.A., Rouse, B.A., and Bakewell, W.E. Alcohol use in a student population. Presented at 29th International Congress on Alcoholism and Drug Dependence, Sydney, NSW, Australia, Feb. 6, 1970; Rouse, B.A., and Ewing, J.A. College drinking and other drug use, Chapter 11 in Ewing, J.A., and Rouse, B.A. (eds.), *Drinking: Alcohol in American Society—Issues and Current Research.* Chicago: Nelson-Hall, 1978.
5. McClelland, D.C., Davis, W.N., Kalin, R., and Wanner E. *The Drinking Man.* New York: The Free Press, 1972.
6. Wilsnack, S.C. Femininity by the bottle. *Psychol. Today,* April 1973, p. 39.
7. Marlatt, G.A., Kosturn, C.F., and Long, A.R. Provocation to anger and opportunity for retaliation as determinants of alcohol consumption in social drinkers. *J. Abnormal. Psych.* 84:652-659, 1975.
8. Goodwin, D.W., Schulsinger, F., Hermansen, L., Guze, S.B., and Winokur, G. Alcohol problems in adoptees raised apart from their alcoholic biological parents. *Arch. Gen. Psychiat.* 28:238-243, 1973.
9. Hill, S.Y., Cloninger, C.R., and Ayre, F.R. Independent familial transmission of alcoholism and opiate abuse. *Alcoholism: Clin. Exper. Res.* 1:335-342, 1977.
10. Bohman, M. Some genetic aspects of alcoholism and criminality—a population of adoptees. *Arch. Gen. Psychiat.* 35:269-276, 1978.
11. Cadoret, R.J., and Gath, A. Inheritance of alcoholism in adoptees. *Brit. J. Psychiat.* 132:252-258, 1978.
12. Kaij, L., and Dock, J. Grandsons of alcoholics: a test of sex-linked transmission of alcohol abuse. *Arch. Gen. Psychiat.* 32:1379-1381, 1975.
13. Goodwin, D.W., Schulsinger, F., Hermansen, L., Guze, S.B., and Winokur, G. Alcoholism and the hyperactive child syndrome. *J. Nerv. Ment. Dis.* 160:349-353, 1975.
14. Tarter, R.E., McBride, H., Buonpane, N., and Schneider, D.U. Differentiation of alcoholics: childhood history of minimal brain dysfunction, family history and drinking pattern. *Arch. Gen. Psychiat.* 34:761-768, 1977.
15. Ewing, J.A., Rouse, B.A., and Mueller, R.A. Alcohol susceptibility and plasma dopamine *B*-hydroxylase activity. *Research Commun. Chem. Path. and Pharmacol.* 8:551-554, 1974.
16. Ewing, J.A., Rouse, B.A., and Mills, K.C. Dopamine *B*-hydroxylase activity as a predictor of response to alcohol. *Japan J. Stud. Alc.* 10:61-69, 1975; Ewing, J.A., Rouse, B.A., Mueller, R.A., and Mills, K.C. Alcohol as a euphoriant drug: searching for a neurochemical basis. *Ann. N.Y. Acad. Sciences* 27:159-166, 1976.
17. Amit, Z., Brown, W., Levitan, D.E., and Ogren, S.O. Noradrenergic mediation of the positive reinforcing properties of ethanol: 1. Suppression of ethanol consumption in laboratory rats following dopamine-beta-hydroxylase inhibition. *Arch. Internat. Pharmacodyn. Ther.* 230:65-75, 1977.
18. Ahtee, L., and Eriksson, K. Dopamine and noradrenaline content in the brain of rat strains selected for their alcohol intake. *Acta. Physiol. Scand.* 93:563-565, 1975.
19. Davis, V.E., and Walsh, M.J. Alcohol, amines and alkaloids: a possible biochemical basis for alcohol addiction. *Science* 167:1005-1007, 1970.

20. Cohen, G., and Collins, M. Alkaloids from catecholomines in adrenal tissue: possible role in alcoholism. *Science* 167:1749–1751, 1970.

21. Turner, A.J., Baker, K.M., Algeri, S., Frigerio, A., and Garattini, S. Tetrahydropapaveroline: formation *in vivo* and *in vitro* in rat brain. *Life Sci.* 14:2247–2257, 1974.

22. Collins, M.A., and Bigdeli, M.G. Tetrahydroisoquinolines *in vivo:* rat brain formation of salsolinol, a condensation product of dopamine and acetaldehyde, under certain conditions during ethanol intoxication. *Life Sci.* 16:585–601, 1975.

23. Myers, R.D., and Melchior, C.L. Alcohol drinking: abnormal intake caused by tetrahydropapaveroline in brain. *Science* 196:554–556, 1977.

24. Myers, R.D. Tetrahydroisoquinolines in the brain: the basis of an animal model of alcoholism. *Alcoholism: Clin. Exper. Res.* 2:145–154, 1978.

25. Barnett, M.L. Alcoholism in the Cantonese of New York City, in Diethelm, O. (ed.) *Etiology of Chronic Alcoholism.* Springfield, Ill.: Charles C. Thomas, 1955, p. 179.

26. Singer K. Drinking patterns and alcoholism in the Chinese. *Brit. J. Addict.* 67:3–14, 1972.

27. Ewing, J.A., Rouse, B.A., and Pellizzari, E.D. Alcohol sensitivity and ethnic background. *Am. J. Psychiat.* 131:206–210, 1974.

28. Ewing, J.A., Rouse, B.A., and Aderhold, R.M. Studies of the mechanism of Oriental hypersensitivity to alcohol, in Galanter, M. (ed.), *Currents in Alcoholism.* V:45–52, 1979.

29. Von Wartburg, J.P., Papenberg, J., and Aebi, H. An atypical human alcohol dehydrogenase. *Canad. J. Biochem.* 43:889–898, 1965.

30. Von Wartburg, J.P. Personal communication, April, 1975.

CHAPTER 2

The Pharmacology Of Alcohol: Some Clinical Aspects

DONALD W. GOODWIN

Entire books have been written about the pharmacology of alcohol and new information on the subject continues to flood the journals. This chapter is confined to certain aspects of the pharmacology of alcohol which appear to have clinical relevance.

First, however, a word or two about where it all begins: with yeast.

When yeast grows in sugar solutions without air, most of the sugar is converted (fermented) into carbon dioxide and alcohol. When the alcohol concentration reaches about 12 or 13%, the process stops. This is why unfortified wines have alcohol concentrations of no more than 12 or 13%.

As a rule, people do not drink just alcohol. They drink alcoholic beverages. Alcoholic beverages are mostly water and ethyl alcohol. Tiny amounts of other chemicals are present, providing most of the taste and smell and all of the color, if any. Called congeners, these chemicals include amino acids, minerals, vitamins, methanol, and the "higher" alcohols, know as fusel oil.[1]

Beverages differ according to the sugar source: from grapes, wine; from grain and hops, beer; from grain and corn, whiskey; from sugarcane, rum; from the potato, vodka.

Man discovered distillation about 800 AD in Arabia (alcohol comes from the Arabic *alkuhl,* meaning essence). Distillation boils away alcohol from its sugar bath and recollects it as virtually pure alcohol. The water is then put back, so that instead of 100% alcohol, the result is, perhaps, 50% alcohol or 100 proof alcohol (percent being one-half of proof).

ALCOHOL'S FATE IN THE BODY

What happens to alcohol when you drink it? Essentially the same thing that happens if you don't drink it. It turns to vinegar. When alcohol sours in open air, bacteria are responsible. To become vinegar (acetic acid) in the body, two enzymes are required: alcohol dehydrogenase (ADH) and aldehyde dehydrogenase (AldDH).

The first is located in the liver in surprisingly large supply. Surprisingly because, as far as we know, alcohol dehydrogenase does nothing except metabolize alcohol. A minute amount of ethyl alcohol is produced in the gastrointestinal tract by bacteria, and perhaps this accounts for alcohol dehydrogenase in the liver. Infinitesimal amounts of alcohol may also be produced by normal metabolic processes in the body. If these sources are the reason the alcohol enzyme is present in such large quantity, it is clearly a case of biologic overkill. It disposes of 86 proof distilled spirits at about the rate of one ounce per hour. Fed into the body's normal metabolic machinery, acetic acid becomes carbon dioxide and water, burning or storing 7 cal/g of alcohol.

Between alcohol and acetic acid, there is an intermediate step, which is why a second enzyme is required. The intermediate chemical is an aldehyde and very toxic. The enzyme that destroys the aldehyde is found not just in the liver but throughout the body. It quickly turns the aldehyde into harmless acetic acid. This enzyme, aldehyde dehydrogenase, is inhibited by disulfiram (Antabuse). This results in an accumulation of acetaldehyde and a toxic reaction characterized mainly by vasodilation and hypotension.

Alcohol is almost entirely oxidized in the liver. A small amount is expired in the breath and excreted in urine and sweat. In the oxidation of alcohol, two molecules of nicotinamide adenine dinucleotide (NAD) are changed to reduced NADH.

$$\text{C}_1\text{H}_5\text{OH} + \text{DPN} \xrightarrow{\quad\text{ADH}\quad} \text{CH}_3\text{CHO} + \text{DPNH}$$

$$\text{CH}_3\text{CHO} + \text{DPN} \xrightarrow{\quad\text{AldDH}\quad} \text{CH}_3\text{COOH} + \text{DPNH}$$

Vinegar may be harmless, but how it is produced may not be. In being oxidized, alcohol is stripped of hydrogen atoms, which must go somewhere. Where they go results in some interesting biochemical changes that may or may not be harmless (Fig. 1).[2] Here are some:

1. There is an increase in lactic acid. This is interesting because increased lactic acid has been associated with anxiety attacks, and heavy drinking is also associated with anxiety attacks.
2. There is an increase in uric acid. This is interesting because increased uric acid is associated with gout, and gout, for centuries, with alcohol.
3. There is an increase in fat—not the slow increase that comes from calories (those 7 cal/g) but a rapid increase from the oxidation of alcohol. The fat is seen mainly in the liver or blood. One night of serious drinking—say, six or seven highballs—discernibly increases the fat content of the liver. The liver will be fattier still if fatty food is eaten.[3]

Is a fatty liver bad? Admittedly it doesn't sound good, but on the other hand, the connection between fatty liver and liver diseases, such as hepatitis and cirrhosis, is undetermined. For one thing, the fat goes away soon after the drinker stops drinking. Also, most people drink but most do not develop liver disease. Among those very heavy drinkers called alcoholics, perhaps only 5 or 10% develop liver disease. On the other hand, most people who develop a particular type of liver disease, Laennec's cirrhosis, are heavy drinkers.

Many disorders connected with heavy drinking are believed to be due to malnutrition, but this may not be true of cirrhosis. Laennec's cirrhosis has been produced in well-nourished baboons after 4 years of drunkenness.[4] Most of the drunk baboons, however, only developed a fatty liver, and controversy still thrives about whether alcohol alone causes cirrhosis. Obviously it doesn't in everybody.

Intoxicating amounts of alcohol increase fat in the bloodstream. In high enough dose, particularly combined with a fatty meal, alcohol may even produce visible fat in the blood (chylomicrons).

It is possible, of course, that the so-called medical complications of alcoholism are not due to alcohol at all. Alcoholics are almost universally heavy smokers and many are malnourished. Even alcoholics who have a normal dietary intake may have nutritional deficiencies, because alcohol in large quantities inhibits the absorption of amino acids, vitamins, and other nutrients. Damage to the nervous system associated with alcoholism— e.g., peripheral neuropathy, Wernicke-Korsakoff encephalopathy, cerebellar degeneration—is almost definitely related to vitamin deficiency, particularly vitamins of the B group.[5] There is no direct evidence that alcohol alone, in the amounts consumed by even alcoholic individuals, damages the brain.

Many things have been tried—insulin, caffeine, exercise—to speed up the elimination of alcohol. Fructose in large doses does this, but the dose is so large it is sickening, and most people prefer to stay drunk.[5]

Alcohol behaves similarly to water, travels everywhere that water travels, and, because of its waterlike properties, can be accommodated by the body in vastly greater amounts than any other drug. A person's blood can consist of one-half of one percent alcohol without producing death or even unconsciousness.

THE EFFECTS OF ALCOHOL

The effects of alcohol do not depend on how much a person drinks, but on how much gets into the bloodstream. This in turn depends on many things.

1. Some alcohol is absorbed through the stomach wall but most reaches the bloodstream through the small intestine.
2. For rapid absorption, it is important that alcohol reach the small intestine in the highest possible concentration in the shortest possible time. People who have had their pyloric valve removed surgically, as for ulcers, find they get drunk faster than previously.
3. Other factors affecting absorption include the presence of food in the stomach and the type of beverage. With the same amount of alcohol consumed over the same length of time, the blood alcohol concentration may vary greatly. Gin on an empty stomach has a far different effect from beer combined with a meal.

In addition to how much alcohol is in the blood, it matters how quickly the alcohol is absorbed. In general, the faster the rate of absorption, the more striking the effect. Also, as alcohol remains in the blood over longer periods, its effects become less. In practical terms, if you make five errors per minute while typing sober, you may make 15 errors per minute while typing with X blood alcohol concentration after one hour of drinking, but only seven errors at the same X concentration after five hours of drinking.

In general, people feel better getting drunk than they do sobering up. That is, as the blood alcohol level climbs from A to B to C, a person may feel euphoric at B and C, but as the blood level falls from C to B to A, not only is there no euphoria at B, but the person feels discomfort, presaging the hangover to come at A. This "slope" effect is closely related to and hard to separate from the duration effect. As people drink more over days, months, and years, they gradually need to drink more to obtain the same effect. The importance of "tolerance," however, is often exaggerated. A seasoned alcoholic at the prime of his drinking capacity may be able to drink, at most, twice more than a teetotaler of similar age and health. Compared to tolerance for morphine, which may be manifold, tolerance for alcohol is modest.

More striking than "acquired" tolerance may be inborn tolerance. Individuals vary widely in the amount of alcohol they can tolerate, independent of drinking experience. Some people cannot drink more than a small amount of alcohol without developing a headache, sick stomach, or dizziness. They rarely become alcoholic but deserve no special credit: they just can't drink much.

Differences in tolerance for alcohol apply not only to individuals, but to racial groups. For example, some Oriental groups develop flushing of the skin, sometimes with nausea, after drinking a little alcohol.[7] Alcoholism is rare in these groups.

Tolerance is reversible. People who have had encephalitis, brain tumors, or other damage to the brain commonly experience at least a temporary decrease in tolerance for alcohol. Alcoholics, after many years of heavy drinking, also may lose tolerance as they grow older. Older people, in general, have less tolerance for alcohol than do younger people.

Any drug response that involves thinking and mood is bound to be influenced by expectation (set). If a person believes alcohol will improve his mood, diminish fatigue, or make him feel sexy, the chances of these occurring may be improved. If he believes alcohol will make him sleepy or produce a headache, these also may occur.

Set is linked to setting. Where is the person drinking? With whom? If he enjoys the people he is with, he may also enjoy the alcohol more. If the occasion is a celebration, a drink may have a livelier effect than would the same amount taken routinely before dinner.

Alcohol is said to make people talk louder, and it often seems true. On the other hand, two men in a duck blind, having a little bourbon to warm up, may talk more softly than usual.

THE "FOUR STAGES" OF INTOXICATION

There is an old saying that alcohol affects a person in four ways. First, he becomes jocose, then bellicose, then lachrymose, and finally comatose.

Comatose he does indeed become, if he drinks enough, but the other three stages are not all that inevitable. Some people hardly feel jocose at all. Many become argumentative and some combative, but these responses are strongly influenced by social circumstances. The legendary barroom fight usually occurs in lower class bars. Countless parties are held nightly in middle class suburbia, and although drinking is common, fighting is not.

One of the paradoxes about alcohol is that people do cry sometimes when they drink. They become anxious and depressed. This challenges the assumption that people drink mainly to feel less anxious and depressed. The motives for drinking are complex, with no single explanation sufficing.

Alcohol is often described as a "depressant" drug that depresses first the "higher" centers in the brain and then downwardly anesthetizes the "lower" centers until finally, in lethal dosage, it snuffs out life itself by depressing the respiratory center at the base of the brain. This is an oversimplification.

What is alcohol "depressing"? Many people get a lift from alcohol and become animated and energetic. Nerve fibers fire about as readily in an alcohol solution as they do otherwise, unless the concentration is far above what most people can drink. It is sometimes said that by depressing the "higher" centers of the brain, alcohol releases the "lower," and this is why people are more animated or uninhibited when they drink. The problem is that studies do not support the top-to-bottom action of alcohol. Coordination, a "lower" function, often is impaired at lower doses of alcohol than is memory, a "higher" function.[8]

Dosage is crucial. Alcohol in rather small doses improves certain types of performance, perhaps because it reduces anxiety. Apparently this is most likely to occur in activities where the person is not very proficient. If he does poorly hitting the target on a firing range, he may improve somewhat after several drinks of alcohol. On the other hand, if he does well normally, his performance may fall off after small amounts of alcohol. Nevertheless, in moderate-to-high amounts, alcohol generally diminishes function across the board. Alcohol has been shown (in cats, at any rate) to dampen activity of the reticular formation before it does other areas of the brain, and this may be the reason.

An interesting exception to the above has emerged in several recent studies. If a person learns certain things while intoxicated—even severely intoxicated—he will remember them better when reintoxicated than when sober, a phenomenon that has been well demonstrated in man as well as animals.[9] Called state-dependent learning, this is one of the few exceptions to the overall impairing effect of alcohol at moderate and high doses.

Alcohol does something else almost unique among drugs. It produces a classic amnesia called blackout. While drinking, the drinker does highly memorable things and cannot remember them the next day. Many social drinkers have had this experience, but it occurs most frequently in alcoholics.[10]

These are mental effects. There are also physical effects which should be mentioned, if only because there are misconceptions about them.

1. It is known that alcohol increases urination by inhibiting antidiuretic hormone. It is generally not known that the increase is temporary, and that after a fairly short period of drinking, the need to urinate decreases.
2. It is commonly believed that alcohol causes dehydration. It does not. When a person has a dry mouth and thirst after an evening of drinking, it may be due partly to the astringent effect of alcohol on the mucous membranes of the mouth. If anything, heavy drinkers may be slightly overhydrated because of the large volume of fluid they consume.
3. It is generally known that alcohol produces a feeling of bodily warmth and, therefore, is just the thing for St. Bernards to carry around their necks in casks and to have at a frosty football game. Alcohol produces a feeling of warmth because it dilates blood vessels in the skin, which is why some drinkers have red noses. However, the warmth is subjective and can be harmfully illusionary. A person's resistance to the effects of severe cold, such as frostbite, in no way is increased by alcohol, although the victim may temporarily think it is.

WHEN ALCOHOL IS CONTRAINDICATED

Alcohol is contraindicated in alcoholism. Follow-up studies indicate that a small proportion of individuals diagnosed as alcoholic return to "normal" drinking for extended periods, but the consensus is that this occurs rarely and that total abstinence is the best policy for most alcoholics. Temporary abstinence is well-nigh obligatory, if only because it is almost impossible to diagnose other psychiatric and sometimes medical conditions when a person is intoxicated or during withdrawal.

Epileptics probably should not drink, or if they do so, with caution and moderation. Drinking is related to an increased frequency of seizures in epileptics.[11] There is no evidence that alcohol causes epilepsy, although grand mal seizures (rum fits) may occur during withdrawal.

Since antiquity, alcohol has been associated with gout. There is evidence that alcohol does indeed increase blood levels of uric acid but only at high blood alcohol levels, and even then the increase is slight. Patients with gout can probably drink moderately with no ill effects. It may be well to avoid large amounts of beer, since beer is rich in purines.

Ever since Beaumont gave alcohol to his gastrostomized patient Alexis St. Martin, a century and a half ago, it has been recognized that alcohol produces inflammation of the gastric mucosa. However, more recent studies indicate that the inflammation disappears after continued use of alcohol.[12] Nevertheless, there is general agreement that patients with gastritis, gastric cancer, and bleeding in the upper digestive tract should not drink.

There is less agreement about whether a patient with gastric and duodenal ulcers should drink. There seems no question that alcohol stimulates acid secretion in the same manner as that produced by histamine, the secretion being rich in acid and low in pepsin. There is also evidence that alcohol produces changes in the mucosal barrier of the stomach that might predispose to ulcers. On the other hand, there is no convincing evidence that ingestion of alcohol alone causes gastric mucosal hemorrhage in man. One investigator found that peptic ulcer was diagnosed in only 5% of 430 consecutive alcoholics surveyed for symptoms of peptic ulcer.[13] This incidence is comparable to the 5 to 10% lifetime incidence of peptic ulcer in the general population. Therefore, whether an ulcer patient is discouraged from drinking depends on the patient and his physician. If alcohol produces local irritation, then he will probably abstain without any advice. Some physicians encourage modest use of alcohol on the grounds that it has a tranquilizing effect. In addition, alcohol reduces hunger contractions, at least in dogs. In view of these factors, no definitive advice can be given.

With regard to alcohol and coronary artery disease, a "fact" accepted by physicians since Heberden's days—namely, that alcohol was good for heart patients and relieved angina pectoris—has recently been challenged by studies in man and animals indicating that alcohol reduces cardiac contractility and may indeed be contraindicated in patients with heart disease. This may occur for a number of reasons, one being that ethanol increases osmolarity of the serum and extracellular fluid, which, in turn, leads to a loss of electrolytes from cardiac muscle cells. On the other hand, alcohol in modest amounts has been prescribed to cardiac patients for a long time, and there is no direct evidence that it increases the incidence of myocardial infarction or cardiac failure. The effect of alcohol on the heart is usually dose related. There is certainly no absolute contraindication against heart patients using alcohol in small amounts.

During withdrawal from heavy drinking, the blood pressure is commonly elevated. However, alcohol apparently does not produce chronic hypertension and because of the tranquilizing effects from alcohol, it may indeed have a kind of phenobarbital effect on blood pressure and lower it slightly.

Alcohol is definitely contraindicated in pancreatitis.

The role of alcohol in liver disease, even with respect to the three liver diseases associated with alcoholism (fatty liver, alcoholic hepatitis, and portal cirrhosis), remains controversial. No one questions that patients with acute hepatitis should abstain from alcohol. The disagreement arises from the question, "How long should they abstain after laboratory tests and other indicators of the disease have returned to normal?" Some clinicians believe they should abstain practically forever, particularly if alcohol appears to be the prime offender. Others believe it makes little difference. One investigator reported that patients consuming large amounts of alcohol during convalescence after acute hepatitis showed no more evidence of posthepatitic liver damage than did those who drank little or no alcohol.[14] Since recurring bouts of alcoholic hepatitis may result in irreversible cirrhosis, the question is hardly trivial, but the clinician must base his advise on evidence that is less than conclusive.

Patients with acute kidney disease should not drink. Those with chronic nephritis can probably drink in moderation but should avoid beer, since beer contains considerable sodium.

Nobody knows why, but apparently alcohol worsens prostatitis. At the very least, where prostatic hypertrophy is present, the diuretic effect of alcohol may result in urgency and urinary retention.

Alcohol has additive or synergistic effects with other drugs. Relatively

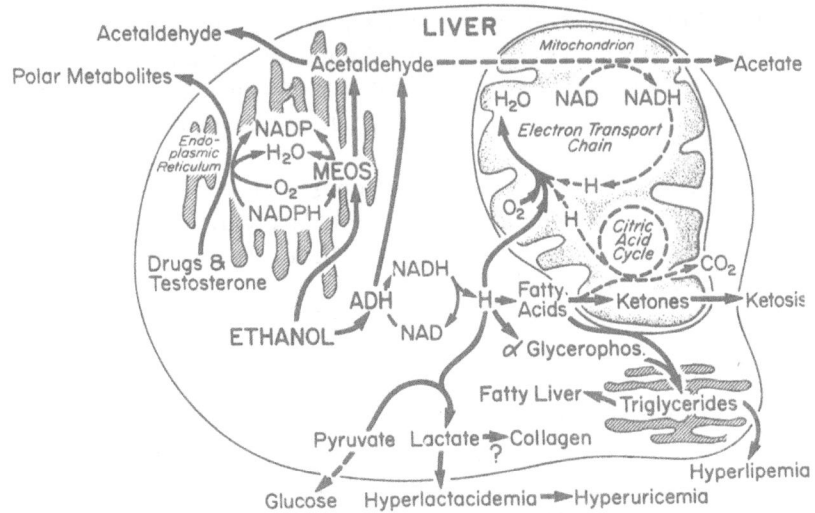

Figure 1. Oxidation of Ethanol in The Hepatocyte

modest amounts of alcohol in combination with halogenated compounds (such as dry-cleaning agents, insecticides, and pesticides) can have devastating effects on the liver. The "accidental" suicides resulting from mixing alcohol with barbiturate and barbituratelike hypnotics have been well publicized. The minor tranquilizers, particularly the benzodiazepine group, apparently have less damaging effects in combination with alcohol, but caution naturally should be exercised, if only because these drugs make people sleepy and so does alcohol. Other drugs may interact with alcohol to produce distressing, if not disastrous, effects. Among these are the oral antidiabetic agents, such as tolbutamide and chlorpropamide. Metronidazole may also produce mildly unpleasant effects in people drinking alcohol, although this is less well documented.

Shown above is the presumed link between oxidation of ethanol in the hepatocyte and fatty liver, hyperlipemia, hyperuricemia, hyperiactacidemia, ketosis, hypoglycemia and testosterone and drug metabolism.

NAD denotes nicotinamide adenine dinucleotide, NADH reduced NAD, NADP nicotinamide adenine dinucleotide phosphate, NADPH reduced NADP, MEOS the microsomal ethanol oxidizing system, and ADH alcohol dehydrogenase. The broken lines indicate pathways that are depressed by ethanol.

It is not clear whether the ketosis has clinical significance. The hypoglycemia apparently only occurs when the patient has been fasting and the liver is depleted of glycogen. It is generally agreed that ADH is primarily responsible for oxidizing alcohol to acetaldehyde. Whether MEOS *in vivo* contributes significantly to the metabolism of alcohol is uncertain, but it may explain cross-tolerance of alcohol with other drugs (e.g., sedative-hypnotics) by enzyme induction. Alcohol produces an increase in smooth endoplastic reticulum, which apparently contributes to a lowering of plasma testosterone, but, again, the biological importance of this is not known.

The hyperlipemia may not be as ominous as it seems. Recent reports (15) indicate that moderate drinkers have relatively high plasma levels of high density lipoproteins (HDL). High HDL levels are associated with a reduced risk of coronary artery disease.

Other events shown above are discussed in the text.

ACKNOWLEDGMENTS

I want to thank Charles S. Lieber, M.D. for permission to use his diagram of the liver cell (Fig. 1). It originally appeared in the *New England Journal of Medicine* 298:888–893, April 20, 1978. Dr. Lieber and his colleagues have contributed meritoriously to our understanding of the metabolism of alcohol and its clinical ramifications.

REFERENCES

1. Leake, C.D., and Silverman, M. Alcoholic Beverages in Clinical Medicine. *Chicago Year Book,* 1966.
2. Lieber, C., and Davidson, C.S. Some metabolic effects of ethyl alcohol. *Am. J. Med.* 33:319–327, 1962.
3. Wallgren, H., and Barry, H. *Actions of Alcohol,* New York; Elsevier, 1970, Chap. 9.
4. Lieber, C., and Rubin, E. Fatty liver, alcoholic hepatitis and cirrhosis produced by alcohol in primates. *N. Engl. J. Med.* 209:128–135, 1974.
5. Victor, M., Adams, R.D., and Collins, G.H. *The Wernicke-Korsakoff Syndrome.* Philadelphia; Davis, 1971.
6. Pawan, G.L.S. Alcohol metabolism in man: acute effects of physical exercise, caffeine, fructose and glucose on the rate of ethanol metabolism. *Biochem. J.* 109:19, 1967.
7. Wolff, P.H. Ethnic differences in alcohol sensitivity. *Science* 175:449–450, 1972.
8. Goodwin, D., Crane, J.B., and Guze, S.B. Alcoholic blackout: a review and clinical study of 100 alcoholics. *Am. J. Psychiat.* 126:77–85, 1969.
9. Goodwin, D.W. Alcoholic blackouts and state-dependent learning. *Fed. Proc.* 33:1833–1835, 1974.
10. Goodwin, D.W., Powell, B.E., Bremer, D., et al. Alcohol and recall: state-department effects in man. *Science* 163:1358–1361, 1969.
11. Lennox, W.G. Alcohol and epilepsy. *Q.J. Stud. Alcohol.* 2:1–11, 1941.
12. Wolff, G. Does alcohol cause chronic gastritis? *Scand. J. Gastroenterol.* 5:289–298, 1970.
13. Bingham, J.R. Precipitating factors in peptic ulcer. *Can. Med. Assoc. J.* 83:205–208, 1960.
14. Gardner H.T. Hepatitis among American occupation troops in Germany: follow-up study with particular reference to interim alcohol and physical activity. *Ann. Intern. Med.* 30:1009–1019, 1949.
15. Castelli W.P. Alcohol consumption and high density lipoproteins. *Lancet* 2:153, 1977.

CHAPTER 3

Screening Techniques and Prevalence Estimation in Alcoholism

DEMMIE G. MAYFIELD
ROBERT G.M. JOHNSTON

For an affliction so pervasive and persistent, alcoholism is notoriously elusive in terms of definition, detection, and diagnosis. A great deal has been written over the years about the "covertness" of the disorder followed by pleas for more diligence in identifying individuals in need of treatment. In recent years, there has been a marked increase in efforts to systematically survey populations for the presence of alcoholism.

In the past three years there have been at least eight reports of reputable national studies estimating the number of excessive drinkers in the United States.[1] The estimates range from 18 million "heavy drinkers" to 14 million "problem drinkers," to 6 million "alcoholics."

While these studies reveal some uncertainty about what should be counted, there is clearly considerable pressure to make a count of the prevalence of alcohol problems. If there is to be a publicly supported program to deal with alcoholism, then more reliable counts should be available, and basic to any program to alter the prevalence of the problem should be baseline and follow-up counts.

Even more insistent than the pressure to obtain epidemiological data has been the exhortation to seek out early cases of alcoholism so they may be more easily and effectively treated.[2] The assertion that alcoholism is more treatable early in its course is supported by little, if any, evidence. It goes without saying, however, that early recovery is preferable to late recovery and more effective methods of treating alcoholism in the early stages will only be developed after we devise more effective methods of case finding.

The methods used to find individual cases are frequently similar to those used in prevalence studies. However, prevalence studies are carried out in a representative sample of the population being studied, whereas case finding is usually carried out in a particular group where there is a known concentration of alcoholics. The method used in case finding will depend in part on the particular setting and will usually be closely associated with treatment programs.

In planning a search for purposes of either a prevalence estimate or to locate cases, three things must be known. (1) What is being searched for; (2) Where it will be sought; and (3) How to go about searching for it.

What is being searched for in this instance proves to be surprisingly difficult to define.[3] In the alcoholism literature a great deal of attention is devoted to debates over definitions of alcoholism. There is no consensus about what alcoholism includes or excludes and there is even disagreement about whether it is an entity, an "ism", or a disease which can be said to include or exclude anything. There is a great yearning for a sine qua non of alcoholism and a real need for a practical defining system.

Fortunately, resolution of the dilemma of the universal, comprehensive definition is not essential to a systematic search for cases. We can have useful definitions of alcoholism which fall far short of a universal definition. In fact, all surveys which have been conducted have focused on a variety of rather circumscribed entities. These entities have been derived from theoretical constructs, from experience with problems presented by alcoholics and from the availability of populations and institutions to the researchers.

The alcoholism which is sought is, more often than not, defined by the problem it presents to the eye of the searcher. Pathologists are apt to see alcoholism as cirrhosis, while sociologists are likely to say this preoccupation with the liver seriously underestimates the incidence of the disorder. Physicians say the pathologists identify the disorder too late. They see alcoholism as a complicator of every other disorder and as a great masquerader. Those in the criminal justice system see alcoholism as a frequent concomitant of almost all forms of misbehavior and as a correlate of recidivism. In industry, alcoholism is seen as a covert cause of default in productivity. Public health epidemiologists see alcoholism as deaths due to liver disease, suicides or accidents, or as chronically institutionalized individuals. Those with broader contact with social institutions say this ignores the much more common and much more expensive societal manifestations of domestic turmoil, community disturbance and occupational impairment which do not leave footprints in vital statistics. Everyone has his own idea of what the real alcoholism is depending on how it impinges upon his area of concern.

Where the searchers are able to look influences what they look for. Physicians have access to sick people and have hospitals and clinics available to them in which to conduct their search. Sociologists may have the community at large available to them but much less of a captive population.

The expertise of the discipline determines to a large degree how the search is conducted and consequently what is found. Sociologists know how to examine large groups, how to draw samples, and how to cover large numbers of subjects with questionnaires and one-shot interviews. Cultural anthropologists, on the other hand, are better able to insinuate themselves into the fabric of the smaller group they are studying and obtain richer but softer data.

Thus, the alcoholism which is sought and found has a lot to do with the discipline of the searchers for this determines what they think it is, where they are able to look, who will do the looking and with what skills and instruments. Studies which have been done all bear the stamp of the what, where, who, and how peculiar to the experience of the investigators. No one has done a study which comprehensively counts all species of alcoholism; indeed such a study is probably impractical and inefficient, and perhaps unnecessary. Problems arise only if what is sought and found as alcoholism is misrepresented or misunderstood as being more universal than it is. This, of course, does frequently happen leading to misinterpretation of the findings and ultimately to inappropriate policy decisions.

In an effort to clarify this issue for ourselves, we reviewed the entire spectrum of alcohol syndromes and manifestations and found that they could be reduced to four categories for purposes of survey studies. These four categories are: (1) Somatopathic Manifestations — physical or organic pathology; (2) Dependency Manifestations — psychological as well as physiological tolerance/addiction phenomenon; (3) Disruptive Social Manifestations — problems in psychosocial areas; and (4) Deteriorative Social Manifestations — decline in social status.

Somatopathically manifest alcoholism is conceptually the simplest and is the most objectively measurable of the several varieties of alcoholism and for that reason this data has always been heavily relied upon in surveys. Dependency manifest alcoholism is less objectively measurable, the manifestations being both behavioral and physiological in nature as well as transient in their occurrence. The dependency aspect of drinking, however, is integral to the loss of control/impairment of control concept which is felt by many to be the essence of alcoholism.[4]

The two categories of social manifestations, though interrelated in a number of ways, do represent different consequences of excessive drinking which must be covered for a complete count. The disruptive category includes most of the acute behavioral manifestations (acute intoxication, problems with the legal system, domestic turmoil, etc.) as well as a variety of default manifestations (occupational failure, under-achievement, etc.). The deteriorative category refers to the decline in social status associated with prolonged excessive drinking, the decline to skid row being the classical example. The deteriorative is distinguishable from the disruptive in that, in the latter, there is impairment in meeting social expectations but there has not been a descent to a lower level of social status.

Any alcoholic may have manifestations in all four categories and many do. It is possible but more unusual to have the manifestations limited to only one category. For most alcoholics, the alcoholism is most prominently manifest in one or two categories and is best detected by inquires directed at these areas. Most surveys, because of the who, how, and where factors have focused on one or two categories, and have, therefore, limited their search and their count.

We feel that these four categories are comprehensive, i.e., all manifestations of all alcoholisms fall into one or more of these areas, and that they are essential. A complete inventory of alcoholics could not omit a search in any of these areas.

The interest in general population prevalence studies is occasional and limited to those with specialized epidemiological interests. Much more commonly, the interest in surveys is for purposes of case finding. The appropriate strategy for this is to search among subpopulations known to have a high prevalence of alcoholism. Thus, effective case finding and treatment has been carried out among drivers arrested for drunken driving and among employees with poor work performance.

General hospitals are also areas with a high traffic of undetected alcoholics.[5] Though studies have regularly uncovered a large number of unsuspected alcoholics in general hospitals, surprisingly few systematic efforts have been made to screen for and treat alcoholism in the general hospital population. In addition to the obvious value of identifying alcoholics for proper treatment, more complete detection of alcoholism is of particular value in the medical setting in that it helps reduce inefficient expenditure of diagnostic procedures and inappropriate treatment of conditions which are really unrecognized symptoms of excessive drinking.

Ideally, alcoholics could be detected if hospital personnel approached the patients with a high index of suspicion for the problem and gathered a wide range of information to verify the diagnosis. This is a time consuming process and is probably not be be achieved in any setting. Thus, a simple screening procedure has considerable appeal.

For this reason we planned a study in a general hospital attempting to determine the most effective and most efficient procedure for alcoholism screening. We were particularly interested in finding a combination of instruments or tests which in complimentary fashion might yield the best detection rate with the least effort.

In terms of categories of manifestations, the hospital setting should be ideal for detecting somatopathic manifestations, to a considerable degree dependency manifestations and to a lesser extent socially disruptive manifestations. The general hospital setting would not be a fertile area for the identification of socially deteriorative manifestations.

In a hospital we do not have easy access to collateral informant sources such as court records, work records or family informants, but we do have a somewhat captive population of cooperative individuals who are readily available for questioning and testing. In particular, we have license to perform a variety of biological tests not possible in most other settings. For screening techniques we have questionnaires and laboratory tests which can be incorporated into the existing routine of admission and evaluation of the individual patient.

Questionnaires are simple to use, may reflect many aspects of drinking behavior and can cover a long period of the patient's life span. The main problem with questionnaires is that they are subject to all the distortions inherent in the public reporting of private events.

The laboratory tests are, at best, biological "markers". These tests have an attractive objectivity which is lacking in questionnaires but inevitably such "markers" indicate only the occurrence of a certain degree of exposure to alcohol. The "markers" must have sufficient specificity and sensitivity and to be really useful they must remain abnormal long enough after the insult by ethanol to reveal excessive drinking but revert to normal after a period of sobriety.

Clearly both questionnaires and biological markers have advantages and limitations. There is reason to hope that these measures would be complementary when employed for screening.

For our study we selected what we felt were the most promising questionnaire and laboratory marker measures to compare with a comprehensive clinical procedure for the identification of alcoholics.

The study was conducted in the Providence VA Medical Center, a 353 bed general hospital which serves as a major medical, surgical, and psychiatric teaching service for Brown University Medical School.

METHOD

Subjects:

A sample of 126 male inpatients was examined. Patients were drawn from all services—medical, surgical, and psychiatric. The first 100 patients of this sample were picked on a random basis at the time of admission.

Questionnaires

A composite drinking questionnaire was drawn up consisting of three separate scales that have already been described in the literature.

1. *The CAGE Questionnaire.*[6] A screening instrument remarkable for its brevity—only four questions. A score of two or more positive responses was taken as a positive test result.

2. *The MAST—Michigan Alcoholic Screening Test.* This was used in a recently modified version[7] that consists of 24 questions. A score of seven or more was considered positive. A subset of 13 of these questions was scored to give the SMAST or Short Michigan Alcoholic Screening Test. A score of three or more on this subscale was considered positive.

3. *The ASIS—The Alcoholic Stages Index Subscales.*[8] This consists of 27 questions arranged into four subscales: (1) "Trouble due to Drinking"; (2) "Personal-Effects Drinking"; (3) "Preoccupied Drinking"; and (4) "Uncontrolled Drinking".

This scale was included in order to examine whether it may be possible to detect alcoholism in the early stages. However, for the purposes of this study, a qualifying score on any one subscale was taken as a positive score for the whole scale.

Laboratory Measures

1. *Blood Alcohol Level (BAL)* was measured using an Alcolmeter,® a small breath sampling device that uses a fuel cell as a sensor. Any positive reading was taken as a positive test result.

2. *Mean Corpuscular Volume (MCV)* was noted from the patients'

admission blood work, this measurement having been performed on a Coulter Counter. This simple measure has been noted as a potential indicator of alcohol usage.[9] The upper limit of normal is considered to be 96 cu microns in a male population.

3. *Gamma Glutamyl Transpeptidase (GGTP)* has been recommended as the liver enzyme most sensitive to alcohol metabolism.[10] Analysis was carried out at 25° C, the upper limit of the normal range at this temperature is 29 IU/L.

Procedure

At admission, patients were approached in the admitting area and asked to take part in the study. Whenever possible, a BAL measure was taken at this time. Later, on the ward, the drinking questionnaire was administered and the patient was then interviewed in order to ascertain his past and present drinking habits. Time and quantity of last consumption was noted as well as estimated average consumption. Whenever possible, a family member or other significant figure in the patient's life was questioned in order to corroborate the patient's history.

The patient was diagnosed as exhibiting alcoholism or not on the basis of: (1) interview data; (2) a full review of the patient's medical records, both current and past; and (3) a knowledge of the BAL and MCV, but without knowledge of the GGTP or the questionnaire scores.

The definition of alcoholism used was that of the alcohol dependence syndrome as described in a recent WHO publication.[4] In this definition the key concept is "loss or impairment of control over drinking." The National Council on Alcoholism Criteria[11] were used as a general guide as to the information pertinent to making this diagnosis. However, it was understood that the syndrome may be present in varying degrees and that the position of the boundary between "normal" drinking behavior and the syndrome is to some extent arbitrary. We tended to include cases in which the syndrome appeared to be relatively mild since we were interested in being able to detect these "early" alcoholics. Finally, patients were diagnosed as alcoholic if there was evidence that they had suffered from the syndrome at any time in the past, thus, we included those alcoholics who were in remission.

Statistical Measures

The statistics most commonly used to describe the effectiveness of a biomedical test are: (1) the Sensitivity—that is the proportion of the patients with the disease, who have a positive response to the test; (2) the Specificity—the proportion of patients who do not have the disease, who have a negative response to the test. However, for practical use of the test in unselected populations, three further statistics are important:[12] (1) the Predictive value of a Positive test result—that is the proportion of those patients who score positive on the test, who have the disease; (2) The Predictive value of a Negative test result—that is the proportion of those patients with negative test results, who do not have the disease; (3) the Efficiency of the test—that is the proportion of all patients tested who are correctly assigned as having the disease, or not having the disease. These last three measures will vary according to the prevalence of the disease in the population, a fact that is frequently overlooked and can seriously limit the utility of a test.

The statistics used may be summarized as follows:

		Test		
		+	−	
Disease	+	a	b	a+b
	−	c	d	c+d
		a+c	b+d	
				a+b+c+d

Sensitivity = a/a+b
Specificity = d/c+d
    Then provided the prevalence of the disease is a+b/a+b+c+d
Predictive value Positive = a/a+c
Predictive value Negative = d/b+d
Efficiency = a+d/a+b+c+d

Results

We used the initial random sample of 100 patients to estimate the prevalence of alcoholism among all hospital admissions, 47 of these patients were diagnosed as alcoholic. This prevalence of 47% is unusually high for any disease and will tend to make the tests used in this study appear more favorable. The total sample of 126 patients consisted of 54 alcoholics and 72 nonalcoholics.

Sensitivity and Specificity were calculated for each test alone and then, after correcting for the fact that the prevalence in the total sample was different from that in the initial random sample, Predictive value Positive and Negative, and Efficiency were calculated. Results are presented in Table 1. It will be noted that all the biological tests were more Specific than

TABLE 1.-Detection of Alcoholics with Questionnaire or Laboratory Test

Tests	Sensitivity %	N₁	Specificity %	N₂	Predictive + %	Predictive – %	Efficiency %
MCV	41	(54)	87	(70)	74	62	65
GGTP	26	(46)	85	(54)	61	57	57
BAL	13	(45)	97	(61)	78	56	58
CAGE	72	(50)	79	(57)	75	76	76
MAST	86	(50)	81	(57)	80	87	83
SMAST	80	(50)	77	(57)	76	81	79
ASIS	80	(50)	73	(56)	73	81	76

N_1=Number of patients on which Sensitivity is based. N_2=Number of patients on which Specificity is based. $N_1 + N_2$=Number of patients for which test results were obtained.

the questionnaires, but they were much less Sensitive, and, the Predictive value of Positive and Negative test results, and overall Efficiency were lower.

Each biological test was paired with each questionnaire test. If either test was positive then the combination test was considered positive. Table 2 presents the same statistics calculated for each pair of tests.

In nearly every case the Sensitivity of the combination of tests was higher than each test used alone. However, this was at the price of a reduction in Specificity. One combination, BAL with MAST, produced an increase in Sensitivity with no reduction in Specificity as compared with

TABLE 2.-Detection of Alcoholics with Questionnaire and Laboratory Test in Combination

Test Combinations		Sensitivity %	N₁	Specificity %	N₂	Predictive + %	Predictive – %	Efficiency %
MCV	CAGE	86	(50)	65	(55)	69	84	75
	MAST	96	(50)	69	(55)	73	95	82
	SMAST	90	(50)	65	(55)	70	88	77
	ASIS	88	(50)	64	(55)	68	86	75
GGTP	CAGE	76	(46)	66	(51)	67	76	71
	MAST	89	(46)	66	(51)	70	87	77
	SMAST	84	(46)	66	(51)	69	83	75
	ASIS	84	(46)	64	(50)	68	83	74
BAL	CAGE	79	(44)	75	(53)	74	81	77
	MAST	90	(44)	81	(53)	81	91	86
	SMAST	84	(44)	77	(53)	77	85	81
	ASIS	86	(44)	69	(52)	71	85	77

N_1=Number of patients on which Sensitivity is based. N_2=Number of patients on which Specificity is based. $N_1 + N$=Number of patients on which both test results were obtained.

the MAST used alone. There was also a gain in Efficiency, this being the highest of any of the tests alone or in combination.

Discussion

This study was not an effort to clarify the understanding of the syndrome or to improve upon the ability to make a diagnosis of alcoholism by clinical methods. The study was designed to find a more efficient way to do the same thing which can already be done but only with a considerable expenditure of costly manpower.

The study demonstrates that screening procedures are effective in identifying alcoholics, many of whom would probably go undetected or unidentified without some systematic inventory. All of the questionnaires are reasonably effective for screening purposes; effective enough to argue for their inclusion in the general procedure of a medical center; limited enough to argue for continued efforts to improve on present screening techniques.

The results also support the premise that biological tests can detect subgroups of alcoholics missed by questionnaires and vice versa. This increase in Sensitivity by use of combinations of tests was, however, offset in most cases by a considerable loss in Specificity. The combination of BAL and MAST was an exception with no loss at all in Specificity. Since measurement of BAL with the Alcolmeter® was simple and inexpensive, it is encouraging that this combination yields such good results.

The inclusion of alcoholics in remission in the alcoholic group undoubtedly biased against the Sensitivity of the biological tests since these tests can only reflect the recent consumption of alcohol. Thus, the low Sensitivity figures for the biological tests are somewhat misleading.

It seems unlikely that any major breakthrough will occur in the content and design of alcoholism screening questionnaires. However, their effectiveness can be improved by making minor variations in their structure. The cut-off values for the tests that were used in this study were the conventional divisions between normal and abnormal result and in the case of the questionnaires, represent an optimum for the questionnaires used alone. However, the optimum cut-off point may be different if tests are used in combination. Also, individual questions or sets of questions from the questionnaires may be more effective than the published questionnaires when used in combination with biological tests.

It is, however, in the area of biochemical tests that we have the real need for and the real possibility of a breakthrough. As we have learned more about the effects of alcohol on hepatic function, it has seemed likely that an insult to the liver by excessive drinking would be accompanied by a biochemically detectable derangement in function that persisted for weeks but was short of the irreversible cirrhotic damage caused by prolonged excessive drinking. If such a derangement were specific to alcohol it would constitute a biological signature of excessive drinking and would be of enormous value, not only in detection, but in definition of the syndrome of alcoholism.

The alpha-amino-n-butyric acid/leucine ratio was proposed as such a highly specific marker for alcoholism.[13] More recently, investigators[14,15] have been unable to verify the specificity reported by its originators and it appears that this biochemical test is not the hoped for biological marker.

Nevertheless, discovery of such a marker remains a distinct possibility for the future. In the meantime, the adroit use of combinations of tests and questionnaires can be a very effective and efficient means of detecting alcoholism in a variety of clinical settings.

REFERENCES

1. Malin, H.J., Munch, N.E., and Archer, L.D. A national surveillance system for alcoholism and alcohol abuse. In Proceedings at the 32nd International Congress on Alcoholism and Drug Dependence (In press).
2. *Manual on Alcoholism of the American Medical Association.* Robert J. Shearer, M.D. (Ed.), American Medical Association, 1968, pp. 9 and 38.
3. Cahalan, D. *Problem Drinkers: A National Survey.* San Francisco: Jossey-Bass, 1976, pp. 1-17.
4. Edwards, G., Gross, M.M., Keller, M., et al. *Alcohol-Related Disabilities.* WHO offset Publication No. 32, World Health Organization, Geneva, 1977.
5. Gomberg, E.S. Prevalence of alcoholism among ward patients in a Veterans' Administration medical center. *J. Stud. on Alcohol* 36:1458-1467, 1975.
6. Mayfield, D., McLeod, G., and Hall, P. The CAGE questionnaire: validation of a new alcoholism screening instrument. *Am. J. Psychiat.* 131:1121-1123, 1974.
7. Selzer, M.L., Vinokur, M.D., and van Rooijen, L. A self-administered short Michigan alcoholism screening test (SMAST). *J. Stud. on Alcohol* 36:117-126, 1975.
8. Mulford, H.A. Stages in the alcoholic process: toward a cumulative nonsequential index. *J. Stud. on Alcohol* 38:563-583, 1977.
9. Unger, K.W., and Johnson, D. Red blood cell mean corpuscular volume: a potential indicator of alcohol usage in a working population. *Am. J. Med. Sci.* 267:281-289, 1974.
10. Rosalki, S.B., and Rau, D. Serum gamma-glutamyl transpeptidase activity in alcoholism. *Clin. Chem. Acta.* 39:41-47, 1972.
11. Criteria Committee, National Council on Alcoholism, New York, N.Y., Criteria for the diagnosis of alcoholism: diagnosis and treatment. *Ann. Intern. Med.* 77:249-258, 1972.
12. Galen, R.S., and Gambino, S.R. *Beyond Normality: The Predictive Value and Efficiency of Medical Diagnosis.* New York: Wiley, 1975.
13. Shaw, S., Stimmel, B., and Lieber, C. Plasma alpha amino-n-butyric acid to leucine ratio: an empirical biochemical market of alcoholism. *Science* 194:1057-1058, 1976.

14. Morgan, M.Y., Milsom, J.P., and Sherlock, S. Ratio of plasma alpha amino-*n*-butyric acid to leucine as an empirical marker of alcoholism: diagnostic value. *Science* 197:1183–1185, 1977.

15. Ellingboe, J., Mendelson, J.H., Varamelli, C.C., et al: Plasma alpha amino-*n*-butyric acid: leucine ratio; normal values in alcoholics. *J. Stud. on Alcohol* 39:1467–1476, 1978.

CHAPTER 4

Stages In The Development Of Alcoholism

ALEX D. POKORNY
THOMAS E. KANAS

INTRODUCTION

In this chapter we want to review the history of the concept of alcoholism as a progressive disorder with successive emergence of alcoholic behaviors and experiences in a predictable order. We will first review a few key studies which have exerted a marked influence in this area, particularly the early studies of Jellinek. We will then report a study of our own, giving findings for a sample of alcoholics and also for a sample of moderate to heavy drinkers not identified as alcoholics. We will then discuss the implications of this for the concept of alcoholism as a progressive disorder with a regular succession of symptoms.

BACKGROUND

Alcoholism has long been regarded as a progressive disorder. For example, in the *Lectures on Clinical Psychiatry* by Emil Kraepelin,[1] it is stated,

The life history which I have brought before you here shows quite the usual course of things in numberless cases of chronic

45

TABLE 1.–Original Grapevine Questionnaire
(Jellinek 1946)

At what age did you first:
1. Get drunk
2. Experience a blackout
3. Start sneaking drinks
4. Begin to lose control
5. Rationalize
6. Change pattern
7. Go on the wagon
8. Act in financially extravagant manner
9. Start weekend drunks
10. Start mid-week drunks
11. Start daytime drunks
12. Take a morning drink
13. Start going on benders
14. Develop indefinable fears
15. Experience remorse
16. Develop unreasonable resentments
17. Commit antisocial acts
18. Sense friends', relatives' urges to stop
19. Become indifferent to liquor type, quality
20. Experience uncontrollable tremors
21. Resort to sedatives
22. Seek medical aid
23. Seek psychiatric aid
24. Have to be hospitalized due to drinking
25. Lose a friend from drinking
26. Lose work time from drinking
27. Lose a job from drinking
28. Lose advancement from drinking
29. Use alcohol to lessen self-consciousness re sex
30. Seek comfort in religion
31. Seek to escape by geographic change
32. Start solitary drinking
33. Start protecting supply
34. Admit to self drinking was beyond control
35. Admit to others drinking was beyond control
36. Reach lowest point.

alcoholism—temptation in youth through our drinking customs, the gradual growth of a taste for drink in a good natured and rather weak willed man, the degradation of his conduct and family circumstances, the good resolutions which are always abandoned in temptation, and the rapid improvement on total abstinence.

In spite of the generally moralistic and voluntaristic tone of this paragraph, the idea of progression emerges clearly.

The publication in this field which has been highly influential and which we want to use as a starting point is the lengthy article, also published as a monograph, on "Phases in the Drinking History of Alcoholics" published by Jellinek in the *Quarterly Journal of Studies on Alcohol* in 1946.[2] This 88 page article was based on Jellinek's analysis of a questionnaire which he had not designed but which he was asked to analyze after the data had been collected. This 36 item questionnaire (Table 1) was developed and published in May, 1945, in the *Grapevine*, the official organ of Alcoholics Anonymous, and was intended to gather information on the ages of alcoholics at the time of certain events which the designers of the questionnaire "assumed to be of significance in the drinking history of the alcoholic". One hundred and fifty-eight members of AA returned the forms but only 98 questionnaires of male alcoholics could be used in the analysis. Dr. Jellinek wrote an exhaustive and detailed interpretation of this data. He also expressed dissatisfaction with many of the questions, and at the end of this report he presented a tentative revised questionnaire of 111 items. This included questions about family attitudes, attitudes of spouse and friends, work experiences, and then approximately 75 questions on drinking behavior and complications.

Jellinek's 1946 article was followed up by a second publication in 1952 on the phases on alcohol addiction,[3] also published in the *Quarterly Journal* and published separately by the World Health Organization. This article was based on an administration of the more detailed questionnaire to some 2,000 alcoholics. The article is a summary of lectures presented by Jellinek at the Yale Summer School of Alcohol Studies and at a European seminar on alcoholism held in Copenhagen in October, 1951. Unfortunately, the summary omits certain key pieces of information. For example, the 1952 article reports on 43 alcoholic "symptoms" (or behaviors or experiences) as shown in Table 2. Most of these are recognizably represented in the earlier list of 111 but many have been considerably reworded. In some instances two or more appear to have been collapsed into one. Finally, a few totally new items appear to have been added.

The 1952 Jellinek article numbered the 43 symptoms and thereby implied that they appear in that order. Jellinek also subdivided the "course" into four phases: the prealcoholic phase, the prodromal phase, the crucial phase, and the chronic phase. Jellinek also identified three key symptoms which were viewed as "markers", indicators of the onset of each of the last three phases: the onset of "alcoholic palimpsests" (blackouts) signaled the start of the prodromal phase; the onset of loss of control signaled the start of the crucial phase; the onset of prolonged intoxications signaled the start of the chronic phase.

Each of these 43 symptoms is described clearly and they are discussed successively in a plausible and persuasive narrative. It is probably because

TABLE 2.–Jellinek Chart of Alcohol Addiction (1952)*

Prealcoholic Phase
    a. Occasional relief drinking
    b. Constant relief drinking
    c. Increase in alcohol tolerance

Prodromal Phase
    1. Onset of blackouts
    2. Surreptitious drinking
    3. Anticipatory drinking
    4. Gulping drinks
    5. Guilt feelings
    6. Avoiding reference to alcohol
    7. Frequent blackouts

Crucial Phase
    8. Loss of control
    9. Rationalized drinking
    10. Social pressures
    11. Grandiose behavior
    12. Aggressive behavior
    13. Persistent remorse
    14. Periods of total abstinence
    15. Changing drinking pattern
    16. Dropping friends
    17. Quitting jobs
    18. Behavior becomes alcohol-centered
    19. Loss of outside interests
    20. Reinterpretation of interpersonal relations
    21. Marked self-pity
    22. Geographic escape
    23. Change in family habits
    24. Unreasonable resentments
    25. Protecting supply
    26. Nutritional neglect
    27. First hospitalization (alcoholism)
    28. Alcoholic jealousy
    30. Regular morning drinking

Chronic Phase
    31. Onset of benders
    32. Marked ethical deterioration
    33. Impairment of thinking
    34. Alcoholic psychoses
    35. Drinking down (socially)
    36. Drinking technical products
    37. Loss of alcohol tolerance
    38. Indefinable fears
    39. Tremors
    40. Psychomotor inhibition
    41. Obsessive drinking
    42. Religious needs
    43. Admitting defeat

*Items reworded by Park, 1973

of these features that the notion of a regular procession of symptoms has become deeply imbedded in the prevailing beliefs about alcoholism, in spite of the fact that Jellinek himself stated that not everyone would have all the symptoms, nor would they necessarily occur in that exact order.

There have been many subsequent studies following up Jellinek's work. We will review selected ones, primarily those influential in the design of our study.

Joan Jackson[4] developed two scales from the items in the Jellinek Drinking History, one measuring preoccupation with alcohol and the other measuring psychological involvement. She showed that these items were scalable using Stouffer's H-technique. The fact that this was possible favored the hypothesis of a progression of symptoms, from least to most deviant alcoholic behavior. She found, however, that the appearance of individual symptoms was not always in the expected order.

Trice and Wahl[5] used 14 of the Jellinek Drinking History items with two groups of alcoholics. They found that there were four clusters of symptoms in terms of grouping around the same onset age. They suggest that clustering is more typical than a steady progression.

Peter Park has published a series of studies related to this issue. In 1962[6] he compared the drinking histories of 806 Finnish alcoholics with those of 192 English alcoholics, using a modified Jellinek Drinking History of 105 items. He found many similarities in the sequence of events but notable differences in the rate of development, in that the progression of symptoms occurred at a slower pace in the English sample.

In 1973 Park[7] compared the ordering of symptoms in Finnish alcoholics with the order reported by Jellinek. He found a typical developmental order in the Finnish group but it was somewhat different from Jellinek's order. However, he felt that his findings supported the general notion that there is an order in the development of symptoms of alcoholism.

In 1973 Park and Whitehead[8] compared the drinking histories of Finnish alcoholics with a new group of American alcoholics. They found that significant experiences develop in essentially the same chronological order in both groups. The rank order correlation coefficients with Jellinek's order were about .55 for the Finnish alcoholics and .74 for American alcoholics. They suggest that the stronger correlation with American alcoholics was due to the fact that Jellinek's study was also done with American alcoholics. They established four separate dimensions of alcoholic problems: economic problems, family problems, social problems, and core symptoms. They point out that alcoholics may not proceed in all dimensions at the same pace.

Orford and Hawker[9] gave Jellinek Drinking Histories to 59 alcoholics and studied the sequencing by a special statistical approach. They found three significant clusters which they interpret as: (1) onset of psychological dependence; (2) tremor, morning drinking and amnesia; and (3) alcoholism psychosis. They consider that the first two clusters correspond with the concepts of psychological and physical dependence, with the latter following the former by an average of around three or four years. The third cluster appeared on the average of two to four years after the onset of physical dependence. These authors felt that there was little purpose to be served in attempting to conceive of the two processes, the dependence and the damage processes, as part of a single process which unfolds in predictable sequence. They also pointed out that alcoholism treatment events, such as hospitalization for drinking or attendance at AA, do not have any necessary relationship to the other events.

There have been a number of studies focusing on the "blackout" aspect of the Jellinek studies. (The term "blackout" in this chapter always refers to amnesia following a drinking episode, even though the person was conscious and seemingly in touch with his surroundings at the time.) Jellinek gave blackouts a key position in the ordering of symptoms. He considered that blackouts were an early indicator of the onset of alcoholism, and also expressed the view that, in future alcoholics, blackouts might occur after ingestion of only a modest amount of alcohol. Goodwin, Crain and Guze[10] point out that it is not clear where Jellinek got the idea that having blackouts after a few drinks would predict future addiction, since the questionnaire did not touch on that point. They suggest that Jellinek's views on alcoholism were derived not only from the questionnaire results but from his extensive reading and his conversations with alcoholics.

Goodwin and associates considered that a simple questionnaire was unsatisfactory, and they substituted group interviews, using a 78 item structured interview form. Through this procedure, items which might have unclear meanings to subjects, such as "blackout" or "blank", could be clarified. Their subjects were 100 alcoholics at two St. Louis treatment centers, with 85% of the sample being male and 71% white, mean age of 44. Of their 100 subjects 64 had experienced one or more blackouts. The blackout group reported a significantly larger number of manifestations of alcoholism and included a higher proportion of subjects with severe alcoholism. All but one of the 64 individuals reporting blackouts stated that these were associated with consumption of large amounts of alcohol, frequently over a period of several days. Seven percent of the group attributed blackouts to drinking for several days and 70% to drinking "more than usual". Goodwin and associates ranked 12 of the leading manifestations of alcoholism according to mean age at onset. They found that blackouts on the average were a relatively late manifestation of alcoholism and were preceded by benders, tremulousness and often severe social repercussions from drinking. They cited Roe's study of 30 middle-aged social drinkers which indicated that 30% had experienced blackouts. They also cited an additional study of their own in which 40% of young men had experienced a blackout at least once and at an average age of 23, an age at which fewer than 8% of the alcoholic sample had experienced a blackout. These authors suggest that blackouts might therefore predict not alcoholism, but nonalcoholism.

In 1973 Curlee[11] repeated Goodwin's study, using 100 hospitalized VA patients. She found that in her sample blackouts were reported more commonly (83%) and also at an earlier age of onset (age 30 compared to age 35 in the Goodwin study). The sequence of symptoms differed significantly from the order of Jellinek, although the difference was less marked than in the Goodwin study.

ISSUES ADDRESSED IN OUR STUDY

We initially set out to administer the complete set of items in Jellinek's Drinking History, along with those additional items included in any one of the other studies cited, to a new sample of alcoholics. In addition, we decided to administer this same battery to a nonalcoholic but drinking control or comparison group, to see how they would respond on these items. The reason for specifying that the control group be composed of drinkers was that a great many of the questions make no sense if given to lifetime abstainers. Our goal was to evaluate how specific the various symptoms were to alcoholism, and whether or not they might also occur in nonalcoholic drinkers.

The stages in the development of alcoholism are of particular interest in the diagnosis of alcoholism, particularly early diagnosis and detection. Alcoholism is often unrecognized and generally underdiagnosed. In many instances we do not identify it until late stage complications occur. One reason is that no simple clear-cut laboratory diagnostic criterion exists so that we have to depend on a summation of indicators, no single one of which is diagnostic. It is in this context that Jellinek's list of experiences is important. If an alcoholic blackout were an early predictor of alcoholism, this would be a very useful thing to know. If morning drinking or a DWI arrest or drinking nonbeverage alcohol or any other of the alcoholism history items were a clear indicator then this would be very useful.

The criteria for diagnosis of alcoholism of the National Council of Alcoholism[12] do make use of a great many drinking history items. The NCA criteria set up certain items as definitive indicators of alcoholism,

TABLE 3.–Comparison of Alcoholic Subjects With Borderline Control
Group and Purified Control Group
(Per cent of total group)

	Alcoholic (N=102)	Borderline Control (N=19)	Pure Control (N=34)
Marital Status			
Never married	4.9 (%)	5.3	5.9
Living with wife	29.4	52.6	55.9
Separated	18.6	10.5	8.8
Divorced	41.2	26.3	26.5
Widowed	5.9	5.3	2.9
Living Alone	38.2	31.6	17.6
Definite Place to Live	57.8	63.2	82.4
Recent drinking pattern			
Mild controlled	0.0	84.2	97.1
Weekend regular	0.0	0.0	2.9
Periodic heavy	28.4	5.3	0.0
Daily heavy	71.6	10.5	0.0
Times hospitalized for drinking	4.8 (mean)	0.8	0.1
Times arrested for drinking	14.6 (mean)	1.5	0.4
Life Pattern of Drinking			
Drinking ever burden	99.0 (%)	63.2	14.7
Drinking ever affect health	78.4	26.3	2.9
Unable to control drinking	64.7	10.5	0.0
Needs to drink to perform task	56.9	15.8	8.8
Ever feel need to cut down	95.1	57.9	20.6
Drinks to point of incapacitated	78.4	47.4	8.8
Deliberately abstains	87.3	57.9	41.2
Experiences withdrawal symptoms	87.3	26.3	0.0
Drinks until supply exhausted	80.4	36.8	8.8
Has experienced morning shakes	95.1	73.7	8.8
Has taken morning drink to steady	94.2	57.9	8.8
Alcohol Dependency Score			
0	3.9	15.8	85.3
1	0.0	0.0	2.9
2	3.9	36.8	8.8
3	2.9	5.3	0.0
4	89.2	42.1	2.9
Items from SAAST			
Blackouts	83.3 (%)	84.2	26.5
Relatives worry, complain	94.1	63.2	35.3
Feels guilty about drinking	96.1	63.2	29.4
Always able to stop	33.3	73.7	100.0
Attended AA	85.3	15.8	0.0
Lost friendships drinking	61.8	26.3	5.9
Lost job drinking	70.6	36.8	5.9
Ever drink in morning	99.0	84.2	41.2
Told have liver trouble	29.4	0.0	2.9
Ever had DTs	29.4	0.0	0.0
Ever hallucinations, shakes	54.9	10.5	0.0
Arrested DWI	66.7	42.1	8.8

others as probable, and still others as possible. As one might expect, the definitive ones are all late-stage manifestations and are therefore not helpful in early identification. In the probable and possible groups we are dependent upon an accumulation of evidence. One or two positives would not be very convincing but five or ten certainly would. Since many of these behaviors are the same as in the Jellinek Drinking History list, it is important to evaluate them for specificity and frequency.

METHOD

The questionnaire was individually administered in the form of a structured interview. The questionnaire included all 111 items in Jellinek's 1946 recommended questionnaire plus 40 items included in the several related studies cited earlier.

The sample consisted of 102 alcoholics and 53 controls. The alcoholics were white, male patients in a VA inpatient alcoholism treatment program, all sober and detoxified, in the age range 30–59, without psychosis or organic brain syndrome, without a history of drug abuse or drug addiction or any severe reaction to prescribed drugs. The control or comparison group consisted of 53 male, white inpatients in the same VA Hospital who had never been diagnosed as alcoholic nor had been treated for alcoholism, but who were not teetotallers or minimal drinkers (defined as drinking once a month or less frequently), in the age range 30–59, without psychosis or organic brain syndrome, without any history of drug abuse or drug addiction, without any history of severe reaction to prescribed drugs, and without any medical or surgical illness so severe as to interfere with cooperation in a structured interview.

Even though the control group members had never been diagnosed as alcoholics nor had they been treated for alcoholism, we later reviewed their answers to the items in the structured interview and separated out 19 individuals because their answers indicated possible alcoholism by the NCA criteria. These 19 were called our "borderline group". This left a group of 34 "pure controls", those who did not qualify for the label of alcoholism even after this second screening.

RESULTS

Table 3 compares the alcoholic group with the borderline group and with the "pure control" group. It is clear that in most respects the borderline group fell in between the two others. This is true with respect to

TABLE 4.–Comparison of Alcoholic and Control Groups on Items in Jellinek Revised Drinking History Questionnaire (Omitting Some Demographic, Background, and Repetitive Items)

	Alcoholics (N=102)			Controls (N=34)		
	Percent Reporting	Mean Age	S.D. of Age	Percent Reporting	Mean Age	S.D. of Age
1. Present Age	100.0	47.8	7.0	100.0	45.8	10.3
15. Age parents first reproached	76.4	30.7	10.5	14.7	25.0	6.8
16. Age first supported by family	15.6	29.8	8.8	11.7	31.0	9.4
19. Age first marriage	97.0	23.1	3.4	94.1	22.3	3.7
19a. Age first divorce	66.6	32.5	7.2	58.8	30.6	10.1
22. Age wife supported	7.8	37.1	9.0	8.8	46.7	5.5
23. Age turned money over to wife	28.4	36.7	9.6	17.6	39.5	11.3
24. Age wife first reproached	84.3	33.3	8.6	20.5	31.1	10.1
25. Age wife's family reproached	28.4	32.5	10.0	5.8	20.5	2.1
26. Age embarrassed wife	50.9	34.2	8.6	8.8	29.7	8.6
27. Age wife complained re money	39.2	35.4	10.2	8.8	34.3	13.6
28. Age wife complained re children	48.0	36.2	7.5	11.7	32.5	10.9
29. Your age when wife jealous	49.0	29.3	7.8	41.1	26.9	8.8
30. Age family changed living habits	35.2	37.1	7.9	2.9	39.0	0.0
34. Age began losing time at work	72.5	34.5	9.4	5.8	28.0	11.3
35. Age first walked off job	50.9	34.4	8.3	2.9	35.0	0.0
36. Age first lost job/drinking	58.8	37.1	9.1	5.8	31.5	6.4
37. Age lost advancement drinking	31.3	34.6	8.3	0.0	—	—
39. Age unemployed over 3 months	50.9	40.8	7.9	0.0	—	—
40. Age changed to periodic drinking	33.3	35.9	9.1	17.6	31.3	9.9
41. Age changed to steady drinking	56.8	31.9	11.5	8.8	29.7	16.7
42. Age first drink	100.0	17.2	3.4	100.0	18.1	2.8
43. Age first drunk	100.0	18.7	5.6	91.1	19.9	4.9
44. Age drank 1x/mo., not drunk	59.8	20.2	6.4	73.5	22.0	6.1
47. Age drank 1x/wk., sometimes drunk	77.4	25.6	8.4	47.0	26.3	9.1
50. Age first weekend drunk	89.2	25.9	9.6	26.4	22.7	6.3
51. Age first blackout, "pulling a blank"	73.5	30.8	10.2	20.5	22.0	3.8

52. Age frequent blackouts, "blanks"	49.0	35.1	10.6	0.0	—	—
53. Age first sneaked drinks	69.6	34.3	10.0	0.0	—	—
54. Age wondered would there be enough	51.9	30.6	8.3	2.9	16.0	0.0
55. Age first gulped drinks	74.5	32.2	10.8	11.7	27.5	14.7
56. Age refused to discuss drinking	47.0	33.2	9.4	5.8	28.5	10.6
57. Age felt more efficient drinking	53.9	33.9	11.2	5.8	26.0	8.5
58. Age mixed better drinking	74.5	24.5	8.8	47.0	25.0	9.9
59. Age began to need more alcohol	94.1	33.2	9.9	32.3	26.5	9.5
60. Age needed less alcohol	48.0	41.7	8.3	5.8	37.5	16.3
61. Age first lost control	93.1	36.2	10.1	2.9	25.0	0.0
62. Age daytime drinks	80.3	36.1	10.6	8.8	32.3	10.7
63. Age interfered with recreation	75.4	39.0	9.7	8.8	31.7	6.4
64. Age first bender	69.6	34.1	10.2	2.9	17.0	0.0
65. Age first morning drinking	89.2	35.5	11.1	17.6	36.2	14.3
67. Age first solitary drinking	79.4	20.5	9.5	20.5	41.4	9.0
68. Age neglected meals	90.1	39.4	9.6	5.8	33.5	16.3
69. Age became indifferent to brands	55.8	25.4	10.8	2.9	18.0	0.0
70. Age drank non-beverage alcohol	17.6	32.4	9.0	2.9	19.0	0.0
71. Age thought friends stuffed shirts	28.4	35.3	8.6	26.4	32.8	9.7
72. Age walked out on friends	31.3	35.2	9.1	8.8	35.3	4.7
73. Age friends walked out	38.2	38.4	8.4	2.9	39.0	0.0
74. Age made alibis re drinking	80.3	35.3	10.6	8.8	26.0	8.7
75. Age first went on wagon	90.1	38.0	8.9	20.5	33.3	13.0
76. Age began making drinking rules	44.1	39.8	9.0	2.9	22.0	0.0
77. Age aggressive when drinking	49.0	31.8	9.9	14.7	28.4	11.0
78. Age first DWI arrest	68.6	35.5	10.0	8.8	46.0	9.8
79. Age justified neglect of family	38.2	34.1	8.4	0.0	—	—
80. Age resented inconsiderate world	33.3	36.1	10.8	17.4	37.2	7.8
81. Age suspected contempt in others	55.8	38.3	9.7	14.7	37.2	10.8
82. Age felt others "sitting" on one	32.3	37.0	7.9	0.0	—	—
83. Age ideas of jealousy	40.1	31.2	8.3	38.2	28.4	10.4
84. Age diminished sex potency	59.8	43.6	7.4	41.1	42.0	8.6
85. Age developed sleeplessness	61.7	38.2	8.9	0.0	—	—

TABLE 4.–Comparison of Alcoholic and Control Groups on Items in Jellinek Revised Drinking History Questionnaire (Omitting Some Demographic, Background, and Repetitive Items) (continued)

	Alcoholics (N=102)			Controls (N=34)		
	Percent Reporting	Mean Age	S.D. of Age	Percent Reporting	Mean Age	S.D. of Age
86. Age developed self pity	48.0	35.9	10.5	50.0	39.0	11.8
87. Age thought best solution death	39.2	39.6	7.9	52.9	35.2	12.4
88. Age contemplated suicide	31.3	39.7	7.9	52.9	38.2	11.8
89. Age changed environment	64.7	38.4	9.8	2.9	41.0	0.0
90. Age accepted services of intermediary	25.4	41.2	7.7	23.5	37.6	12.4
91. Age persistent remorse	81.3	38.4	9.0	14.7	34.4	16.6
92. Age behaved resentfully	51.9	34.5	10.8	55.8	35.9	12.3
93. Age stopped trying to control drinking	52.9	41.6	8.3	0.0	—	—
94. Age first convulsion/drinking	15.6	41.3	9.4	2.9	30.0	0.0
95. Age uncontrolled tremors	87.2	38.7	10.3	2.9	34.0	0.0
96. Age vague fears	50.0	38.9	9.1	11.7	31.7	16.3
97. Age periods of despondency	62.7	40.1	8.6	64.7	36.7	12.0
98. Age "what's the use" attitude	56.8	40.4	8.2	35.2	37.9	12.0
99. Age feared alcohol would let down	39.2	41.7	7.9	5.8	28.5	4.9
100. Age began to protect supply	72.5	37.7	10.4	2.9	34.0	0.0
101. Age sought medical aid/drinking	72.5	40.5	9.2	2.9	41.0	0.0
102. Age volunteered for psychiatric advice	72.5	45.1	7.8	2.9	41.0	0.0
103. Age family urged psychiatric advice	31.3	39.9	8.5	44.1	35.4	9.3
104. Age psychiatric advice for fears	24.5	37.3	8.3	97.0	36.9	12.5
105. Age hospitalized/intoxication	75.4	43.4	8.0	2.9	20.0	0.0
106. Age hospitalized—ailments from drinking	46.0	42.3	8.7	5.8	30.0	15.6
107. Age felt religious need	53.9	41.1	6.9	26.4	36.6	9.9
108. Age admitted to self drinking out of control	94.1	42.4	8.2	2.9	30.0	0.0
109. Age admitted to others drinking out of control	82.3	43.0	7.4	2.9	30.0	0.0
110. Age reached lowest point	93.1	44.1	7.9	88.2	44.2	9.8
2. Age attended A.A.	84.3	41.5	7.7	2.9	32.0	0.0

marital status, living alone at present, having a definite place to live after leaving the hospital, as well as recent drinking pattern, times hospitalized for drinking and times arrested for drinking. A similar relationship holds true with respect to the several items under Life Pattern of Drinking, having experienced morning shakes, drinking in the morning to steady one's self, and with respect to classification by alcohol dependency score. The alcohol dependency score is based on the work of Griffith Edwards and associates.[18]The degree of dependence is based on a summation of scores on morning shakes and morning drinks, with score zero for none, score 1 for "once or twice", and score 2 for "more often"; the possible range of scores is from 0 to 4.

Table 3 also includes a comparison of these same three groups on 12 items from the 31 item Self-Administered Alcoholism Screening Test (SAAST), which is a refinement of the Michigan Alcoholism Screening Test.[14] Note that blackouts are as common in the borderline group as in the alcoholic group, but in most other respects the borderline group falls between the alcoholic and the pure control group.

The responses of the 102 alcoholic subjects and the 34 "pure controls" on the 111 item 1946 Jellinek recommended questionnaire are given in Table 4. We have omitted from this already long table certain demographic and family environment items, as well as a few items which appeared to be repetitious.

Table 5 presents the responses of these same two groups to 40 questions which were added to the Jellinek items by one or another of the authors, earlier cited, who repeated or extended Jellinek's work.

A perusal of Tables 4 and 5 brings out several interesting points: (1) the great majority of the items are reported not only in the alcoholic group but in at least a small percentage of the control group. The only exceptions are those items which clearly enter into the definition of alcoholism, such as losing job advancement due to drinking, having frequent blackouts, sneaking drinks, abandoning attempts to control drinking, stealing, pawning, or begging in order to get alcohol, having hallucinations or DTs, and ever sleeping outdoors after drinking. (2) A few members of the control group report behaviors which would ordinarily be considered to be highly indicative of alcoholism. This includes items such as losing a job from drinking, weekend drunks (26%), beginning to need more alcohol (32%), daytime drinking, morning drinking, solitary drinking, going on the wagon, making rules to control drinking better, having a convulsion associated with drinking, protecting one's supply, attending an AA meeting, hiding of drinking, experiencing physical craving, experiencing a separation from spouse due to drinking, feeling dependent on alcohol, and drinking a fifth per day (12% of control subjects). In almost all of these

TABLE 5.–Comparison of Alcoholic and Control Groups on Items Used by Other Authors as Supplements to Jellinek Drinking History Questionnaire

	Alcoholics (N=102)			Controls (N=34)		
	Percent Reporting	Mean Age	S.D. of Age	Percent Reporting	Mean Age	S.D. of Age
1. Age drinking became a burden	100.0	28.6	9.5	26.4	25.1	5.4
2. Age drank at specific time	77.4	30.9	11.0	29.4	31.7	13.3
3. Age passed out/drinking	61.7	25.8	10.1	32.3	19.3	6.7
4. Age drank to relieve hangover	92.1	31.7	11.0	11.7	24.5	4.2
5. Age felt tense after drinking	93.1	32.9	10.7	26.4	23.3	6.5
6. Age depressed after drinking	82.3	34.9	10.3	26.4	26.0	6.5
7. Age memory not as sharp	70.5	42.4	7.2	52.9	43.0	9.1
8. Age began to hide drinking	75.4	34.9	9.1	2.9	35.0	—
9. Age experienced physical craving	92.1	36.1	10.2	8.8	21.6	4.6
10. Age began to wander off	36.2	34.3	9.3	2.9	28.0	—
11. Age began stealing to drink	10.7	32.2	9.1	0.0	—	—
12. Age began to pawn for drink	49.0	35.0	9.1	0.0	—	—
13. Age began to beg to drink	11.7	38.8	7.4	0.0	—	—
14. Age began to borrow to drink	52.9	33.4	9.2	2.9	18.0	0.0
15. Age began to feel superior drinking	26.4	24.9	8.0	14.7	28.8	11.6
16. Age felt could work better drinking	52.9	34.7	10.5	0.0	—	—
17. Age felt mentally alert drinking	54.9	34.7	10.6	14.7	42.6	5.9
18. Age first arrested/drinking	88.2	30.5	10.9	26.4	35.9	13.5
19. Age wife threatened to leave	60.7	36.0	9.9	8.8	26.3	11.0
20. Age first separated/drinking	53.9	37.0	8.7	2.9	39.0	0.0
21. Age family life unsatisfactory	77.4	34.1	8.1	11.7	33.2	17.6
22. Age took non-prescribed drugs	27.4	33.7	12.1	23.5	28.2	9.0
23. Age combined tranquilizers/alcohol	29.4	37.0	9.0	11.7	31.7	13.9
24. Age first accident/drinking	70.5	34.8	10.3	11.7	29.2	10.0
25. Age achieved highest work level	100.0	34.8	8.8	100.0	38.1	9.1
26. Age lost sleep/drinking	61.7	37.7	8.7	0.0	—	—
27. Age auditory hallucinations	33.3	38.7	8.2	0.0	—	—

28. Age visual hallucinations	29.4	38.9	8.0	0.0	—	—
29. Age first DTs	29.4	38.5	8.6	0.0	—	—
30. Age employment declined	86.2	39.9	8.4	64.7	39.0	9.2
31. Age work became sporadic	66.6	40.3	7.9	32.3	39.2	9.2
32. Age felt dependent on alcohol	87.2	39.9	8.4	11.7	31.2	13.7
33. Age drank to forget disappointments	60.1	33.6	9.8	14.7	39.4	9.0
34. Age became broke/drinking	55.8	34.5	10.0	8.8	28.0	10.8
35. Age slept outdoors	34.3	37.7	7.0	0.0	—	—
36. Age daily drinking without intoxication	82.3	28.9	10.9	29.4	35.2	12.7
37. Age drank fifth/day	89.2	32.7	10.6	11.7	22.0	3.4
38. Age usually became drunk	93.1	34.2	11.6	38.2	26.6	11.3
39. Age resented comments on drinking	67.6	34.1	10.6	17.6	28.0	13.2
40. Age forgot things/drinking	78.4	33.1	11.1	20.5	23.6	7.6

instances the average age at which the controls reported this behavior was far lower than for the alcoholic subjects. For example, the 70% of alcoholics who report a first bender give an average age of 34.1 years, whereas the one control subject who reports a first bender was age 17 at the time. Similarly, the drinking of nonbeverage alcohol is reported at an average age of 32.4 by the alcoholic subjects, whereas the one control subject who reports this was age 19 at the time. (3) It seems evident that some of the items are being answered not just in relation to alcoholism, but in relation to other psychiatric or medical illnesses or to life experiences in general. The following items in particular suggest this process: ideas of jealousy were reported by 38% of the controls and 40% of the alcoholics; diminished sex potency was reported by 41% of the controls and 60% of the alcoholics; self pity was reported by 50% of the controls and 48% of the alcoholics; thinking that the best solution was death was reported by 53% of the controls and 39% of the alcoholics; contemplation of suicide was reported by 53% of the controls and 31% of the alcoholics; accepting the services of an intermediary was reported by 24% of the controls and 25% of the alcoholics; behaving resentfully was reported by 56% of the controls and 52% of the alcoholics; periods of despondency were reported by 65% of the controls and 63% of the alcoholics; family urging psychiatric advice was reported by 44% of the controls and 31% of the alcoholics; and so on. The questions are so worded that they do not constantly mention "in relation to alcoholism," or "as a direct result of alcohol use". The subjects are therefore likely to answer positively if they have had this experience from any cause. This process is undoubtedly at work in the alcoholic group as well as in the control group. We conclude that we should not view every positive response by an alcoholic subject as necessarily indicating an experience which is a direct result of alcoholism.

Table 6 shows how the alcoholic group compares with the "pure controls" in terms of 35 items in the 1952 Jellinek scale. This table shows both the percent of subjects reporting a particular symptom and the mean age at onset. The symptoms are at times repeated; for example, symptom 1 is "first blackout", whereas symptom 5 is "frequent blackouts". You will note that 20% of the pure control group reported a blackout as against 74% of the alcoholic group, but that the mean age at which this is reported is 22 years in the pure controls compared with 30.8 in the alcoholics, a difference much like that reported by Goodwin. In general there is a tendency for the symptoms to appear at earlier ages in the control group (for those individuals who do experience that particular symptom). There are relatively few of the symptoms which are not experienced by at least one or two members of the pure control group, individuals who fairly clearly do not have alcoholism.

TABLE 6.–Frequency and Age of Onset of Twenty-Eight Selected* Jellinek Items

	Alcoholics (N=102)		Pure Controls (N=34)	
	Percent Reporting	Mean Age at Onset	Percent Reporting	Mean Age at Onset
PRODROMAL PHASE				
1. First blackout	74 (%)	30.8 (yrs)	20 (%)	22.0 (yrs)
2. Sneak drinking	70	34.3	0	–
3. Freq. anticipatory drink- ing	50	31.0	3	16.0
4. Evasion	47	33.2	6	28.5
5. Freq. blackouts	50	35.1	0	–
CRUCIAL PHASE				
8. Loss of control	93 (%)	36.2 (yrs)	3	25.0
9. Rationalization	80	35.3	9	26.0
10. Freq. grandiose behav.	49	31.2	9	30.3
12. Freq. aggressive behav.	32	31.2	9	30.3
13. Remorse	81	38.4	15	34.4
15. Control attempts	90	38.0	20	33.3
16. Freq. avoid friends	17	35.9	3	39.0
17. Freq. quitting jobs	32	36.2	0	–
19. Loss of interests	75	39.0	9	31.7
22. Geographic escape	65	38.4	56	40.0
25. Supply protection	72	37.7	3	34.0
26. Freq. neglect	90	40.4	3	45.0
27. Hospitalization	75	43.4	3	20.0
28. Sexual decline	60	43.6	41	42.0
29. Jealousy	40	31.2	38	28.4
30. Freq. morning drinking	81	38.3	15	39.8
CHRONIC PHASE				
31. Freq. Benders	63	37.0	0	–
35. Drinking down	0	–	0	–
36. Freq. technical products	7	37.6	0	–
37. Tolerance decline	48	41.7	6	37.5
39. Freq. tremors	78	39.5	0	–
42. Religious needs	54	41.1	26	36.7
43. Admitting defeat	94	42.4	3	30.6

*Parks, *J. Stud. Alc.,* 34:473–488

Table 7 gives 27 of the 43 Jellinek variables arranged in order of onset in our sample of 102 alcoholics. Note that "first blackout" comes first, thus fitting Jellinek's assertion that this is an early symptom of alcoholism; on the other hand, in the pure control group the first blackouts occurred an average of 8 years earlier.

Table 7 gives, in the next to last column, the order of onset in the

TABLE 7.–Chronological Order and Phasing of 27 Alcoholism Experiences:
Comparison with Jellinek Order and Phasing

VARIABLE	Mean Age of Onset in Alcoholic Sample (N=102)	Our Phase	Order of Onset in Jellinek System (43 items in all)	Jellinek Phase
First blackouts	30.8	Early	1	Prodromal
Freq. anticipatory drinking	31.0	"	3	Prodromal
Freq. grandiose behavior	31.0	"	11	Crucial
Freq. aggressive behavior	31.2	"	12	Crucial
Jealousy	31.2	"	29	Crucial
Evasion	33.2	"	6	Prodromal
Sneak drinks	34.3	"	2	Prodromal
Freq. blackouts	35.1	"	7	Prodromal
Rationalization	35.3	"	9	Crucial
Freq. avoids friends	35.9	"	16	Crucial
Loss of control	36.2	Middle	8	Crucial
Freq. quit jobs	36.2	"	17	Crucial
Freq. benders	37.0	Late	31	Chronic
Freq. technical products	37.6	"	36	Chronic
Protect supply	37.7	"	25	Crucial
Control attempts	38.0	"	14	Crucial
Freq. morning drinking	38.3	"	30	Crucial
Remorse	38.4	"	13	Crucial
Geographical escape	38.4	"	22	Crucial
Loss of interest	39.0	"	19	Crucial
Freq. tremors	39.5	"	39	Chronic
Freq. neglect	40.4	"	26	Crucial
Religious need	41.4	"	42	Chronic
Tolerance decline	41.7	"	37	Chronic
Admitting defeat	42.7	"	43	Chronic
Hospitalization	43.4	"	27	Crucial
Sexual decline	43.6	"	28	Crucial

Rank order correlation between our order and Jellinek's=.74

Jellinek system (only 27 of the 43 ranks are included). The last column shows how these 27 experiences were classed in Jellinek's phases. Although there is some intermixture of the three phases, there is generally good correspondence with Jellinek's grouping.

When we converted our mean age of onset and Jellinek's order to ranks (1 to 27), the rank order correlation coefficient between the two was .74.

DISCUSSION

There have been more recent conceptualizations of the progression of alcoholism. DSM-II has categories for drinking problems which imply a progression. This system has been tightened up and clarified in a publication by Sheldon Miller and associates.[15]

Benjamin Kissin[16] has offered a conceptualization of the long term process of the development of alcoholism which divides this into three phases: (1) emergent development of the susceptible individual; (2) the induction phase with exposure to alcohol and beginning dependency; (3) the phase of deep rooted alcoholism in which new physical, self-perpetuating mechanisms develop. Kissin's view is much more phar-macological in nature and places less stress on psychological, subjective and interpersonal behaviors.

In our sample of 102 alcoholics, first blackouts was the earliest symptom of the 21 shown in the Table. Also, frequent blackouts occurred reasonably early, eight in order of the 27. So for alcoholics these are early manifestations.

On the other hand, we saw on the SAAST scale that 26% of the pure controls reported blackouts as compared to 83% of the alcoholics. Those controls who reported blackouts reported the first occurrence at a mean age of 20.0 years, as compared to a mean age of 30.8 years for the first blackout reported by alcoholics. Therefore the occurrence of an alcoholic blackout *early in life* might even be said to predict nonalcoholism, more in line with Goodwin's findings than with Jellinek's.

In answering the Jellinek history question, 20% of our control group reported a (first) blackout, as against 74% of the alcoholic group. It is generally accepted that about 10% of drinkers become alcoholics. If we therefore picture a group of 1,000 young people beginning to drink, we could assume that roughly 100 would later become alcoholics. Seventy-four of these 100 will have a first blackout, whereas 20% of the other 900, or 180, will also have a first blackout. Therefore only 74/254, or 29% of those who report a first blackout will become alcoholics. Clearly this is not a very specific indicator for alcoholism.

The idea of a progression, a typical succession of symptoms is certainly a familiar one in relation to diseases. Even acute illnesses typically have an incubation period, prodromal or early signs of symptoms, an acute phase, perhaps a crisis or turning point, a resolution phase and a convalescent phase, possibly ending with residuals. Textbooks usually describe and list the whole range of signs and symptoms that may appear in one of these phases, but it is not expected that every patient will have all of them or that they will always follow a particular order.

There are also disorders with exacerbations and remissions, such as multiple sclerosis, in which advances of the disease are followed by retreats, although never to the beginning point. There is therefore a step-wise, long-term progression. Again, there is a wide variety of ways in which this disorder can start, develop, and progress. Although textbooks list all of the possibilities, it does not seem to bother us that a particular patient may show only one or a few of the range of possible manifestations. There is no reason why alcoholism could not be fitful in progression in some cases as well as uniformly progressive in others.

The physical damage aspect of alcoholism would usually follow the chronic disease or intermittently progressive disease models. For example, the earlier or milder stages of liver damage, such as fatty liver, appear to be reversible if drinking stops, whereas the advanced degrees of liver damage such as hepatitis and particularly cirrhosis may become irreversible. The "landmarks" in physical disorder progression can be simply the diagnostic tests to establish presence and severity of a disorder of some organ system.

One major conceptual problem in the disease concept of alcoholism is related to the presence of a range of "normal drinking" at the proximal end of the "scale". Up to some point we want to consider drinking as nonmaladaptive, nondisease, and nonpathological. All of the rating scales for alcoholism tend to dip into this area: they inquire into age at first drink, age at time of first intoxicated episode, etc. According to Goodwin, it is possible that the first alcoholic "blackout" lies within the normal drinking part of the range. The presence of this normal drinking phase puts an extra burden on diagnostic schemes: they have to draw the line between normal drinking and problem drinking. This may be why the concept of "progression" creates different problems in alcoholism than with other diseases. The notion of "progression" includes some (presumed) first decisive step from the range of normal drinking into that of pathological drinking. Since at least nine out of ten social drinkers do not make this step, there cannot be an inevitable or built-in progression. What is it then, that leads the other 1/10 to "progress"? We typically postulate some kind of mechanism which takes hold or comes into play in this minority. The theories range widely and include genetic predisposition, some biochem-cial difference, possibly a biochemical change after sustained exposure to alcohol, possibly early organ damage or physical change, possibly a conditioning or habit reinforcement mechanism, possibly the presence of personality problems, neurosis or psychosis such as depression, and possibly the workings of social and cultural pressures and influences.

Another possibility is that one or another of these may be operative in different alcoholics, so that there may not be a single alcoholism from an etiological or development standpoint. This point of view has been well developed by Kissin:[17] in the early stages, problem and excessive drinking may be due to a variety of causes, but as the disorder becomes established and becomes more of a "pharmacological" condition (with psychic dependence, tolerance, physical dependence, withdrawal syndromes) it thereafter becomes more of a single disorder, a "final common pathway".

Many of the earlier writings in the area of progression of symptoms seem to ignore the pharmacological aspects of alcohol. This is not surprising since many of these concepts were developed and put forth before the development of the current pharmacological knowledge of alcohol. Jellinek's initial paper was published in 1946, where as the fact that DTs represented the withdrawal reaction from physical dependence on alcohol was only established by the work of Victor and Adams in 1953 and Isbell and associates in 1955. In the otherwise excellent paper by Trice and Wahl,[5] published in 1958, there is the statement: "About 1/3 of the alcoholics agreed that the first convulsions, tremors and protecting supply belong together; here, the appealing explanation is a causal one, e.g., pathological anxiety, which reflects itself in three symptoms." A more modern explanation would be that such a person has physical dependence and is protecting his supply to insure that withdrawal will not be absolute.

An important complication in viewing alcohol as a progressive disorder is the existence of various possibilities regarding continued or further use of alcohol. The simplest case is where the subject never quits using alcohol, so that both the drinking behavior and the complications tend to get uniformly worse. The next simplest case is where a subject stops drinking completely, never to resume. Here the condition may reverse or stablize at some impaired level, but in some instances (as in cirrhosis) may progress anyway. The most common situation, however, is that the alcoholic individual will alternate periods of abstinence with periods of heavy drinking. Since the damaging influence is being applied intermittently, this will certainly be reflected in the resulting complications and secondary effects. This will clearly interfere with any simple and predictable scheme of gradual progression.

With respect to alcoholic "blackouts", it appears to us that a "blackout" is simply a manifestation of high blood levels of alcohol or rapidly rising blood levels of alcohol. We question the assertion by Jellinek that in the early stages of alcoholism a blackout may occur after only two or three drinks. It is likely that persons who report this are simply hiding the actual amount and rate of their alcohol ingestion.

More recently, research has been reported which has considerably illuminated the alcoholic "blackout". Direct observations of alcoholics during drinking episodes indicate that blackouts occur after heavy alcohol intake and at high blood levels, [18-21] that persons who are in an intoxicated state for which they will be amnesic can be identified by an impairment in short-term memory,[18] and that the impairment in short-term memory in alcoholic blackouts is similar to that found in Korsakoff's syndrome,[22,23,24] although this last relationship is still being worked out in detail. None of this work suggests that blackouts would occur at low blood alcohol levels (after three or four drinks and without evidence of intoxication). It is tempting to speculate that the advanced drinker who might have a "subclinical Korsakoff's syndrome" might develop amnesia on smaller doses of alcohol. Even if this occurred, it would be a late sign of alcoholism.

Tabulating the first occurrence of a symptom or behavior by age at the time seems to be of limited significance in differentiating alcoholics from nonalcoholics. In fact, it appears that virtually any of the symptoms listed may occur in an isolated fashion, perhaps only once, even in our purified control group, persons who clearly have not developed alcoholism. Yet in looking at the individual symptoms and behaviors they do clearly suggest alcoholism. What may be missing from this approach is the quantitative factor. Regarding blackouts, for example, the occurrence of a single blackout may not mean anything except that a person drank excessively on one occasion. (The inexperienced drinker might be more likely to do this than the experienced one.) It is when blackouts begin to occur *frequently* that they assume diagnostic and prognostic significance. The same argument can be applied to most of Jellinek's list of symptoms and, in fact, to drunkenness itself.

CONCLUSIONS

1. We have generally confirmed the order of appearance of the symptoms of alcoholism, as described by Jellinek. Our order of appearance of 27 leading symptoms yielded a rank order correlation coefficient of .74 when compared with Jellinek's order.
2. Most of the other attempts to repeat Jellinek's work have come to the same conclusion, confirming the order in general but differing in many details.
3. Although blackouts appear early in the drinking history of alcoholics, they appear even earlier in the drinking history of 1 out of 5 nonalcoholic drinkers.
4. It is estimated that 7 out of 10 drinkers who experience a first blackout will not become alcoholics.
5. Blackouts seem to occur only after heavy and/or rapid drinking, with visible intoxication.

6. Most of the drinking behaviors are also found in some nonalcoholic drinkers, the exceptions being those items which indicate marked tolerance, physical dependence, withdrawal reactions, and physical damage.

7. The 111 items in Jellinek's expanded 1946 questionnaire appear to be composed of a mixture of moderate to heavy drinking behaviors, habituation, psychological dependence, altered pattern of drinking, family problems, work problems, social problems, legal problems, evidence of increased tolerance, physical dependence, withdrawal reactions, physical damage, and treatment and restitutive efforts. Subsequent work has done much to identify and clarify these underlying processes. We consider that it is better to work with each of these processes separately, establishing their presence, degree of progression, reversibility, etc., rather than combining all of them into a single scale of progression of alcoholism.

REFERENCES

1. Kraepelin, E. *Lectures on Clinical Psychiatry.* Translated by Johnstone, T. New York: William Wood and Company, 1912.

2. Jellinek, E.M. Phases in the drinking history of alcoholics: analysis of a survey conducted by the official organ of Alcoholic Anonymous. *Q.J. Stud. Alcohol.* 7:1–88, 1946.

3. Jellinek, E.M. Phases of alcohol addiction. *Q.J. Stud. Alcohol.* 13:673–684, 1952.

4. Jackson, J.K. H-technique scales of preoccupation with alcohol and of psychological involvement in alcoholics: time order of symptoms. *Q.J. Stud. Alcohol.* 18(1); 451–467, Jan.-Dec. 1957.

5. Trice, H., and Wahl, R. A rank order analysis of the symptoms of alcoholism. *Q.J. Stud. Alcohol.* 19:636–648, 1958.

6. Park, P. Drinking experiences of 806 Finnish alcoholics in comparison with similar experiences of 1922 English alcoholics. *Acta Psychiat. Scand.* 38:227–246, 1962.

7. Park, P. Developmental ordering of experiences in alcoholism. *Q.J. Stud. Alcohol.* 34:473–488, 1973.

8. Park, P., and Whitehead, P.D. Developmental sequence and dimensions of alcoholism. *Q.J. Stud. Alcohol.* 34:887–904, 1973.

9. Orford, J., and Hawker, A. Note on the ordering of onset of symptoms in alcohol dependence. *Psychological Med.* 4:281–288, 1974.

10. Goodwin, D., Crane, B., and Guze ,S. Alcoholic "blackouts": a review and clinical study of 100 alcoholics. *Am. J. Psychiat.* 126(2): 191–198, Aug. 1969.

11. Curlee, J. Alcoholic blackouts: some conflicting evidence. *Q.J. Stud. Alcohol.* 34:409–413, 1973.

12. Criteria Committee of the National Council on Alcoholism: Criteria for the diagnosis of alcoholism. *Am. J. Psychiat.* 129:127–135, 1972.

13. Edwards, G., Hensman, C., and Peto, J. Drinking problems among recidivist prisoners. *Psychological Med.* 1:388–399, 1971.
14. Swenson, W., and Morse, R. The use of a self-administered alcoholism screening test (SAAST) in a medical center. *Mayo Clin. Proc.* 50:204–208, 1975.
15. Miller, S., Helmick, E., Berg, L., Nutting, P., and Shorr, G. Alcoholism: a statewide program evaluation. *Am. J. Psychiat.* 131:210–214, 1974.
16. Kissin, B. The pharmacodynamics and natural history of alcoholism, in *The Biology of Alcoholism, vol 3: Clinical Pathology.* New York: Plenum Press, 1974.
17. Kissin, B. The use of psychoactive drugs in the long-term treatment of chronic alcoholics. *Ann. N.Y. Acad. Sci.* 252:835–395, 1975.
18. Goodwin, D., Othmer, E., Halikas, J., and Freemon, F. Loss of short-term memory as a predictor of the alcoholic "blackout." *Nature* 227:201–202, July 11, 1970.
19. Ryback, R. Alcohol amnesia. *Q.J. Stud. Alcohol.* 31:616–632, 1970.
20. Goodwin, D. Two species of alcoholic "blackout." *Am. J. Psychiat.* 127:1665–1670, 1971.
21. Tamerin, J., Weiner, S., Popper, R., Steinglass, P., and Mendelsohn, J. Alcohol and memory: amnesia and short-term memory function during experimentally induced intoxication. *Am. J. Psychiat.* 127:1659–1664, 1971.
22. Cermak, L., and Butters, N. Information processing deficits of alcoholic Korsakoff patients. *Q. J. Stud. Alcohol.* 34:1110–1132, 1973.
23. Cermak, L., and Ryback, R. Recovery of verbal short-term memory in alcoholics. *J. Stud. on Alcohol* 37:46–52, 1976.
24. Goodwin, D., Hill, S., Hooper, S., and Viesselman, J. Alcoholic blackouts and Korsakoff's syndrome, in Gross M.M. (ed.) *Alcohol Intoxication and Withdrawal.* New York: Plenum Press, 1973.

CHAPTER 5

Neurological Syndromes Associated with Alcohol

STANLEY H. APPEL

NEUROLOGICAL SYNDROMES ASSOCIATED WITH ALCOHOL

The abuse of alcohol has definite effects on the nervous system of man. Some of these effects are due to acute intoxication; others are due to withdrawal, to associated nutritional deficiency, or to toxic effects of alcohol metabolites on the central and peripheral nervous system. In Table 1, we have listed the range of neurologic syndromes associated with alcohol. Although thiamine or other B vitamin deficiencies have been clearly implicated in the pathogenesis of several of these syndromes, they are not responsible for all of them. In conditions such as alcoholic myopathy, we suspect that the muscle plasma membrane may be the fundamental target of the insult, but there are no unequivocal data as to its specific cause. In conditions such as diffuse cortical atrophy, we have no knowledge either of the etiological factor or the subcellular locus of the injury. Alcohol itself has been implicated as a specific toxin and nutritional deprivation is thought to play essentially no role in the deficit. However, further data are required to implicate alcohol itself in any neurologic syndromes in man. In the discussion which follows we have selected several of the syndromes of Table 1 which are best understood, and have described their characteristic neurological features.

TABLE 1.–Neurological Diseases Associated with Alcohol

1. Acute intoxication

2. Alcohol withdrawal syndrome (time of appearance after cessation of drinking)
   Tremulousness (7–24 Hours)
   Hallucinosis— visual or auditory (12–48 Hours)
   Delerium tremens (36–96 Hours)
   Withdrawal seizures (7–48 Hours)

3. Nutritional diseases of the nervous system
   Polyneuropathy
   Wernicke-Korsakoff Syndrome
   Amblyopia

4. Possible nutritional or toxic effects of alcohol or metabolites
   Alcoholic myopathy
   Cerebellar degeneration
   Central pontine myelinolysis

5. Secondary to cirrhosis
   Hepatic coma
   Hepatocentral degeneration

ALCOHOLIC MYOPATHY

A spectrum of muscular abnormalities has been associated with alcoholism. Some patients may be essentially asymptomatic with respect to the musculoskeletal system and have an elevated serum creatine phosphokinase (CPK) level. Other patients may have muscle tenderness as well as an elevation of serum CPK. A few patients have been observed to have a severe acute illness characterized by striking muscle cramps with trace amounts of myoglobin in the urine. A more severe form of the same illness is characterized by the sudden onset of severe muscle pain and cramps, exquisite muscle tenderness, and gross myoglobinuria. Some of these patients may develop considerable atrophy, especially in the proximal distribution, accompanied by muscle tenderness and creatinuria. Occasionally the chronic myopathy may appear without any preceding acute syndrome (Figure 1).

When patients have severe cramps or gross myoglobinuria, their serum enzymes are usually elevated. However, CPK may be increased in a substantial number of alcoholic patients in the absence of abnormalities on clinical muscle examination or on muscle biopsy examination. When severe clinical syndromes are present, intracellular edema, cellular disruption and hyaline and granular changes may be noted on histological examination of muscle biopsy specimens. The mechanism by which alcohol induces these changes is not known. One prominent possibility is

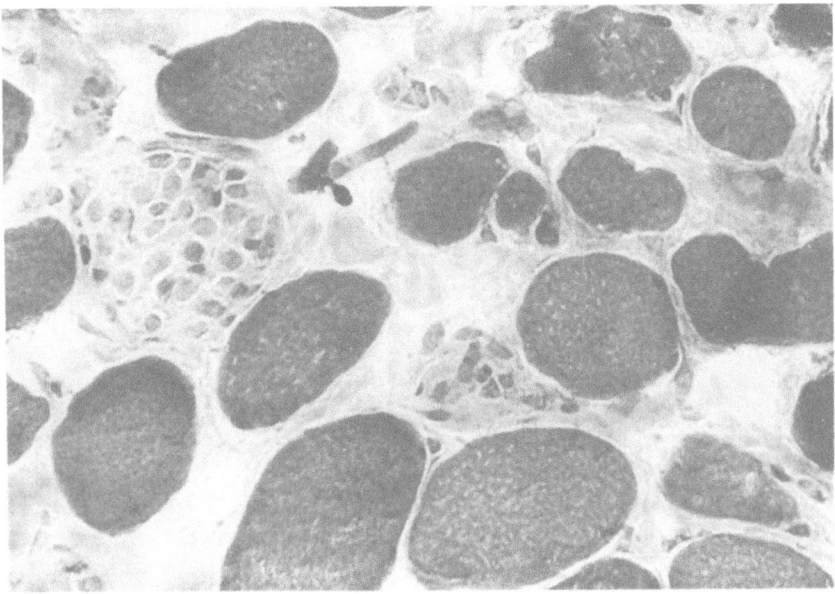

Figure 1. Biopsy from quadriceps muscle of alcoholic patient with severe proximal muscle weakness following an episode of rhabdomyolysis with very high CPK. Biopsy was taken one month after this episode and shows necrotic fiber (arrow) and rounding of fibers. In acute phase, necrosis of fibers is commonly seen. In severe subacute cases, such as the present one, necrosis and other myopathic changes are also seen. (Courtesy of Dr. Y. Harati.)

that leakage of myoglobin occurs by direct damage of the cell membrane by alcohol.

Nutrition per se has not been shown to play an important role, although patients are more likely to develop rhabdomyolysis and myoglobinuria if they use alcohol in conjunction with a low carbohydrate diet. Ischemia may also play a role, or some abnormal metabolite of alcohol may be responsible. All forms of the alcohol-induced disorder appear to be reversible when drinking is stopped.

ALCOHOLIC POLYNEUROPATHY

Patients with alcoholic polyneuropathy usually have complaints of weakness, paresthesias, and pain. The symptoms usually begin slowly and progress just as slowly. Weakness and pain commonly begin distally in the lower extremities and progress proximally. The pain may take the form of a dull ache in the feet and legs, and complaints of coldness and occasionally

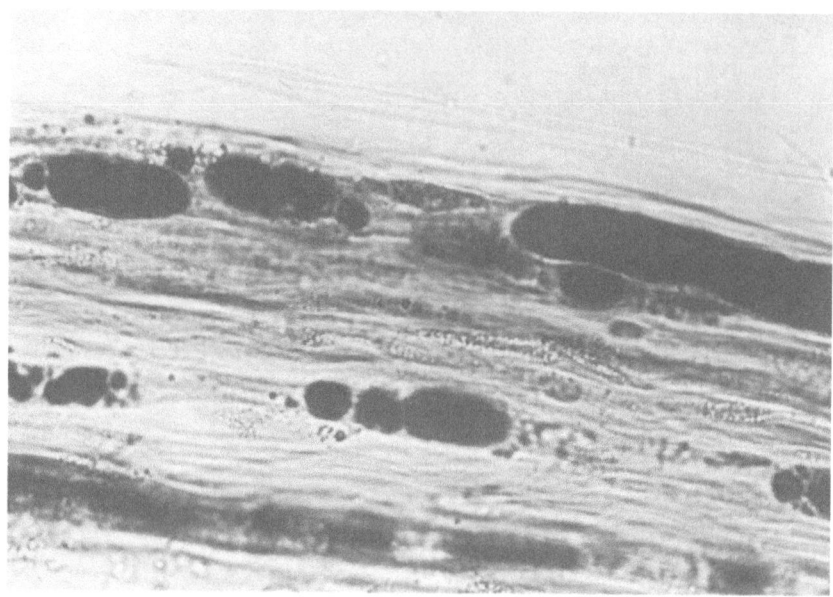

Figure 2.   Sural nerve biopsy showing breakdown of myelinated fibers into myelin ovoids and balls, a sign of axonal degeneration usually seen in alcoholic neuropathy. This is a teased nerve fiber and stained with osmic acid. (Courtesy of Dr. Y. Harati.)

burning sensations may be present. When the burning sensations are prominent, the patients cannot stand to have anything touch their feet and walking becomes extremely difficult. Gradually the hands may become involved, but usually less significantly than the legs. The cranial nerves are usually spared except for occasional involvement of the optic and vagus nerves. Deep tendon reflexes may be lost in the legs even when only slight weakness is present. Reflexes in the arms are usually present. The sensory impairment usually involves all modalities, but in the presence of burning dysaesthesias, position and vibration sense may be particularly impaired. When the vagus nerve is involved, patients may have difficulty phonating. Their voice is husky, they may have actual vocal cord palsy, and they may complain of difficulty swallowing.

When the optic nerve is involved in alcoholic amblyopia, patients complain of blurring of vision for near and distant objects. Visual acuity is reduced, and large centrocecal scotomas may be present bilaterally. With good nutrition and vitamin B supplementation, improvement may occur in most acute and subacute cases.

The primary pathologic changes are confined to peripheral nerve degeneration while nerve roots may be involved in advanced cases. Both myelin and axis cylinders may be involved secondary to Wallerian Degeneration. The anterior horn cells of the spinal cord demonstrate "axonal reaction" secondary to the axon damage in peripheral nerves and roots. This deficit has been related to thiamine deficiency since restoring thiamine to patients who continue to consume alcohol results in improvement of the polyneuropathy. However many other vitamins may also contribute to the pathology. Recovery from nutritional polyneuropathy is usually slow with restoration of motor function in several weeks. In severe disease, recovery may take several months to a year (Figure 2).

ALCOHOLIC CEREBELLAR DEGENERATION

One of the most characteristic syndromes associated with alcoholism is that of transient ataxia associated with acute inebriation. In acute intoxication, the cerebellar involvement is only one of function and rarely progresses to involve structural changes. In the chronic form, cerebellar dysfunction is characterized by widebased stance and gait, varying degrees of instability of the trunk, and ataxia of the legs. The arms are involved to a much lesser extent than the legs, with very little dysmetria, decomposition of movement, or increased rebound. The general rule to be followed is that alcoholic cerebellar degeneration involves gait more than legs, and legs more than arms. Often the patient may be markedly ataxic while erect and walking, and have minimal deficits of legs and arms when tested in a recumbent position on an examining couch or bed. In most patients the cerebellar syndrome evolves subacutely over a period of several weeks, and may subsequently remain unchanged for many years. In others, the disease evolves over a period of many months but eventually stabilizes. The disorder is far more frequent in men than in women.

The involvement of the cerebellum in alcoholic cerebellar degeneration is identical to its involvement in Wernicke's Disease, and probably represents the same disease process. Thus the cerebellar involvement is probably nutritional in origin, possibly related to a deficiency in thiamine. However the data supporting this proposition are at best circumstantial, and a direct toxic effect of alcohol cannot be ruled out. Purkinje cells are dramatically compromised in the cerebellar cortex, especially in the midline portion of the cerebellum including both the anterior and superior aspect of the vermis and the anterior portion of the anterior lobes. When the cerebellar degeneration appears with ocular and mental signs, we consider the syndrome to be that of Wernicke's Disease. However, when the ataxia and gait disturbances appear by themselves, we consider the disorder to be that of alcoholic cerebellar degeneration.

THE WERNICKE-KORSAKOFF SYNDROME

Wernicke's Disease is a neurologic disorder characterized by the acute onset of nystagmus, ataxia of gait, ocular palsies, global confusion and polyneuropathy, occurring together or in various combinations. Korsakoff's Psychosis may be defined as an abnormal mental state in which memory and learning are affected out of all proportion to other cognitive functions. According to Doctors Victor, Adams and Collins,[1] Wernicke's Encephalopathy and Korsakoff's Psychosis are two facets of the same syndrome in the alcoholic nutritionally deprived patient. Both disorders appear in the same clinical setting and the mental symptoms which may start with mild delirium may progress to global confusion, apathy, and subsequently pass through a stage of amnesia and confabulation. In its severest form the memory and learning defect may be present without confabulation, and this syndrome has been termed alcoholic dementia. However, both the clinical characteristics of the dementia and the pathologic changes are identical to those noted in the Wernicke-Korsakoff Syndrome and do not justify a separate designation. From a pathological point of view Wernicke's Disease and Korsakoff Psychosis are the same, differing only with respect to the age of the glial and vascular reaction.[2]

The characteristic presentation of the patient with Wernicke-Korsakoff Syndrome includes ataxia, confusion, and ocular motor palsies. On examination patients commonly have a tachycardia as well as evidence of nutritional deficiency such as a red depapillated tongue, discoloration or increased pigmentation of the skin, and evidence of liver disease manifested by hepatomegaly, jaundice, ascites, and spider angiomta.

The most characteristic derangement of mental function is that of a global confusional state. Patients are usually disoriented and apathetic. Their attention span is markedly limited, and they have minimal spontaneous speech. In this stage memory function is extremely difficult to assess. When such patients become alert and responsive, it is apparent that memory and learning are significantly disturbed. The characteristic

TABLE 2.–Amnesic Defect in Wernicke-Korsakoff's

1. Immediate and remote memory intact—verbal and non-verbal

2. Recent memory impaired—cognitive deficit, decreased attention

   A. Impaired use of semantic encoding—use associative and acoustic cues normally

   B. More sensitive to proactive interference

   C. Perseveration, inappropriate strategy

*Adapted from Butters and Cermak [4].

defect in memory function is that of impaired recent memory.[3] Immediate and remote memory are intact for verbal and non-verbal tasks. However, in the analysis of the impaired recent memory, Butters and his colleagues have demonstrated increased perseveration and the use of inappropriate strategies to encode the memories.[4] The primary defect appears to be an impaired use of semantic encoding while associative and acoustic cues are employed normally. This deficit is quite distinct from that noted in other encephalopathies with impaired memory function such as Huntington's Chorea or Alzheimer's Disease.

The most common ocular abnormality noted in the Wernicke-Korsakoff Syndrome is that of nystagmus. This usually takes the form of horizontal nystagmus on lateral gaze, together with a vertical nystagmus on upward gaze. Horizontal nystagmus may also appear by itself whereas vertical nystagmus alone is less common. Weakness of abduction is the next most common ocular abnormality noted, and is often bilateral. A large percentage of patients may also have weakness of conjugate gaze.

As mentioned in the section on alcoholic degeneration, the ataxia seen in Wernicke-Korsakoff is clinically and pathologically identical to that noted in alcoholic degeneration. An intention tremor of the limbs is rather unusual, whereas a marked disorder of gait and locomotion is more characteristic. Similarly, cerebellar speech is rather uncommon in these disorders. The polyneuropathy in Wernicke-Korsakoff patients is identical to that noted clinically and pathologically in patients who present only with peripheral nerve disease. Often patients have no complaint referable to the limbs, but the signs of polyneuropathy are evident on examination. In these situations, the polyneuropathy is usually mild and consists only of loss of muscle bulk and the presence of tenderness in the legs, a depression of the ankle jerks and often of the knee jerks, and patchy and variable decrease in pinprick and touch sensation over the feet and legs. Patients with Wernicke-Korsakoff Syndrome usually have impaired sensory and motor function together with impaired reflexes. Approximately 25% of patients may have only a loss of reflexes, whereas approximately 20% of the patients have impaired reflexes and a loss of sensation.

On laboratory examination patients usually have an abnormality in liver function tests, as well as an anemia, possibly of nutritional origin. Electroencephalograms (EEG) are abnormal in a significant number of cases with no characteristic pattern being noted. Cerebrospinal fluid (CSF) examination usually demonstrates a slightly elevated protein, but essentially no other changes unless trauma and/or infection are present.

Confabulation has been generally regarded as a specific feature of Korsakoff Psychosis and a requisite for diagnosis. However, in no sense is it specific for this disorder and many patients with this syndrome do not confabulate. Usually confabulation takes place in a setting of confusion and a possible gross perceptual disorder. Later in the disease during convalesence, the patient may relate past events and experiences with no regard for proper temporal sequence, and this has been interpreted as confabulation. As a rule, confabulatory content is consistent with the patient's occupation or usual activities. In no sense is confabulation a deliberate attempt to hide the memory defect out of embarrassment, but rather it represents the patient's sincere effort to fill in the gap in his memory with whatever statement possible.[3]

The major pathological changes of Wernicke-Korsakoff Syndrome involve the periaqueductal regions, the floor of the fourth ventricle, the mammillary bodies, and portions of the thalamus including medial dorsal nuclei, anterior medial nuclei, and pulvinar. In addition the anterior lobe of the cerebellum as well as the vermis may be involved as are the peripheral nerves in the lower extremities. At the light microscopic level, blood vessels are extremely prominent as the result of proliferation of cellular element in their walls. Myelinated fibers appear to be more involved than nerve cells. The lesions of the closed medial nuclei of the thalamus have been specifically implicated in the amnestic-confabulatory syndrome, but other lesions in the limbic system are commonly present and these may be equally important in the memory deficits.

Nutritional supplementation of the patient with Wernicke-Korsakoff demonstrates that thiamine may improve the ocular palsies within several days to weeks. The nystagmus and cerebellar signs take longer to return, and may persist in a substantial number of cases. The confusional state usually is quite responsive to thiamine, and any patient with a past history of alcoholism or nutritional deprivation who presents in the emergency room with a confusional state should be given thiamine intravenously. When patients with a more chronic Korsakoff Psychosis are administered thiamine, the results are not striking. Usually the majority of patients have incomplete recovery of their memory function, even though they may have good recovery of their ocular palsies, ataxia, and peripheral neuropathy.

SUBACUTE NECROTIZING ENCEPHALOMYELOPATHY (LEIGH'S DISEASE)

Thiamine has been well recognized as an important vitamin which participates as a cofactor in a number of enzymatic reactions primarily concerned with energy metabolism in cell. It participates in oxidative decarboxylation of pyruvate to acetyl CoA. In addition it participates in the pentose phosphate pathway. Although such reactions are important in the central nervous system, data with thiamine antagonists suggest that these enzyme systems may be normal at a time when neurologic deficits are present. For this reason thiamine has also been postulated to play a structural role in the nervous system, perhaps as a vital constituent of the axon membrane which regulates sodium flux and nerve conduction.

Leigh's Encephalopathy is an inherited disorder in which muscle weakness, hypotonia, and mental deterioration appear within the first two years of life.[5] Involvement of vision, motor function, cerebellar function, and respirations are usually present as is lactic acidosis. The disease is progressive and usually leads to death in several months to a year. Pathologically the lesions are quite similar to those noted in Wernicke's Disease with the exception that the mammillary bodies are usually involved in Wernicke's Disease and are spared in Leigh's encephalopathy.

These pathological similarities suggest a potential role for thiamine in the disorder. In Leigh's there is no nutritional deficiency of thiamine; however, thiamine triphosphate is greatly reduced in the brain.[6] An inhibitor has been demonstrated in the urine of Leigh's patients which prevents the conversion of thiamine diphosphate to thiamine triphosphate. The effects of this inhibitor have been overcome by the administration of large doses of thiamine, thereby providing some definite benefit on reversing the devastating clinical syndrome.

The importance of this inborn error of metabolism in man is to suggest that thiamine may play a role within the central nervous system other than as a cofactor in well-recognized enzymatic reactions. Whether such a role is primarily as a structural component of nerve cell membranes or some other specific function is presently unclear. Nevertheless, this syndrome has been quite important for its ability to generate new insights with respect to the pathogenesis of the various alcoholic nutritional states and the molecular mechanism by which thiamine deficiency impairs neurological function. Further study of this rare condition may not only shed light on molecular defects noted in the alcoholic patients, but may also contribute to a greater understanding of the normal structure and function of central and peripheral nervous system of Man.

REFERENCES

1. Victor, M., Adams, R.D., and Collins, G. H. *The Wernicke-Korsakoff Syndrome.* Philadelphia: F.A. Davis, 1971.
2. Victor, M., and Silby, H. Thiamine deficiency, in Goldensohn, E.J. and Appel, S.H. (eds.), *Scientific Approaches to Clinical Neurology.* Philadelphia: Lea & Febiger, 1977.

3. Talland, G.A. *Deranged Memory.* New York: Academic Press, 1965.
4. Butters, N., and Cermak, L. Some Analyses of Amnesic Syndromes, in Issacpan, R.L., and Pribram, K.H. (eds.), *Brain-Damaged Patients in the Hippocampus,* Vol. 2, New York: Academic Press, pp. 377–410.
5. Leigh, D. Subacute necrotizing encephalomyelopathy in an infant. *J. Neurol. Neurosurg. Psychiat.* 14:216, 1951.
6. Cooper, J.R., and Pincus, J.H. Thiamine triphosphate deficiency in Leigh's disease (subacute necrotizing encephalomyelopathy), in Hammes, F.A., and Van Den Berg, C.J. (eds.), *Inborn Errors of Metabolism.* New York: 1973.

CHAPTER 6

Can Anyone Become Alcoholic?

ROY B. MEFFERD, JR.
JOHNE M. LENNON
NANCY E. DAWSON
LAUREN BOEHME

In conceptualizing alcoholism as a disease,[1,2] several questions must be considered:

1. Is everyone susceptible to alcohol addiction—as is the case with heroin—or are only certain people susceptible?
2. Is the addiction alcohol-specific, a special case of a broader range of possible addictions, or is it merely an expression of extreme general susceptibility to habit formation and maintenance?
3. Does prolonged exposure to alcohol induce permanent physiological and/or psychological changes, such that "once an alcoholic, always an alcoholic"?
4. Does the development of alcoholism follow the predictable course described by Jellinek?
5. Does the compulsion of alcoholics to re-commence drinking after a period of sobriety result from a physiological *need,* a psychological *craving,* or simply a generalized *desire* for motivational-emotional relief?
6. Do Jellinek's categories of drinkers merely differ in levels of motivation, emotional control, learning speed and the like?

7. Is there *an*"alcoholism" personality, or are there different kinds or types of alcoholics?

The answers to all of these questions are uncertain and doubtless none are completely true! Yet all may be somewhat true.

There is persuasive evidence[3] about the first three questions. First, all primates, in quite small samples, suffer common effects of prolonged involuntary infusion of alcohol. Due to the small sample size, the question of universal addictability, therefore, remains open.

The story is quite different, however, with voluntary imbibing. Most animals avoid alcohol like poison and must be enticed to drink it. Having sampled alcohol, some primates become steady drinkers. However, relative to Question 2, other primates began drinking *only* in combination with a powerful "reinforcing" drug such as cocaine. This suggests that there may be an "addictive" mechanism common to alcohol and other habituating drugs. Finally, some individuals could not be induced to imbibe at all. This suggests that drinkers have a particular genotype that places them at high-risk relative at least to alcohol, and/or perhaps to the acquisition of powerful habits relating to motivation and emotions.

Just as with primates, some humans start drinking readily with few preliminaries, while others steadily limit their intake or refrain entirely. Given situations sufficiently traumatic and prolonged, some in the latter group succumb to drinking. Relative to question 3, this suggests that there are individual differences in factors that serve as deterrents to drinking.

What about the progressive development of addiction once drinking has started (i.e., Question 4)? The precision at critical points of Jellinek's description has been questioned.[4] Furthermore, a significant relationship has been noted between the age of onset of drinking and the severity and duration of the addiction (Question 3 above). Early versus late onset of alcoholism appears to relate to childhood adjustment: poor adjustment, unstable emotions, immaturity and low social competency versus stable adjustment, respectively. Many of the alcoholics who had a well adjusted childhood apparently started their drinking as adults secondary to some psychopathology. Some of the latter readily quit drinking as soon as the situation or condition improved. Conversely, the alcoholics who had started drinking early in life appeared to have developed a life-long problem. The two types were denoted as essential versus relative alcoholics.[5,6]

Recently, these early and late onset drinkers were found to differ markedly in the proportions of those who evidenced minimal brain dysfunction (MBD) in childhood.[7] The childhood symptoms of MBD are almost identical to those of the early onset drinkers. However, drinking appears to be independent of intelligence.[8] The early onset of drinking also appears to be related to a familial history of alcohol usage.[7,9] This promising lead needs exploration.

Question 5 is especially difficult. It deals with a phenomenon that persists after prolonged sobriety must have removed all residual by-products of alcohol. It involves powerful motivational and emotional arousal, and, in turn, ergotropic activation. Whether or not this drive results from an alcohol induced physiological change at some receptor site or in some synthesizing system is as yet unknown. A theory based on this premise must explain peculiar features of the phenomenon—its irregular periodicity, its varying intensity and duration in different people, and above all its basic similarity to the development in some people of cravings during abstinence for various drugs, tobacco, caffeine, chocolate, eating (as opposed to food), etc. A psychological explanation seems more persuasive, but the phenomenon has received little direct attention since the brief symposium on craving in 1955.[10]

Question 6 is asked primarily to emphasize that Jellinek's behaviors have implicit motivational elements of self-determination, conformity, and self-control.[11,12] His drinking behavior typology has been examined experimentally mainly in this light. This will be discussed as a special case of the nosological aspects of Question 7. Whether the data are observed behaviors, self-inventories, or what, the question reduces to whether alcoholism is or is not a unitary addiction or disease.

The resolution of this basic question is confused, but some of these tangled threads can be unraveled at present. By necessity almost all of the nosological research has been done during sober periods of *de facto* (chronic) alcoholics, usually while they were receiving therapy. Active alcoholics have many things in common regardless of their personality, intelligence, socioeconomic background—the drunkenness problem, the therapy, and the milieu. Such a confounded state-trait situation yields *both* differences (i.e., there are different kinds of alcoholism)[13] and similarities (i.e., there is *an* alcoholism personality).[14]

The situation is confused: (1) by the large variety of measuring instruments and constructs used by different authors. Fortunately, sufficient factor analyses are becoming available to permit educated guesses at transposing various results to a common base. (2) Another point of confusion is methodological, and perhaps it is insurmountable at present—the obvious difficulty of classifying people who are *average* on the two (or more) dimensions being contrasted. With these *average* people, slight change of a few points in scores is sufficient to shift them across the mean on either side. Only people well-removed from the central (NO TYPE) position can be reliably classifiable in terms of a dimension. Thus, there appears to be a technical limit of around half of a sample who are classifiable, even on two dimensions, as will be validated by actual data below.

As a first step we have attempted (with apologies to the various authors, if we erred) to gain some common base by transposing their results into Eysenck's[15] secondary level, biologically-based typology: Neuroticism (below and above average = emotionally stable, S, and neurotic or unstable, N, respectively) and Introversion (I) and Extraversion (E).

Turning first to the efforts dedicated to defining different kinds of alcoholism — Brown[16] attempted to distinguish Jellinek's delta and gamma alcoholics, but he succeeded in classifying only about 25% of his sample. The larger group were neurotic introverts (NI), while the smaller group were categorized as psychopaths (i.e., moderate N and high E, in Eysenck's typology). Until recently, this weak result has remained at about the same level in all studies.

Even the best actuarial interpretative systems using personality measures, such as the MMPI, have been found to classify *only about a fourth* of the alcoholics into reliable types.[17-22] This ambiguous situation led to a virtual rejection of the possibility that an alcoholic personality existed at all "... aside from uncontrolled drinking behavior, alcoholic patients may be little different from other types of psychiatric patients".[23]

A major recent effort to establish reliable types of alcoholics[24] is noteworthy. The sample was large (N = 366). Major personality and need assessment instruments were used along with sophisticated multivariate techniques. Seven types of alcoholics were established. The largest type included only 14.5% of the total sample, and all seven types combined included only 53% of the sample.

When Nerviano's seven types are translated, as best we can from his system to that of Eysenck's system: (1) relative to neuroticism, N, Nerviano's Types C, E, and F were clearly N, 17.5% of the alcoholics — and it may be inferred that Type B is somewhat N: a total of 25.6% of the alcoholics; (2) Types A and G are clearly stable, S — 17.5% — and it may be inferred that Type D is moderately S: 23.5% of the alcoholics; (3) relative to the other dimension — Types C and G are clearly Extraverted, E, and Type A is slightly E: 25.5%; and (4) Types E and F are clearly Introverted, I, and Types B and D may be inferred to be somewhat I: 23.5% of the alcoholics. Thus, of the alcoholics whom Nerviano was able to categorize (about 50%), half were high and half were low neuroticism, and on the other independent dimension, half were extraverted and half were introverted.

If we take advantage of the fact that the N and I-E dimensions are essentially not correlated, we may graph them at right angles with the dimensions crossing at the mean of each dimension. The expected

TABLE 1.–Discrimination of Controls and Four Psychiatric Categories of Males by Means of the Ten Primary Personality Constructs of the Birkman Method[1]

Sample Category[2]	Percent of Sample Currently Classified[3]				
	Categories				
	C	Al	Ad	SP	SS
Controls (C)	XX				
Alcoholics (Al)	83	XX			
Addicts (Ad)	95	72	XX		
Schizophrenics Paranoid (SP)	85	66	75	XX	
Schizophrenics Simple (SS)	89	64	73	58[4]	XX
N	100	117	87	68	55

[1]See Footnotes 1 and 2 of the Chapter.
[2]The schizophrenics were veterans comparable to the sample of alcoholics; the addicts were receiving methadone therapy at a large free medical clinic; and the controls were a sample of industrial workers with educations and ages comparable to the other groups.
[3]Pairwise multiple discriminant function analysis with constant parameters (Nie, et al., 1975). All results are concurrent validities only.
[4]Not significant.

proportion of alcoholics in each of the four quadrants formed in this way (NE, NI, SE, SI), is 25% of the total, or 12.5% of those typified by Nerviano. Actually, Types A and G appear to be SE – 17.6%; Types E and F (plus a tentative Type B) appear to be NI – 17.5%; Type C is probably NE – 8%; and Type D is possibly categorized as SI – 6%. The 47% NO TYPES are presumed to be *average* on both of Eysenck's dimensions.

Thus, from early work to this recent comprehensive and sophisticated effort, the numbers of alcoholics categorizable *vis-à-vis* types of alcoholism only doubled, and about half are left dangling as NO TYPES. This ability to classify only half of the samples of *admitted* alcoholics places the burden of proof that there are distinct kinds of alcoholism upon the proponents of this typological persuasion. With present techniques, classification of these NO TYPES as other than *average* is mainly a matter of random assignment, which is not helpful in the least.

A significant conclusion from this summary of indirect classification efforts is that the various types of alcoholics simply collapsed into two of the high order dimensions of one of the major personality systems. We approached this question directly with a sample of 129 hospitalized male chronic alcoholic veterans. We found that they were almost equally distributed in the four Eysenck quadrants established with both his questionnaire and his mean values:[25] SE (24.8%); SI (17.8%); NE (29.5%); and NI (27.9%). Thus, it is clear that people of any broad personality type *can* become alcoholic.[24,26-31]

This brings us to a perplexing anomaly—in spite of the preceding review it is abundantly clear that alcoholics *can* be identified at rates far greater than chance by using personality measures. This fact has fueled speculation that there is an "alcoholism" personality. A large literature has developed supporting the view that people of this postulated personality type are peculiarly prone to cope with life's stresses with behaviors and situations that are conducive to developing and maintaining alcohol addiction and its cravings.[32-38]

What makes alcoholics identifiable? Some authors have suggested that this identification is possible because a prolonged addiction *per se* causes people to begin to look alike.[39] However, the extremely rare longitudinal studies belie such naiveté—those who become alcoholic seem to have had unique identifiable personality traits well before they had even sampled the panacea.[40-43]

In spite of the uniform distributions on the major personality dimensions, when we resorted to the underlying primary dimensions of personality, alcoholics were significantly different from controls as well as from several psychiatric categories[44] (Table 1).* Does this mean that there is *an* alcoholism personality? The answer is: not necessarily.

In spite of the demonstrated discriminability at the primary construct level of the alcoholic veterans from other groups, the differences are based on relatively small mean differences.† A major feature of many problem-groups is the common reflection in several constructs of low self-esteem—elevated depression and self-consciousness, and depressed sociability. Unfortunately, for classification purposes, all such groups with problems may reflect the same state changes to greater or lesser extents——addicts, schizophrenics, prison inmates.

Another pervasive effect is due to the fact that scaled scores such as Depression, Sociability, and so on, are the sums of answers to a variety of correlated (usually at low levels) questions. A given sum (score) can be

---

*This study was made possible by permission to use data from a large private data base owned by Birkman and Associates, Inc. Houston, Texas. The Birkman Method used here is a proprietary system of Questionnaire and Reports owned by Birkman and Associates, Inc., and made available for public use through the non-profit Birkman-Mefferd Research Foundation (3200 Audley, Suite 101, PO Box 27545, Houston, Texas).

†All clinical groups differed significantly (i.e., p<.05 *t* test) from the control groups on most constructs, but there were few such differences between the clinical groups—descriptively they "looked" alike.

TABLE 2.–Discrimination of Controls and Four Psychiatric Categories by Means of Item Scales[1] Developed From the Personality Items of the Birkman Method[2]

| Sample Categories | Percent of Sample Correctly Classified[3] | | | | |
| | Categories | | | | |
	C	Al	Ad	SP	SS
Controls (C)	XX	88	87	80	78
Alcoholics (Al)	97	XX	76	91	88
Addicts (Ad)	99	85	XX	88	86
Schizophrenics Paranoid (SP)	92	90	85	XX	68
Schizophrenics Simple (SS)	96	92	76	78	XX

[1]Scales comparable to MMPI scales such as the *AMac*, SC, etc.
[2]See Footnotes of Table 1.
[3]The "correct" classification rates are shown for both categories of each pair—the rates in the rows are those predicted from the groups in the intersecting columns. All results are significant showing that accuracy is not contingent on a high rate of false negatives in any other group.

obtained from a very large number of different combinations of answers.[45] While these scores reflect common factor (or construct) variance,[46] subtle patterns of responses are lost.

The distinction noted above is highly relevant to this discussion. Regardless of a person's pre-morbid personality—the habitual way a person behaves—value system, perceptions of others, etc., these must be influenced during a serious continuing problem. While primary traits obviously could reflect these changes, the pre-post alcoholism studies cited above suggest that this may not be a major factor. What is more likely to happen is for problem-induced *patterns* of responses to develop that may cut across the underlying factor structure.

Early in the effort to predict alcoholism, authors started developing specific scales from the items of standard personality instruments. This was done by various procedures that maximized the differences between an alcoholic and some reference group. An early scale[47] developed from the Minnesota Multiple Personality Inventory (MMPI) used as its reference group the non-alcoholic psychiatric patients—the *AMac*. Since then it has become apparent that the outpatients used in that reference group differ from inpatient samples, and other efforts have become increasingly concerned with the appropriate people to serve as controls of alcoholics.[48] The report by Pattison,[49] to be discussed later, bears directly on this problem. His work suggests that different basic personality types may require separate item scales.

While we are not addressing the topic directly, the question of the predictability of low base-rate phenomena needs to be mentioned. Despite the tremendous public health costs involved, most distinct psychiatric dysfunctions actually exist at a low base rate (around 5%) within the population — alcoholism,[50] drug addiction, schizophrenia, violence, and even criminality. Any low base rate phenomenon is exceedingly difficult to predict for sampling and statistical reasons. There is an ever present tendency to "over-predict" the targeted dysfunction. For example, when the predictive equation or test is applied to a sample from the general population it is over-inclusive and false positives are inordinately high.[51,52]

It often has been noted that the best way to identify an alcoholic is to ask him directly. This view is counter-productive, and warrants comment. One example has been noted[53] — a particular item response may be unreliable with a random sample, but be highly reliable for a particular class of people. *Admitted* alcoholics almost universally acknowledge that they have had a problem with alcohol. On the other side of the coin, *unadmitted* alcoholics are the problem, and MacAndrew[47] eliminated such direct questions from his *AMac* scale because of the expected strong denial of such questions by *unadmitted* alcoholics. Indirect questions avoid this classification problem.

Another way to improve item scales such as Alcoholism, is to broaden its base beyond the typical self-inventory of personality measures. We have used a nonclinical self-inventory that combines personality and value system measures. Particularly powerful, however, is the combination in this personality instrument directly with one of social perception — the same questions are answered for a person's beliefs and attitudes about MOST PEOPLE and for SELF. Fewer restraints are brought to the appraisal of others than to ones' self. This interaction, SELF versus MOST PEOPLE, adds a powerful *new* dimension to the discrimination task.

The next step in clarifying Question 7 was to determine whether or not there were groups of questions answered by alcoholics in a reliable pattern *that crossed the personality constructs*. Table 2 shows that alcoholics were quite discriminable from a variety of other psychiatric categories. Recall that (1) the alcoholics had representatives from each personality quadrant of a particular high-order typology, and (2) all the psychiatric groups actually "looked" very much alike at the primary construct level. Yet, the identifying item clusters were drawn almost equally from across the ten constructs of the instrument.

This result argues against a unique alcoholism personality. This conclusion would become stronger if it also were possible to classify

TABLE 3.–Discrimination of Controls and Four Psychiatric Categories by Means of Item Scales Developed From the Social Perception Items[1] of the Birkman Method[2]

Sample Categories	Percent of Sample Correctly Classified[3]				
	Categories				
	C	Al	Ad	SP	SS
Controls (C)	XX	71	79	78	80
Alcoholics (Al)	82	XX	79	78	76
Addicts (Ad)	85	84	XX	80	78
Schizophrenics Paranoid (SP)	79	78	79	XX	76
Schizophrenics Simple (SS)	84	78	80	73	XX

[1]No comparable scales are known to us.
[2]See Footnotes of Table 1.
[3]See Footnote 3 of Table 2.

alcoholics on the basis of their social perceptions, and this was clearly possible (Table 3).

We may presume that the general alcoholic situation potentiated a very persistent state of anxiety and depression. Several other groups have similar chronic stressful situations—addicts, schizophrenics, prisoners. After their egos and self-confidence have suffered prolonged insults, all of these groups look more like one another than any of them look like "normal" controls. As groups, they all tend to "over-punish" themselves. Thus, all such groups are readily classifiable as deviant from a functional coping control group. Whether or not there is a common thread that predisposes people toward any one of the problem areas[54] is unresolved. However, this low self-esteem veneer does appear to be a matter of state changes, since some of this commonality disappears with successful rehabilitation.[55]

On the other hand, each of these major problems exerts specific situational effects that cut across factor structures. Patterns of responses and other behaviors become common within the particular problem groups. The lability of such patterns is evidenced by the dramatic shift in behaviors observed between the paranoid, hostile, defensive pre-admitted alcoholic, and the proclamation of "I am an alcoholic", with full acknowledgement of the problem and most of its side-effects.

The persistence of the underlying personality pattern was dramatically illustrated by the exciting results of Pattison.[49] He categorized drinkers who appeared at four types of facilities having different psychiatric milieus (i.e., aversive treatment, outpatient clinics, halfway houses, and police facilities) on the basis of their relative treatment needs in five areas (*viz.* drinking *per se*, vocational, interpersonal relationships, emotional and physical), and the relative effectiveness of the treatment at these different facilities in the five need areas. The clients of the aversive training centers were reported to be functional individuals who simply wanted to stop drinking, and did so with aversive techniques. They had no problems in the other areas (i.e., they were no nonsense, non-neurotics), other treatment was neither sought nor effective. At the other end of the scale were the skid-row "burned-out" alcoholics for whom the police provided a custodial job. Irrespective of their therapy needs, no treatment was desired or was effective—they were living at the bottom of Maslow's[56] hierarchial pyramid of needs and had lost their social status and any drive for self-actualization above that very basic level. Their original personality had become irrelevant. Outpatients appeared to have relatively low social needs (Introverts?) but powerful emotional problems (Neurotics?) that responded to emotional-treatment. Those seeking the halfway house treatment needed social support (Extraverts?) and had emotional problems (Neurotic?) that benefited from this continuous support, and they benefited from any and all treatments offered.

Quite obviously, during drinking, alcoholics likely would have scored high on most scales of alcoholism. However, we found that alcoholics still exhibited their deep-seated personality traits. This basic personality, clouded as it was by the common alcohol-induced commonality, influenced both the selection and the benefit derived from various therapies.

We conclude that given the situation and opportunity, personality appears to play as small a role as intelligence does in whether or not a person *does* become alcoholic. However, alcoholism is predictable in *admitted* alcoholics by means of indirect questions because of the common situation-induced changes. It seems reasonable that the same should be the case with *unadmitted* alcoholics, provided the questions are sufficiently subtle. If we are correct, however, it may be impossible to predict risks of *becoming* alcoholic from such psychological measures. Yet, this view appears to be unrealistic.[57] Both of the major aspects of addiction—the relative ease of habit formation and dissipation, and the relative intensity and tenacity of the craving following the last exposure—must be related to other major behavioral traits. Obviously, more pre-post alcoholism studies directed at these questions are needed.

REFERENCES

1. Jellinek, E.M. Phase of alcohol addiction. *Q. J. Stud. Alcohol.* 13:673-684, 1952.
2. Jellinek, E.M. The Disease Concept of Alcoholism. Highland Park, N.J.: Hillhouse Press, 1960.
3. Altshuler, H.L. Primate studies in alcoholism, in Fann, W., Karacan, I., Pokorny, A., and Williams, W. (eds.), *Phenomenology and Treatment of Alcoholism.* Jamaica, N.Y.: Spectrum Publishers Inc., 1979.
4. Pokorny, A.D. Stages in development of alcoholism, in Fann, W., Karacan, I., Pokorny, A., and Williams, W. (eds.), *Phenomenology and Treatment of Alcoholism.* Jamaica, N.Y.: Spectrum Publishers Inc., 1979.
5. Rudie, R.R., and McGaughran, L.S. Differences in developmental experience, defensiveness, and personality organization between two classes of problem drinkers. *J. Abnorm. Soc. Psych.* 62:659-665, 1961.
6. Sugerman, A.A., Reilly, D., and Albahary, R. Social competence and the essential-reactive distinction in alcoholism. *Arch. Gen. Psychiat.* 12:552-554, 1965.
7. Tarter, R.E., and Buonpane, N. Differentiation of alcoholics. *Arch. Gen. Psychiat.* 34:761-768, 1977.
8. Bergman, H., and Agren, G. *Cognitive style and performance in relation to the progress of alcoholism.* Reports from the Psychological Laboratories, Univ. of Stockholm, 1973, No. 398, p. 18.
9. Templer, D.I., Ruff, C.F., and Ayers, J. Essential alcoholism and family history of alcoholism. *Q. J. Stud. Alcohol.* 35:655-657, 1974.
10. Jellinek, E.M., Isbell, H., Lundquist, G., Tiebout, H.M., Dushene, H., Mardones, J., and MacLeod, L.D. The "craving" for alcohol. *Q. J. Stud. Alcohol.* 16:34-66, 1955.
11. Walton, H. Personality as a determinant of the form of alcoholism. *Brit. J. Psychiat.* 114:761-766, 1968.
12. Brown, R.A. Conformity in gamma and delta alcoholics. *J. Clin. Psychol.* 33:895-896, 1977.
13. Winokur, G., Rimmer, J., and Reich, T. Alcoholism IV. Is there more than one type of alcoholism? *Brit. J. Psychiat.* 118:525-531, 1971.
14. Miller, W.R. Alcoholism scales and objective assessment methods: a review. *Psychol. Bull.* 83:649-674, 1976.
15. Eysenck, H.J., and Eysenck, S.B.G. *The Description and Measurement of Personality.* London: Routledge & Kegan Paul, Ltd., 1969.
16. Brown, M.A. Alcoholic profiles on the Minnesota Multiphasic. *J. Clin. Psychol.* 6:266-269, 1950.
17. Fowler, R.D., and Coyle, F.A. A comparison of two actuarial systems used in classifying an alcoholic outpatient population. *J. Clin. Psychol.* 24:434, 1968.
18. Goldstein, S.G., and Linden, J.D. A comparison of multivariate grouping techniques commonly used with profile data. *Multivariate Behav. Res.* 4:104-114, 1969.
19. Partington, J.T., and Johnson, P.G. Personality types among alcoholics. *Q. J. Stud. Alcohol.* 30:21-34, 1969.
20. Whitelock, P.R., Overall, J.E., and Patrick, J.H. Personality patterns and alcohol abuse in a state hospital population. *J. Abnormal Psych.* 78:9-16, 1971.
21. Lawlis, G.F., and Rubin, S.F. 16 P.F. study of personality in alcoholics. *Q. J. Stud. Alcohol.* 32:318-327, 1971.
22. Nerviano, V.J., and Gross, W.F. A multivariate delineation of two alcoholic profile types on the 16 PF. *J. Clin. Psychol.* 29:371-374, 1973.

23. Skinner, H.A., Jackson, D.N., and Hoffmann, H. Alcoholic personality types: identification and correlates. *J. Abnormal Psych.* 83:658–666, 1974.
24. Nerviano, V.J. A common personality pattern among alcoholic males: a multivariate study. *J. Consult. Clin. Psychol.* 44:104–110, 1976.
25. Eysenck, H.J., and Eysenck, S.B.G. *Manual for the Eysenck Personality Inventory.* San Diego: Educational and Industrial Testing Service, 1963.
26. Gilberstadt, H., and Duker, J. *A Handbook for Clinical and Actuarial MMPI Interpretation.* Philadelphia: W.B. Saunders, 1965.
27. Goldstein, S.G., and Linden, J.D. Multivariate classification of alcoholics by means of the MMPI. *J. Abnormal Psych.* 74:661–669, 1969.
28. Goss, A., and Morosko, T.E. Alcoholism and clinical symptoms. *J. Abnormal Psych.* 74:682–684, 1969.
29. Horn, J.L., and Wanberg, K.W. Symptom patterns related to excessive use of alcohol. *Q. J. Stud. Alcohol.* 30:35–58, 1969.
30. Skinner, H.A., Reed, P.L., and Jackson, D.N. Toward the objective diagnosis of psychopathology: generalizability of modal personality profiles. *J. Consult. Clin. Psychol.* 44:111–117, 1976.
31. Huba, G.J., Segal, B., and Singer, J.L. Organization of needs in male and female drug and alcohol users. *J. Consult. Psychol.* 45:34–44, 1977.
32. Weingold, H.P., Lachin, J.M., Bell, A.H., and Cox, R.C. Depression as a symptom of alcoholism: search for a phenomenon. *J. Abnormal Psych.* 73:195–197, 1968.
33. Tarter, R.E. Personality characteristics of male alcoholics. *Psychol. Repts.* 37(1):91–96, 1975.
34. Lorefice, L., Steer, R.A., Fine, E.W., and Schult, J. Personality traits and moods of alcoholics and heroin addicts. *Q. J. Stud. Alcohol.* 37:687–689, 1976.
35. Manaugh, T.S., and Schoot, E.M. EPPS scores of male alcoholics: a review and cross-validation. *J. Clin. Psychol.* 32:197–199, 1976.
36. Foulds, G.A., and Bedford, A. Personality and coping with psychiatric symptoms. *Brit. J. Psychiat.* 130:29–31, 1977.
37. Pryer, M.W., and Distefano, M.K. Correlates of locus of control among male alcoholics. *J. Clin. Psychol.* 33:300–303, 1977.
38. Donovan, D.M. Radford, L.M., Chaney, E.F., and O'Leary, M.R. Perceived locus of control as a function of level of depression among alcoholics and non-alcoholics. *J. Clin. Psychol.* 33:582–584, 1977.
39. Franks, C.M. Alcoholism, in C.G. Costello (ed.), *Symptoms of Psychopathology.* New York: Wiley, 1970.
40. McCord, W., and McCord, J.A. A longitudinal study of the personality of alcoholics, in Pitman, D.P., and Snyder, C.R. (eds.), *Society, Culture and Drinking Patterns.* New York: Wiley, 1962.
41. Jones, H., MacFarland, J., and Eichorn, D. A progress report on growth studies at the University of California, *Vita Humana* 3:17–31, 1960.
42. Mendelson, W., Johnson, N., and Stewart, M.A. Hyperactive children as teenagers: a follow-up study. *J. Nerv. Ment. Dis.* 153:273–279, 1971.
43. Cantwell, D.P. Psychiatric illness in the families of hyperactive children. *Arch. Gen. Psychiat.* 27:414–417, 1972.
44. Nie, N.H., Hull, C.H., Jenkins, J.G., Steinbrenner, K. and Bent, D.H. *Statistical Package for the Social Sciences,* 2nd ed. New York: McGraw-Hill, 1975.
45. McQuitty, L.L. Elementary linkage analysis for isolating orthogonal and oblique types and typal relevancies. *Educ. & Psychol. Measurement* 17:207–229, 1957.

46. Cronbach, L.J., and Gleser, G.C. Assessing similarity between profiles. *Psychol. Bull.* 50:456–473, 1953.
47. MacAndrews, C. The differentiation of male alcoholic outpatients from non-alcoholic psychiatric outpatients by means of the MMPI. *Q. J. Stud. Alcohol.* 26:238–246, 1965.
48. Atsaides, J.P., Neuringer, C., and Davis, K.L. Development of an institutionalized chronic alcoholic scale. *J. Consult. Clin. Psychol.* 45:609–611, 1977.
49. Pattison, E. M. Differential treatment approaches. In Fann, W., Karacan, I., Pokorny, A., and Williams, W. (eds.), *Phenomenology and Treatment of Alcoholism.* Jamaica, N.Y.: Spectrum Publishers Inc., 1979.
50. Calahan, D., and Cisin, I.H. Navy survey personnel attitudes and behavior concerning alcohol and problem drinking. *J. Alcohol and Drug Educ.* 22:25–28, 1976.
51. Megargee, E.I. The prediction of dangerous behavior. *Crim. Justice & Behavior* 3:3–22, 1976.
52. Mefferd, R.B., Jr., Lennon, J.M., and Dawson, N.E. Violence—an ultimate non-coping behavior. In Hayes, J.R. (ed.), *Violence and the Violent Individual.* Jamaica, N.Y.: Spectrum Publishers Inc., 1980.
53. Suziedelis, A., Lorr, M., and Tonesk, X. Comparison of item-level and score-level typological analysis: a simulation study. *Multivariate Behav. Res.* 15:135–145, 1976.
54. Zimering, S., and Calhoun, J.F. Is there an alcoholic personality? *J. Drug Educ.* 6:97–103, 1976.
55. Edwards, D., Steven, F., and Schuckit, M. Personality and attitudinal change for alcoholics treated at the Navy's Alcohol Rehabilitation Center. *J. Comm. Psychol.* 5:180–185, 1977.
56. Maslow, A.H. *Motivation and personality.* New York: Harper, 1954.
57. Hoffman, H., Loper, R.G., and Kammeier, M.L. Identifying future alcoholics with MMPI alcoholism scales. *Q. J. Stud. Alcohol.* 35:490–498, 1974.

CHAPTER 7

Alcoholism, Borderline and Narcissistic Disorders: A Psychoanalytic Overview

PETER HARTOCOLLIS
PITSA C. HARTOCOLLIS

On the basis of a systematic review of the psychoanalytic literature, we will attempt in this chapter to draw a composite picture of alcoholism and, in the process, show that the condition greatly overlaps with what psychoanalysts and others, clinicians as well as researchers, describe as borderline states or, more broadly, borderline and narcissistic personality disorders.[1] Such a diagnostic coincidence may be particular to psychoanalytic practice or experience with alcoholic patients — the kind of alcoholic patients psychoanalysts are familiar with. It should be also pointed out that psychoanalysts tend to discuss alcoholism concurrently, indeed interchangeably, with drug addiction — the implication being that both conditions represent manifestations of the same basic psychopathology.

That alcoholics may be heavy users of drugs, and vice versa, enhances the impression that the two conditions are governed by similar dynamics. Nevertheless, there are obvious differences in both the use of the two categories of addictive (chemical) substances and their psychophysiology. The abuse of alcohol usually precedes drug addiction. And, characteristically, drug addiction involves more violence than alcoholism, a difference that may be related to sociocultural factors, which undoubtedly play an important role in the development of both conditions.[2]

EARLY PSYCHOANALYTIC FORMULATIONS: REGRESSION AND BORDERLINE PSYCHOSIS

The first psychoanalytic conceptualization of alcoholism (and drug addiction in general) was made by Abraham.[3] He suggested that alcoholics are struggling against latent homosexual wishes — an idea obviously related to Freud's theory of paranoia, with alcoholic delusional jealousy serving as the connecting link. Others stressed the importance of oral narcissistic and depressive personality traits. Pointing out that exhibitionistic and sadomasochistic tendencies might be even more crucial than unconscious homosexuality, Sachs, as reported by Yorke,[4] saw addiction to alcohol as a compromise between the perversions and compulsive neurosis. Rado,[5] on the other hand, described alcoholism as a hypomanic attempt to escape the awareness of narcissistic pain or depression. He proposed the term "pharmacothymia" to describe the mood-lifting effects of chemical substances for a "group of human beings who respond to frustrations in life with a special type of emotional alteration, which might be designated 'tense depression' ... or 'initial depression' marked by great 'painful' tension and, at the same time, by a high degree of intolerance to pain."[6,7]

In considering the dynamics of alcoholism, Glover stressed the importance of sadism and aggression in general. He pointed out that, while orally gratifying, alcohol unbinds aggression so that all object relations are colored by it — oral aggression or, rather, oral ambivalence; but also anal erotism and sadism — and he suggested that such disorders as alcoholism and drug addiction might represent "transitional states," clinically and developmentally related to both the neuroses and the psychoses. Clearly, the characteristics Glover attributed to alcoholics — namely, a "localized" or transient disturbance in reality testing; object relations invested with pre-oedipal aggression, frustration and disappointment; and an archaic, severe and inconsistent superego — coincide with those attributed by contemporary authors, Kernberg[8] in particular, to patients with a borderline personality organization.

Espousing the idea of repressed aggression as its central dynamic, Simmel[9] saw in alcoholism a latent "narcissistic neurosis" controlled by means of obsessional mechanisms. Simmel's ideas, derived from his experience with hospitalized alcoholics and drug addicts in Tegel/Berlin, were developed further by Will Menninger[10] and his brother Karl[11] in Topeka. It was at the Menninger Clinic that Knight[12] explored the early object relations of alcoholics, reconstructing the personality characteristics of parental figures and the developmental determinants of the alcoholic condition from the analysis of adult male patients. He described two types of alcoholism, "essential" and "reactive"—the former, earlier in its onset, often polysymptomatic, involving as a rule serious behavioral maladjustment and responding poorly to psychoanalysis or psychoanalytic psychotherapy; the latter appearing after a more or less successful social and family adjustment, as a reaction to some recognizable external or internal stress, and responding favorably to psychoanalytic treatment.* In agreement with Glover, Knight declared: "alcohol addiction, along with other drug addictions, constitutes a borderline condition psychiatrically."[12]

Curiously, Knight did not follow up on his seminal ideas concerning the dynamics and treatment of alcoholism. Instead, he turned his attention to borderline disorders or, more specifically, "borderline schizophenia"—a development that may be related to his earlier interest in alcoholics in more than a coincidental way. Significantly, it seems to us, in discussing Knight's work in alcoholism, Karl Menninger[13] declared: "I regard it as near a psychosis ... I think that addiction to alcohol is more serious than any neurosis and should be thought of along with the psychoses."

Knight's[12] description of "essential alcoholics" is worth quoting in part, as it unmistakably applies to patients with typical borderline pathology:

They are completely dependent economically and emotionally.... Also one finds lacking the character traits which derive from the second anal stage—those of perseverance, retention and mastery of the object.... The character traits are essentially oral derivatives— oral dependence, oral demanding, pleasure seeking with small regard to reality requirements or possibilities. This lack of reality sense is evidenced by their unreliability, irresponsibility and especially by their lying and general lack of sincerity.

Fifteen years later, Knight[16] conceptualized the "borderline case" as "one in which normal ego functions of secondary process thinking, integration, realistic planning, adaptation to the environment, maintenance of object realtionships, and defenses against primitive unconscious impulses are severely weakened."†

---

*On the basis of genetic research, Winokur and his co-workers[14] have more recently identified two types of male alcoholism, "sociopathic" and "primary", entities phenomenologically equivalent to Knight's "essential" and "reactive" alcoholism, respectively. A third type, "depression-alcoholism," was ascribed primarily to women.[15]

†W. Menninger[10] referred to two more groups of patients who habitually abuse drinking: "neurotic characters" as described by Alexander, and "psychotic personalities" in whom "alcoholism represents only a symptom in a paranoid or schizoid or otherwise psychotic system." Clearly, these represent borderline patients.

CONTEMPORARY VIEWS: AFFECT-TOLERANCE AND STRUCTURAL DEFICIT

The ability of alcohol and drugs, in general, to relieve bad feelings almost instantaneously has led to the hypothesis that addiction is an attempt at self-healing. According to this view, advanced first by Rado,[5] the peremptory nature of the drug use is a reflection of the intensity of the addict's affects; addiction to chemical substances is presumably a defense against affects that have lost the capacity to serve as signals of inner distress or danger, affects that have reverted to their primitive, massive, psychosomatic form normally experienced in a traumatic situation, particularly in early childhood before the establishment of an effective ego structure.[17-19] The idea is implicit in Kohut's[20] assertion that drugs are not symbolic substitutes for missing love objects as traditionally assumed, but replacements for "psychological structure." According to Kohut,[21] drug addiction, and presumably alcoholism, is similar to the narcissistic personality disorders in that both conditions share a developmental defect in the self.

As Khantzian[22] has pointed out in reviewing the contemporary literature on addictive personalities, the emphasis is on ego functions and ego impairments, with attention focused on the areas of affect tolerance and drive defense. Rather than delving into the regressive, acting out aspects of addictive behavior, contemporary workers stress its adaptive functions, the dynamic interaction of the psychopharmacologic effect of chemical substances and the personality organization of the addicted individual in his present environment. In describing the personality of the alcoholic or drug addict, these workers borrow heavily from the literature of borderline and narcissistic disorders. Characteristically, Wurmser[19] concluded that the psychopathology of such patients is "most frequently of the borderline type." His description of their subjective experience corresponds closely to the typical feelings of borderline patients; namely, loneliness, emptiness and depression, meaninglessness and pervasive boredom or hurt, rejection, shame and murderous rage. Alcohol or drugs help to alleviate such feelings or to make them more bearable. The following account of an alcoholic patient, diagnosed also as depressed, underscores the point:

I took pills and became drunk deliberately at times—one, when I could no longer carry on my facade; two, when anger at my mother or father overwhelmed me and I feared I'd express it; three, when I feared my husband would approach me sexually.... When my feelings of frustration, guilt, futility—to cite a few—became too intense to endure, I drank to alleviate the pain. I did not then identify any of the diffuse misery I felt as anger, at least not consciously, and I had no idea that the capacity for hostility is at least as great in a human being as is the capacity for love. This is perhaps not surprising in view of the fact that I had certainly not properly developed the capacity to love; I was emotionally starved because I was unable to express affection in any of the normally acceptable ways—not even to my husband, who naturally misinterpreted this and subsequently rejected me completely.

This patient had been through Alcoholics Anonymous and many attempts at psychotherapy before she came to our hospital. But she still felt that she was not an alcoholic. She said:

I am not—and never have been—powerless over alcohol. Again, morally this makes my apparent behavior all the more reprehensible, but I cannot in good faith pray for God's intervention when I acted deliberately and willfully. I can pray for self-knowledge, strength, and the wisdom to avoid wallowing in remorse or self-pity. I see now that my means of escape was a potentially suicidal act of self-destruction—a 'plea for help' just as 'sick' as lacerating one's wrists or taking an overdose of pills. I am ashamed to say that my drinking also expressed an element of hate—of lashing out at those I loved and hated most in a vicious 'I'll show you I don't care' gesture, which I must have known would offend, hurt and displease them. I, who had spent a misguided lifetime desperately seeking *approval*, could become despicable in the eyes of the world and thereby increase my self-punishment.

Two of the most characteristic clinical features of alcoholism, at least of the global, most commonly encountered type in this country described by Jellinek[23] as *delta* alcoholism—"loss of control" and "craving"—are as typical of borderline patients. "Loss of control," referring to a person's inability to regulate his drinking, is what the literature of borderline disorders describes as "weak impulse control." The symptom of "craving" corresponds to a pervasive experience of unpleasure—what borderline patients describe as emptiness or inner badness—and the urge to obliterate it by compulsively indulging in alloplastic behavior, such as self-mutilation, sexual promiscuity, repeated masturbation, over-eating, or drinking to excess. In this respect, Little[24] has observed that patients with a single pattern of addiction are probably closer to the border of psychosis than patients who can have any one of several objects or modes of gratification, even when they may need them all at once.

BORDERLINE PERSONALITY ORGANIZATION AND PATHOLOGICAL NARCISSISM

Even though by no means universally accepted, the belief that typical personality traits establish themselves before the development of alcoholic addiction is supported by observation of formerly addicted patients after prolonged abstinence, especially in the absence of psychodynamic treatment.[25-27] Put in terms of Kernberg's[28] classificatory system of character pathology, alcoholics display a severe disturbance in object relationships, reflecting inadequate object constancy and identity diffusion; a pathological condensation of genital and pre-genital instinctual strivings with a predominance of pre-genital aggression; a primitive, poorly integrated and largely insufficient superego; and a developmentally mixed picture of ego defenses, predominantly denial, splitting,* projection, and omnipotence. Such structural characteristics, defining Kernberg's lower level of character pathology, are pathognomonic of borderline patients, characterizing as well Knight's "essential" alcoholics.

Whether "reactive" or, in Winokur's[14] more recent terminology, "primary" alcoholics fall within the spectrum of borderline disorders is more difficult to decide. We could imagine someone asking Knight to comment on his later thinking about alcoholism and receiving something like the following response: "But of course, there are no alcoholics, only borderlines who happen to share a common symptom—drinking to excess." He might or might not have limited such a statement to the group of "essential" alcoholics; and that, as far as we are concerned, is a crucial question.

Some persons become publicly identified as alcoholics relatively late in life, following what appears to be a successful personal and social adjustment, their primary problem seemingly being excessive drinking and its debilitating effects. In this connection Kernberg's[30] remarks about a paradoxical discrepancy in the degree of disturbance between the actual interpersonal functioning and the level of character organization that some borderline patients display seem to us relevant. "Reactive" ("primary") alcoholics may for a long time manage to function in an apparently normal way. Narcissistic character traits, obsessive defenses,

---

*The importance of the primitive mechanism of splitting in the psychopathology of drug addiction has been stressed by Rosenfeld.[29]

and a massive use of denial provide such individuals with a protective shield of self-deception, which isolates them from close personal contact with people whom they depend on but cannot trust. They feel empty and angry inside, very much like people with an "as-if personality,"[31] but so far as anyone else is concerned they are pleasant and function adequately. Gradually, however, as the cumulative impact of internal and external frustrations undermines the effectiveness of their protective devices, the level of their functioning begins to suffer. And, wishing to maintain their precarious emotional equilibrium, they resort to increasing amounts of alcohol, which has the power to reenforce denial, even though not performance, which continues to deteriorate, exposing further their borderline pathology.

On the other hand, such patients may be classified more accurately as narcissistic rather than borderline. As Settlage[32] has pointed out, the distinction between the two conditions is not very clear in the literature. In fact, according to Kernberg,[28] a large proportion of narcissistic individuals, if not all of them, share the same borderline personality organization. But narcissistic disorders are generally considered less severe than borderline disorders. Like "reactive" ("primary") alcoholics, narcissistic patients are, according to Settlage again, "usually capable of functioning quite well in the area of work responsibilities. Yet they have major difficulty in regulating affects and self-esteem, in maintaining a cohesive sense of self, and in their capacity for intimacy in full object relations."[32]

The following case illustrates the problem of distinguishing between a narcissistic and a borderline disorder in a patient clearly identified as alcoholic:

A 42-year-old, moderately successful executive came to treatment complaining about obsessive thoughts of a homosexual nature. In addition, he called himself an "alcoholic," even though he had totally abstained from drinking for the past seven years. Handsome, well dressed and well mannered, he expressed himself in a soft-spoken, friendly, articulate but somber way, giving the impression of being mildly depressed. He described his mother as self-centered, domineering and sadistic. Even though feeling better about her now, he still held her responsible for his becoming an alcoholic, recalling that when at the age of 14 he went home drunk, she reacted with indifference, saying nothing about it. He described his father as cold, distant and ineffectual. In spite of his early dependence on drinking, the patient went through high school and managed to finish college; but he could not hold a job for any length of time, invariably being fired because of his drinking behavior. While on a drinking spree, he married a woman he had met only a few days earlier and divorced her as soon as he was sober, a few days later. At the age of 33, he sought a psychiatrist and had once-a-week psychotherapy for two years, until he was offered a promotion to an office in another city. With the consent of his therapist, he accepted the offer, was placed on disulfiram, joined Alcoholics Anonymous, and quit psychotherapy. Thereafter, for nearly seven years, he was able to maintain a stable work adjustment, with a marginal social life revolving around AA meetings and heterosexual relationships of short duration.

His new therapist made the diagnosis of narcissistic personality with obsessive-compulsive features and started him in psychoanalysis, five times a week. Two months later, as he was describing the loneliness of the past weekend, during which he had experienced an intense longing for his analyst, the patient became agitated, got up from the couch and declared that he was going to kill the analyst if he did not take him in his hands. At the analyst's firm suggestion that he could manage to contain himself if he sat on the chair across from him, the patient calmed down and, shortly afterwards, was able to return to the couch. Subsequently, he described feelings of admiration and complete trust for the analyst, only to revert to hateful, murderous fantasies a few days later, but without coming near the point of losing control or abandoning his sense of reality testing again. He revealed perverse sexual fantasies about other men as well as women and wondered about his identity, asking repeatedly the question, "Who am I," and "What do I want from life?" In short, he presented the classical symptoms and signs of a patient with a borderline personality organization.

DRINKING IN THE SERVICE OF DENIAL

The fact that a person is addicted to alcohol indicates that his primary defenses have been weakened on one level, yet strengthened on another. Drinking comes to the rescue of a person whose basic mental mechanisms have begun to lose their adaptive power, being helpful not only by providing relief from psychic pain (literally anesthesia), but by stimulating these mechanisms or defenses as well. The alcoholic whose premorbid personality is typically maintained by denial, splitting, rationalization and projection, finds himself compelled to use these defenses even more extensively, more openly and more or less exclusively after he becomes a heavy drinker.[33] Secondary defenses are built within the context of his premorbid character traits, typically identified as the alcoholic personality and representing a superficial, fragile and maladaptive form of reaction formation and obsessiveness, which shield the individual from the experience of negative, difficult to tolerate affects.

In listing the alcoholic's typical ego defenses, we placed denial first in order to emphasize its uniqueness in the case. Students of alcoholism have observed that denial is one of its more striking features.[34] We believe that the content of his denial is important in understanding the alcoholic patient and his personality development. There is something particular about the alcoholic's denial. On the surface, it is a denial of problems—primarily a denial of the idea that drinking may reflect a personal problem, except for the problem that other people's reaction to it creates. More careful examination, however, will reveal that what the alcoholic denies is a problem for which he needs any help. He may very well admit that he has problems so long as he can deny the idea that he needs help. What he denies is in essence the notion of help, the idea that he needs help. As Kernberg[30] observed with regard to narcissistic individuals, "The greatest fear of these patients is to be dependent on anybody else." And yet, behind this denial there lies a strong wish for help—only that this wish is fraught with anxiety.

The following letter of a woman alcoholic, expressing feelings of distress at the idea that her family did not like her because she was sick, reads like an echo from the past, a revival of childhood feelings regarding her place in the family:

> Mother, you wouldn't believe what a rotten opinion I have of myself—now that I can see it just a little I can hardly believe it myself. The way I appear to others has been the most colossal hoax imaginable. The creation of the bright, charming, witty, efficient and talented personality that you know is the product of a near genius brain with the emotional maturity of a six-year-old. When I start really thinking about how I really, *really* feel about everything—people, situations, achievements, effort, everything—two things come through loud and clear: I'm absolutely frightened to death, and I feel as though I'm such a disappointment to everyone, including myself.... I seem to be *so* sharp and intelligent and yet *no one* could be more naive or guileless than I am when it comes to knowing the difference between how things really are and how I want them to be. I'm so afraid I'll fail. Then I think of you all at home so *angry* with me because I'm sick and bitter because I don't appear to be making

any progress—the agony is too much—and up goes the phony mask
and I become again the person I created and I hate myself even
more.

The same patient returned to the hospital from a town trip late and
drunk. However, she secreted herself in her room, skillfully avoiding the
nursing staff the next day. She also failed to appear for her appointed
session with the therapist. Then she became quite angry, blamed the
nursing staff for not finding her and wrestling from her the secret of her
being upset and drunk.

What makes an alcoholic, especially of the "reactive" type, different
from the typical borderline patient is his or her apparent lack of anger.
Even though psychological testing invariably points to a great deal of inner
aggression and suppressed anger, the alcoholic patient is typically affable,
and denies feelings of anger about anyone. Alcoholics have an extremely
low tolerance for the direct expression of anger and hence they are
constantly leaning over backwards to deny any hostile or aggressive
impulses. Denial is also used extensively in connection with sexual
problems. Drinking serves the purpose of strengthening the denial of
anger or of sexual impulses when the denial becomes weak and the anger
or the sexual impulses come close to awareness.

A DEVELOPMENTAL HYPOTHESIS

In describing his patients' early object relations, Knight[12] speculated
that the future alcoholic is likely to become overindulged by his mother
and to react with rage when faced with the moment of weaning.
Aggressive fantasies, prompted by the mother's efforts to control his
insatiable needs for oral gratification, make him fear that she will retaliate
in anger, hurt him or abandon him. Such a fear prompts him to deny his
oral aggressive needs and to seek satisfaction in omnipotent but passive
fantasies and neurotic behavior, which eventually lead to problem drinking
and alcoholism. Mother's own relationship to the child, on the other hand,
is determined by feeling anxious and resentful in facing her child's needs,
because she perceives them as demands on herself when she feels
deprived in her own need for emotional attention. It is significant that
several investigators describe the fathers of alcoholic patients as cold and
distant and by implication unable to fulfill not only the child's emotional
needs, but those of the mother as well.[12,35]

A survey of over 300 long-term alcoholic patients by the authors
confirmed the impression, derived from personal clinical work with such

patients, that alcoholics have had a child-mother relationship that discouraged the communication of the normal developmental need for help. In a majority of cases, we found that alcoholic patients had more or less serious problems in childhood, including bedwetting, sleep-walking, shyness and withdrawal or excessive aggressiveness. The patients themselves reported having had fewer problems in childhood than what their relatives indicated—a finding that underscores the alcoholic's propensity to deny the existence of psychological difficulties whether in the present or in the past. In the course of treatment, alcoholics will more readily recall having experienced serious emotional problems as children—problems, however, for which they could not find satisfactory help. Alcoholic patients recall asking for help and not finding it, or not asking at all because of the impression that they could not find it. This inability to ask for help, present since childhood, seems to be a function of the personality of the alcoholic's mother. Thus, in a high proportion of our cases, patients described their parents in negative terms, remembering them as aggressive, domineering, possessive, unfriendly, inconsistent, cold or distant. Both men and women alcoholics were more critical of their mothers than of their fathers, men slightly more than women. Such findings point to a mother-child relationship that discouraged the admission of problems and rewarded their denial. The mother lets the child know that what she really wishes is to get rid of his needs, which she perceives as demands upon and complaints against her. Then, rather than helping him satisfy such needs, she encourages him to deny them. She welcomes him with a show of happiness and gestures of love whenever he appears or claims to be happy. She is nice to him so long as he does not voice any wishes for help or any resentment for not getting what he wishes to have from her, the tender unsolicited care that she would like to have for herself.

The following are excerpts from psychotherapy reports, referring to the feelings of chronic alcoholic patients about their parents in childhood:

In a highly intellectualized, sarcastic, cynical way, the patient, a 37-year-old journalist with at least 15 years of alcoholic abuse, family, and social maladjustment, heaped a barrage of accusations at his mother for being hypocritical, rejecting, and cold, and on his father for being domineering, punitive, and tyrannical. His anger was directed most intensely toward his mother, whom he perceived as expecting him to make up for the frustrations she experienced in her relations with his father.

A 43-year-old man, a successful writer with a long history of heavy drinking and brief depressive episodes, described his mother as a woman who felt very sorry for herself, who constantly complained that no one loved her, and who made incessant demands on the patient that he "take care of her."

Another alcoholic patient, a 36-year-old college graduate and mother of four children, acknowledged that, in spite of three years in analysis, she was still unable to experience feelings—except for "knowing" that the feelings were "really there." Yet, she reasoned, if she did something about it, about making contact with her feelings, "even worse hell would break out." It was better to let things go on this way, even if to her own destruction. Referring to herself in the third person, as if talking about someone else (possibly the analyst and ultimately mother), she said: "I can see what she must be feeling, but I can't feel it." She talked about being "encased." She couldn't trust anyone, she never had, she didn't dare to. "Should I want to dare?" she wondered. But if she did trust her analyst, he would find out that there was nothing to her, nothing to be trusted about. And he would ridicule her.

The same patient awakened one morning crying from an unremembered dream, to which she could only associate her lifelong terror and hatred of mother. She wondered, could she, would she talk with her mother about herself and her difficulties in her relationship with mother in all her growing-up years? Would mother attempt to deny it all? Would she herself accept mother's denial?

Following Masterson and Rinsley's[36] suggestion regarding the development of a "split-mother image" in borderline patients, we presume that the origin of the alcoholic's pathognomonic denial is to be found during the "rapprochement" subphase of the "separation-individuation" period of infantile development described by Mahler.[37,38] During this crucial phase in the formation of an autonomous identity, mother and child reach a tacit agreement not to disturb each other with their personal problems— a relationship characterized by a mutual attitude of denial. Regressing to the hypomanic mode of functioning that characterizes the preceding developmental subphase of "practicing," the child denies having any problems that may involve any wish for help; and, in a reciprocal fashion, the mother denies any awareness of such problems on the part of the child. The child's needs may express themselves in psychosomatic symptoms, but these are dissociated from his wishes and treated medically. The child then grows up looking happy and brave, or at least quiet and unassuming, until internal and external pressures begin mounting, family and social responsibilities, competitive strivings and libidinal longings become too heavy to cope with by means of his favorite defense of denial and its superego appeasing variants of rationalization and externalization. At a certain point, he may discover that something so easy to get and so perfectly normal to use in our society—alcohol—can reinforce these defenses and help him carry on with a semblance of competence. And eventually he or she becomes addicted.

What seems to be unique with alcoholics, especially the characterologically more advanced "reactive" ("primary") types, is their ability to suppress the negative side of ambivalence—angry, hateful, depressive and, in short, aggressive tendencies—in favor of a pleasant, friendly, cheerful facade. Such behavior corresponds to the positive "split-mother image" that borderline patients carry within. In fact, one may say that "reactive" alcoholics cannot get openly angry or hurtful unless they get drunk. Alcohol, soothing or not, is the magic potion that converts the Dr. Jekyll-like identity of the "reactive" alcoholic into that of Mr. Hyde's. The same mechanism holds generally true with regard to the alcoholic's sexual identity, which becomes clearly and aggressively homosexual or aggressively seductive, homosexually or otherwise, when he or she becomes drunk.

TREATMENT CONSIDERATIONS

In tracing the psychoanalytic literature on the subject, we have tried to show that inherent in old and new views lies the notion that alcoholism is a developmental disorder akin to borderline states. According to the same literature, treatment should be modified psychoanalysis or expressive-supportive psychotherapy, individually or in groups.

Indications for psychoanalysis should be virtually the same as for borderline patients in general, and more specifically for passive-aggressive personalities, sadomasochistic personalities, the better functioning infantile or hysteroid personalities, and narcissistic personalities that fall into what Kernberg[30] has described as the intermediate level of organization of character pathology, or what Knight[12] classified as "reactive" alcoholics. Modified psychoanalysis, or expressive-supportive psychotherapy, is indicated for the more severe borderline personality disorders, most patients with infantile and severe narcissistic personalities who were never able to make a stable adjustment in their life, whose drinking becomes habitual and is combined with drug addiction or sexual deviation or some other form of antisocial behavior, "as-if personalities," schizoid and paranoid character disorders which more or less coincide with Knight's type of "essential" alcoholism. In addition to modified psychoanalysis or expressive psychotherapy, such patients need a supportive, firmly structured environment that in most cases only a hospital can provide. This point was emphasized quite early by psychoanalysts, beginning with Simmel[9] and Knight[12,13] who, along with William Menninger[10] devised a meticulous treatment milieu and defined a special working relationship between the psychotherapist and the hospital doctor, which, in its essentials, is still in effect at the Menninger Clinic, as one of us has described elsewhere.[39] Knight's[40] description of treatment for borderline patients is but a variant of his earlier description of treatment for alcoholics, and it may apply to them as well.

The basic requirement is to uncover and remove the patient's crippling defenses, beginning with his drinking, which both relieves psychic pain and necessitates the redoubled employment of denial, splitting, rationalization, and projection, which characterize the alcoholic's premorbid personality. The alcoholic's actual or potential wish to drink—appearing more or less undisguised in fantasies and dreams—should be considered, initially at least, within the context of the therapeutic alliance rather than in connection with its putative genetic origin. The point should be made that alcohol is not a substitute for mother or love as the patient may claim, but an end in itself, a primary object affording discharge of tension and signifying the patient's inability to tolerate his feelings of frustration, narcissistic hurt, or loneliness, and to accept the therapist as his helper. Confrontation of the patient's typical defenses is not only the first step in the treatment of alcoholics, but also essential to maintain throughout treatment; for, if exercised consistently, with concern and patience, it promotes and safeguards the therapeutic alliance, which is always fragile with alcoholics, and borderline patients in general, full of mistrust and anxiety.

Dealing with the patient's defenses should be in terms of their current, adaptational meaning rather than their genetic content. The alcoholic's defenses aim at sparing his vulnerable self-esteem. Specifically, they protect him from the experience of anxiety, depression, guilt or, in the more severe, clearly borderline cases, anger, fear, emptiness, self-contempt and other such negative affects, narcissistic in origin. To interpret the patient's defenses—or resistances, including the transference—beyond the here-and-now, to attempt to reconstruct the traumatic oedipal or pre-oedipal childhood, makes little difference to the alcoholic patient, if not making it worse. In one of the cases cited earlier, the patient was able to acknowledge that she had real feelings even though she could still not experience them as such, and she knew that in hating her analyst she was transferring onto him the hatred she harbored for her childhood mother. Yet, in spite of three years in classical analysis, she was not at all ready to give up her alcoholic illness. As her analyst put it, "all [my] interpretative work 'made sense' to her but did not 'click.'" In fact, the analyst's interpretative "pressures" upset the patient to the point that she became delusional for the first time in her life. This bit of psychotic transference, typical of borderline patients in analysis, was also interpreted; and it promptly cleared. Soon afterwards, however, the patient began drinking again. When she was brought back to the hospital she indicated that the analyst was the first one she wanted to see, but also the last one who could help her.

Defenses should be further analyzed within the context of the patient's character traits, typically identified as the alcoholic personality and representing a superficial, fragile and maladaptive form of reaction formation and obsessiveness, which again shields the individual from the experience of unpleasant affects, predominantly anger, boredom, emptiness and sheer narcissistic hurt.

The way an analyst and, in general, a psychotherapist approaches his patient's defenses is bound to determine the kind of transference that develops in the process of treatment. When core defenses are under attack, the patient's aggressiveness is going to surface in the transference, alone or fused with homosexual potential. Oral aggressive and paranoid tendencies may drive the patient back to drinking, and for this reason firm setting of limits and the ready availability of a hospital have been advocated by those who prescribe psychoanalytic psychotherapy or analysis to alcoholic patients.[10,12,13,39]

On the other hand, the alcoholic's oral dependent proclivity to behave properly without complaining can make him look like an ideal patient, resulting in relaxation of vigilance on the part of those concerned with his well-being and of the therapist himself, who may feel that his help is superfluous or no longer necessary. Caught in a transference-countertransference bind, the therapist comes to feel like the patient's childhood mother, all too ready to let him go his own way and forget him, while the patient feels secretly inadequate, misunderstood and deprived of the love and protection that he does not dare demand for the fear that it may be experienced as insatiable, bothersome, or rejectable. And the mere probability of rejection, along with the secret craving of "love"—experienced as emptiness, badness, or alienation—tends to make him angry and revengeful, ready to drive him back to drinking, away from treatment.

The slightest indication of rejection on the therapist's part, a long weekend, a canceled appointment or spending more time with another patient, may become the fatal trigger point. That is why firmness and limit setting should be combined with empathic attention, personal warmth and encouraging comments, even active advice on occasion—what

Winnicott,[41] in referring to the normal early mother-child relationship, has described as "the holding environment." As Knight[40] put it in discussing the treatment of borderline states, "[the patient] needs *proofs* of emotional support, of trusting and trustworthiness, and of genuine human interest rather than merely detached professional interest." Or, as Kohut[20] wrote with reference to addicts, "[their dependence] must be recognized and acknowledged. In fact, it is a clinical experience that the major psychoanalytic task in such instances is the analysis of the denial of the real need; the patient must first learn to replace a set of unconscious grandiose fantasies that are kept up with the aid of social isolation by the, for him, painful acceptance of the reality of being dependent."

Once committed to treatment—or rather to the therapist, to whom he or she is likely to become very dependent, virtually addicted—the patient should be guided along in expanding his or her capacity for genuine object relations beyond the therapeutic situation. The process is inevitably long and arduous, involving the use of transitional objects,[24] inanimate ones like disulfiram, a job, or a hobby; and live people, who may or may not be the ones—spouse, lover, mother—the patient had available at the beginning of treatment.

SUMMARY

This paper traces the psychoanalytic literature on alcoholism from its early conceptualization as a manifestation of oral narcissism, latent homosexuality and repressed aggression, to the current view that defines it in terms of ego deficit and low affect-tolerance. Implicit in old and newer views seems to be the notion that, generally, alcoholism is a developmental disorder of a borderline nature. On evidence from current psychoanalytic reports and our own research, we propose that most alcoholic patients are borderline, narcissistic or both. That some alcoholic patients recover from their dependence on alcohol, with or without treatment, means no more than that some borderline and narcissistic individuals can function indefinitely without apparent need for psychiatric help.

REFERENCES

1. Hartocollis, P. *Borderline Personality Disorders*. New York: International Universities Press, 1977.
2. Zinberg, N.E. Addiction and ego function. *Psychoan. Stud. Child.* 30:567–588, 1975.
3. Abraham, K. The psychological relations between sexuality and alcoholism (1908), in *Selected Papers*. London: Hogarth Press, 1927 pp. 80–89.

4. Yorke, C. A critical review of some psychoanalytic literature on drug addiction. *Brit. J. Med. Psych.* 43:41–159, 1970.
5. Rado, S. The psychoanalysis of pharmacothymia. *Psychoanal. Quart.* 2:2–23, 1933.
6. Glover, E. On the etiology of drug-addiction. *Int. J. Psycho-Anal.* 13:298–328, 1932.
7. Glover, E. *Psychoanalysis,* 2nd ed. New York: Staples Press, 1949.
8. Kernberg, O. Borderline personality organization. *J. Amer. Psychoan. Assoc.* 15:641–685, 1967.
9. Simmel, E. Psycho-analytic treatment in a sanatorium. *Int. J. Psycho-Anal.* 10:70–89, 1929.
10. Menninger, W. The treatment of chronic alcohol addiction. *Bull. Menn. Clinic* 1:101–112, 1937.
11. Menninger, K.A. *Man Against Himself.* New York: Harcourt, Brace and Co., 1938.
12. Knight, R.P. The dynamics and treatment of chronic alcohol addiction. *Bull. Menn. Clinic* 1:233–250, 1937.
13. Knight, R.P. The psychoanalytic treatment in a sanatorium of chronic addiction in alcohol. *JAMA* 111:1443–1448, 1938.
14. Winokur, G., Reich, T., Rimmer, J., and Pitts, F.N., Jr. Alcoholism: III. Diagnosis and familiar psychiatric illness in 259 alcoholic probands. *Arch. Gen. Psychiat.* 23:104–111, 1970.
15. Winokur G., Rimmer, J., and Reich, T. Alcoholism IV: Is there more than one type of alcoholism? *Brit. J. Psychiat.* 118:525–531, 1971.
16. Knight, R.P. Borderline states. *Bull. Menn. Clinic.* 17:1–12, 1953.
17. Schur, M. Comments on the metapsychology of somatization. *Psychoan. Stud. Child.* 10:119–164, 1955.
18. Krystal, H., and Raskin, H.A. *Drug Dependence, Aspects of Ego Functions.* Detroit: Wayne State University Press, 1970.
19. Wurmser, L. Psychoanalytic considerations of the etiology of compulsive drug use. *J. Amer. Psychoan. Assoc.* 22:820–843, 1974.
20. Kohut, H. Introspection, empathy, and psychoanalysis. *J. Amer. Psychoan. Assoc.* 7:459–483, 1959.
21. Kohut, H. Preface, in Blaine, J.D., and Julius, D.A. (eds.), *Psychodynamics of Drug Dependence* (NIDA Research Monograph 12). Washington, D.C.: U.S. Dept. of Health, Education and Welfare, 1977, pp. vii–ix.
22. Khantzian, E.J. The ego, the self, and opiate addiction: Theoretical and treatment considerations, in Blaine, J.D., and Julius, D.A. (eds.), *Psychodynamics of Drug Dependence* (NIDA Research Monograph 12). Washington, D.C.: Dept. of Health, Education and Welfare, 1977, pp. 101–117.
23. Jellinek, E. *The Disease Concept of Alcoholism.* New Brunswick, N.J.: Hillhouse Press, 1960.
24. Little, N. Transference in borderline states. *Int. J. Psychoanal.* 47:476–485, 1966.
25. Armstrong, J.D. The search for the alcoholic personality. *Ann. Amer. Acad. Polit. Soc. Science* 315:40–47, 1958.
26. McCord, W., McCord, J., and Gudeman, J. *Origins of Alcoholism.* Stanford, Calif.: Stanford University Press, 1960.
27. Blane, H.T. *The Personality of the Alcoholic: Guises of Dependency.* New York: Harper and Row, 1968.
28. Kernberg, O. A psychoanalytic classification of character pathology. *J. Amer. Psychoan. Assoc.* 18:800–822, 1970.
29. Rosenfeld, H.A. On drug addiction. *Int. J. Psycho-Anal.* 41:467–475, 1959.
30. Kernberg, O. Factors in the psychoanalytic treatment of narcissistic personalities. *J. Amer. Psychoan. Assoc.* 18:51–85, 1970.

31. Deutsch, H. Some forms of emotional disturbance and their relationship to schizophrenia, in *Neuroses and Character Types*. New York: International Universities Press, 1965, pp. 262–281.

32. Settlage, C.F. The psychoanalytic understanding of narcissistic and borderline personality disorders: advances in developmental theory. *J. Amer. Psychoanal. Assoc.* 25:805–833, 1977.

33. Hartocollis, P. A dynamic view of alcoholism: Drinking in the service of denial. *Dynam. Psychiat.* 2:173–182, 1969.

34. Hartocollis, P. Denial of illness in alcoholism: *Bull. Menn. Clinic.* 32:47–53, 1968.

35. Strecker, E.A., and Chambers, F.T. *Alcohol, One Man's Meat.* New York: Macmillan, 1938.

36. Masterson, J.F., and Rinsley, D.B. The borderline syndrome: The role of the mother in the genesis and psychic structure of the borderline personality. *Int. J. Psycho-Anal.* 56:163–177, 1975.

37. Mahler, M.S. *On Human Symbiosis and the Vicissitudes of Individuation, Vol. I: Infantile Psychosis.* New York: International Universities Press, 1968.

38. Mahler, M.S. A study of the separation-individuation process and its possible application to borderline phenomena in the psychoanalytic situation. *Psychoan. Stud. Child,* 26:403–424, 1971.

39. Hartocollis, P. Psychotherapy and the alcoholic, in Hirsch, J. (ed.), *Opportunities and Limitations in the Treatment of Alcoholics,* Springfield, Ill.: Charles C. Thomas, 1967, pp. 53–75.

40. Knight, R.P. Management and psychotherapy of the borderline schizophrenic patient. *Bull. Menn. Clinic.* 17:139–150, 1953.

41. Winnicott, D. W. *The Maturational Processes and the Facilitating Environment.* New York: International Universities Press, 1965.

CHAPTER 8

The Family In Alcoholism

DONALD I. DAVIS

INTRODUCTION

Alcoholism does not occur as an isolated event affecting one individual. For every case, there are multiple victims. The primary victims are usually the alcoholic and his immediate family, although colleagues, unknown pedestrians, and many others may at times feel the consequences as well. The phenomenology of alcoholism would be seriously incomplete without an inspection of the family issues involved and their implications for application of the growing array of family and marital therapy approaches to the treatment of alcoholism. This chapter will focus, first, on the more compelling reasons for including the family when dealing with an alcoholic and, second, on family oriented approaches to treatment.

FAMILY ISSUES IN ALCOHOLISM

It is becoming common knowledge that only a very small percentage of alcoholics are living on skid-row. The bias toward dealing with alcoholics as isolated individuals persists, nonetheless. Therefore, it seems worth stating that most alcoholics do not live alone. In our own recent survey of the drinking and other drug taking habits of several thousand general medical, surgical and psychiatric patients in a university medical center, we found that the majority of heavy and problem drinkers were still living with at least one family member. Of those who were not, most were living in a stable relationship with at least one significant other and had been for three or more years. Furthermore, most of the problem drinkers either living alone or without such long term relationships were young adults.

A special word is in order about young adult alcoholics, those in their twenties and thirties. Clinically, we usually have found that it is a mistake to assume that young adult problem drinkers, regardless of domicile, are independent of their families of origin. As has been more rigorously documented by Vaillant[1] and Stanton[2] for young adult male heroin addicts, young adult alcoholics are usually found to be in frequent contact with one or both parents, either by telephone or in person. Further, it is common to find that they move back into the home of their parents intermittently. More importantly, even when they do not move back into their parents' home, the degree to which they include their parents in the process of making important decisions about their own lives is often extensive.

The fact that alcoholics live with, or in some important way are in contact with significant others is only one dimension of the rationale for looking to family therapy for help in treating alcoholism. Along more functional dimensions, all aspects of family life are compromised when a member of the family is abusing alcohol. The marital relationships, parenting, and often development of the children suffer.

It is doubtful that there are any good marriages in which one or both spouses are alcoholics and still actively drinking heavily.[3] Studies recently reviewed by Paolino and McCrady have shown that divorce is higher amongst marriages with an active alcoholic than amongst non-alcohol involved marriages ([3], Appendix A). There is no data from which to conclude either that alcoholism causes a greater number of divorces or that bad marriages cause alcoholism. From a treatment standpoint, however, it is enough to know that the family system of an alcoholic has an unusual risk of disruption of lives and of morbidity. Divorce itself has these consequences. Divorce among actively drinking alcoholics leaves a family system less well prepared to weather a marital breakup than are most families. Thus, assessment of the need for help in the marital relationship of married alcoholics seems indicated.

Clinically, what the author and many others who have shared their clinical and personal experiences with the author have found is that chronic alcoholics and their spouses often have great difficulty resolving their differences while the alcoholic continues to drink heavily. This applies not just to issues unique to alcoholism but to any of the broad range of inevitable dilemmas that arise in any marriage. When there is a difference of opinion, and one spouse has the option of an altered state of consciousness, couples do not stay at the task of problem solving until differences are reconciled.

Such a marital deficit can become a serious factor in the early phases of abstinence. The clinician frequently observes a disillusionment during the period just after abstinence is initiated. It seems to have to do with the discovery that, while individuals are recovering and less tense, the marriage remains unsatisfactory or stressful. Lack of mutual problem solving mechanisms is probably a major contributor to this disillusionment. In fact, abstinence is often associated with heightened awareness of interpersonal conflict as the couple carry their talks further, no longer constrained by one partner's falling asleep or becoming uncontrollably angry. Soon they discover that they are truly at an impasse. For example, couples come to realize that they still do not agree, or no longer agree, on such matters as when to have children, how many children to have, whether to buy a house, whether to ask a grandparent to move in or out, when to have sex, and many more issues that are quite significant for that particular family.

Parenting suffers as well as the marital relationship when alcoholism is present in a parent in the family. It is well known that there is a high frequency of alcohol use in association with physical abuse of children by parents. Not all of that use is by chronic heavy drinkers, and not all alcoholic parents physically abuse their children. There are, however, more subtle areas of child neglect that many would say are inevitable consequences of chronic alcoholism. A description of an interview with the mother of a four-year-old girl will help to illustrate this point. The author was asked to interview, as a consultant, a woman in her mid-twenties who had been hospitalized for two weeks for depression of acute onset. The episode had followed abandonment by the man with whom she had been living for several years. He was also the father of her four-year-old daughter. The question for the consultant had to do with understanding the role of alcohol in this woman's depression. It was thought that she had been drinking heavily, a pint of hard liquor a day, since becoming depressed over the few weeks before hospitalization. History indicated a similar pattern abruptly following the same man's departure two years earlier. A brief, purposefully rather repetitive inquiry led to the finding that this young mother had been drinking a pint or so of hard liquor for at least eight years. Subsequent probes readily uncovered the myriad ways in which alcohol had interfered in her life, affecting her performance on her job, driving, socializing, and in fact directly contributing to her mate's two decisions to leave. She was proud, though, that she had protected her little daughter from the ravages of drinking. There she drew the line. She was a good mother and clearly loved her daughter dearly. Still, it soon became apparent that her daughter was being neglected unwittingly. When asked how she, mother, was able to stay awake long enough in the evening to be with her daughter, she replied with genuine pride, "Oh, she's a very independent little girl". It evolved that mother was increasingly taking daughter to be cared for by grandmother, both because she worked later to make up for her poor work in the morning hours and because she could not handle her child to her own satisfaction. Grandmother, however, did not want to care for a small child. After once again claiming of her four-year-old, "She can take care of herself", she began to cry and acknowledged that she was an alcoholic and that her alcoholism even was leading her to be a poor parent.

Children of alcoholics are victims in ways that are even harder to document than neglect.[4,5] Two of these ways were highlighted in a recent panel of alcohol educators.[6] The first is that it is common for the children of alcoholics to take responsibility for their parent's alcoholism (just as children often describe ways in which their behavior is thought to be responsible for their parent's divorce). They feel and act guilty, and they may also feel and act angry at having to bear the burden of this guilt. They may sulk and retreat socially, or they may achieve highly. There are many different reactions to perceiving that one's parent is an alcoholic. What is a frequent common ground for these children, as they describe in therapy sessions and share among themselves in Al Ateen (an organization for teenagers who have an alcoholic parent), is that they believe they are in some ways responsible, that they dwell on the issue, that they sometimes go to great lengths to either make their parent happier or compensate for what that parent can no longer do, and that they are not very happy in their own lives. Research to back up these specific clinical impressions is lacking, though there is ample evidence that there are hardships and high risks of behavioral consequences for the children of alcoholics.[7,8]

A second important consequence of alcoholism to children of alcoholics is only apparent when they become young adults. It has to do with predisposition to either develop some substance abuse problem themselves or to marry someone who has or develops alcoholism. The reference here is to familial, nongenetic factors. Goodwin has reviewed the state of the knowledge of the role of genetics in the development of alcoholism and had concluded that some genetic factor may contribute to at least a predisposition toward alcoholic behavior and severe complications of alcoholism when heavy drinking is present.[9] We cannot do justice here to the issue of the role of genes in the transmission of alcoholism, except to say further that Goodwin and others have also concluded that genes alone do not explain fully the distribution and variety of alcoholism problems arising in the offspring of alcoholics. Environment clearly contributes to the documented increased incidence of alcoholism in children and grandchildren of alcoholics when compared with offspring of nonalcoholic parents.

There are two types of issues to keep in mind in assessing the risks to the next generation. One is that of increased drug use itself. The other deals with behavior that may facilitate or foster alcoholism in the family system of offspring but not necessarily in the child himself. The latter is more of an abstraction as yet. Clinically, it appears that nonalcoholics who grew up with an untreated (and often unacknowledged) alcoholic adult often seem to have a high threshold for concerns over heavy or problem drinking in a spouse. When the spouse of an alcoholic has such a background, the whole family is more ready to deny the existence of alcoholism.

One does not have to postulate deviousness on the part of such a spouse to understand how they came to put up with heavy drinking and drunken behavior for as long as they have. In fact, in their recent extensive review, Paolino and McCrady appear to have debunked theories of disturbed personality in spouses of alcoholics as significant contributors to alcoholism.[3] That does not detract from the impact of alcoholism in the spouse's family of origin on the maintenance of an alcohol problem in the present family. Based on the experiences in their family of origin alone, there is often reason to include the spouse in the educational process of the early phase of intervention with alcoholism without fear that one is necessarily up against a personality in need of basic change.

One more aspect of family life in the family of an alcoholic that may justify inclusion of the family in the treatment of the alcoholic will be examined here. It is the family interactional consequences of alcoholism. There have now been a number of both clinical research and laboratory research studies of the interaction among family members in families which have one or more alcoholics or other drug abusers. Klagsbrun and Davis[10] recently reviewed this literature and concluded that what stands out from these studies is the important role that family interactional processes seem to play in maintaining the alcohol or other drug abuse behavior of an individual.

We are not addressing the issue of causality. There is nothing in this literature to either support or disprove that there is a role for family interaction processes in the etiology of alcoholism. Rather, we are talking about how problem behavior involving the use of alcohol may actually be sustained by family interaction, even after the drinking behavior has become clearly destructive. We are talking about the ways alcohol abuse and drunken behavior seem to come to serve a function for a family regardless of whether the family can be seen to have played a role in the development of the problem in the first place. Davis, et al., have employed the term "adaptive consequences of drinking" to describe these functions alcoholic behavior may come to serve in a family.[11]

A case example of a research situation with a family of an alcoholic will help illustrate the concept of how a family can adapt to a drinking problem and in turn how the family's adaptation can come to serve as a source of resistance to change in the drinking behavior. The father in this family was a chronic heavy drinker of many years duration. He still had his job, however, and continued to live with his wife. Their adult daughter had recently been discharged from a psychiatric hospital for depression. She alternated between living in her parents' home and living on her own, but only a block away. Just prior to taking part in the research, all three had entered family therapy as the last of many attempts, including a trial with Alcoholics Anonymous, to get help for father's drinking problem. One part of the research study involved the use of the largely nonverbal psychodramatic technique of family sculpting. In this case each family member was instructed by a research psychologist, who was not involved in their therapy, to characterize or portray a typical family situation in which each family member was present, using the other two family members and themselves as the characters. They were asked to do this under two conditions, first when alcohol is not present and then, again, when alcohol is introduced into the scene. Only mother's response will be described. Without alcohol in the picture, mother had her husband sit in a chair right next to her, but sitting parallel to her rather than looking directly at her. She further instructed father that he was to "put up a barrier" whenever she either spoke to him or turned to look at him. He was to do so by raising his jacket up and holding it between them. At the same time, daughter was instructed to walk both toward and away from both parents, back and forth, apparently without making conversation or having eye contact with her parents. Then mother was told, "Now alcohol is introduced. What is it like now?" Mother immediately sent father to the farthest corner of the room and said that he was out of the picture. She then moved to the opposite corner of the room from him and had her daughter come sit in a chair right next to her, facing her; and she indicated that she and her daughter were in conversation. Mother also indicated that all three of them were having at least a little something to drink. The family members were asked to describe their feelings in these situations; but even if we ignore the descriptions of their affect, the simple changes in position and activity offer us a poignant example of the differences in this family under drinking and nondrinking circumstances. The most prominent observation is that when alcohol is not present in this family, no one is really in contact with anyone else. When alcohol is introduced, at least the daughter is no longer vacillating between leaving her parents and staying with them.

Both father's and daughter's portrayal of their family with and without alcohol were quite similar to mother's, with the exception that each of them showed daughter becoming more connected with her father, as well as with mother, when father was drinking. We would speculate from this example that father's drinking, regardless of how it got started, has come to serve in this family at least the function of keeping their adult daughter in more direct contact with her parents. We would further speculate that, should father succeed in becoming abstinent, the family would serve as a source of resistance to sustaining his abstinence, unless either (1) mother and father were helped to find an alternative way of keeping daughter connected with them, or (2) mother and father were helped to find new ways to tolerate their relationship together once daughter had finally moved out.

This illustration from a research experience provides us with an example of how we might find evidence that the drinking behavior of an alcoholic has come to serve a significant function within his or her family. The resistance to giving up such a function could be great, even among well intentioned family members, unless the family is helped to either substitute for the function or make the function unnecessary. It should be emphasized that, while the above example was derived from a research experience, within a different context the same experience could have occurred in the course of family therapy, and often does. Of course, the particular role the drinking may have come to serve is likely to be different for each family.

The family and marital issues discussed above provide a theoretical basis for including family interaction in the treatment of the alcoholic. Drawing upon this material, an argument could be that, with such pervasive interpersonal consequences of alcoholism, would it not be productive to treat alcoholism with a family or marital technique most of the time? If these family issues are usually operating, one should be able to accomplish several things through family interaction that one cannot accomplish through treatment of the identified alcoholic patient alone. First, treatment of concomitant marital disturbance can be offered. Second, treatment or prevention of negative emotional and behavioral sequelae in children can be accomplished. Third, resistance from other family members to sustaining effective therapeutic change (abstinence in particular) by the alcoholic can be avoided. The alternative to each of these expectations is that successful treatment of the individual alcoholic alone will just as frequently and effectively deal with each of these concerns. These are all testable arguments. Hopefully, in the future they will be adequately examined. There is only rudimentary direct testing of these alternatives to date. For example, there is evidence from studies with widely used marital inventories that marriages do improve some when an alcoholic simply stops drinking.[12,3] On the other hand, there is evidence that interpersonal stress (such as marital stress) is more likely than other life stresses to lead to a renewed bout of heavy drinking among abstinent alcoholics.[13,14]

Research simply does not yet answer these important theoretical questions. There do appear to be, though, some pragmatic reasons for bringing family approaches to an alcohol problem. For example, working with families, even at the most peripheral level, has been shown to offer benefits in the treatment of alcoholism. It has been shown that, regardless of the type of treatment offered ultimately, just having a family member accompany an alcoholic patient at the time of an initial interview was associated with alcoholics staying in treatment longer.[15]

Experience to date with bonafide family therapy approaches to alcoholism also provides a substantial pragmatic basis for attempting more family work in the field, even in the absence of definitive outcome data. In the past decade, there has been a rapprochement between the two rapidly developing fields of alcoholism treatment and of family therapy that has not always existed. In fact, the widespread adaptation of the many recent advances in family therapy to the field of alcoholism treatment was quite slow in developing.[16] The literature that there is on family therapy for alcoholism has been reviewed recently by several authors. Briefly, all reviewers concluded that methodologically definitive studies comparing the outcome of family therapy with other approaches to the treatment of alcoholism have not yet been done.[16,17,3] However, Steinglass emphasized that there is in the literature a sound basis of support for future more conclusive treatment outcome studies;[16] while Janzen found that there is, at the very least, evidence that family therapy for alcoholism has at times been a successful mode of intervention in and of itself.[17] Paolino and McCrady note that the several behavioral marital therapy studies in the literature provide a combined treatment outcome success rate of 70% or better,[3] which compares favorably with success rates in the range of 60% for alcohol treatment outcome studies in general.[18] These outcome comparisons are based solely on evaluation of drinking behavior of the identified alcoholic. Abstinence and usually also decreased drinking at follow-up are taken as indicators of successful outcome. Family, marital, and child behavior in the family of the alcoholic are not yet a strong part of even our best treatment outcome studies. It need hardly be stated that future problems of children of alcoholics, or transmission of alcohol related behavioral problems to future generations, have never been assessed as outcome variables. What is known is that some family and marital treatment approaches applied to alcoholism have had at least as good effects as more traditional treatment approaches in reducing alcoholic drinking behavior. Therefore, from a pragmatic standpoint, the risk of choosing these approaches does not seem great; while the risk to the family of the alcoholic of not including them may be significant. The latter point remains to be demonstrated by future research.

Going beyond the literature and into the field, Coleman and Davis have found additional support for bringing family therapy into the mainstream of alcoholism treatment.[19] Their report on a National Survey of over 2,000 treatment programs in the United States which offer treatment for abuse of drugs, including alcohol, revealed a high level of enthusiasm for family approaches to addictive disorders among at least some of the staff of most programs surveyed. To summarize briefly, the Survey revealed a high level of intuitive interest in the appropriateness of family therapy approaches to substance abuse, whether alcohol or other drugs were involved. Unfortunately, there was not a comparable consistently high level of family therapy expertise found with which to implement this intuition. Even so, those who were already using some form of family approach answered uniformly that they would continue doing so; and those programs with the least family therapy expertise, rather than being pessimistic about the benefits of family work, indicated a strong desire to be offered family therapy training.

There is even more evidence, though not specifically related to alcohol problems, that family therapy can serve a primary prevention role. Alexander and colleagues[20] conducted a well controlled treatment outcome study with court referred, delinquent adolescents. One of their most remarkable findings was that, two to three years later, there was a significantly lower incidence of court appearances for delinquent behavior among younger siblings of those delinquent adolescents whose families were offered therapy, but not among those whose families were not. Like children in the families of a delinquent, children in the families with an alcoholic member have a high incidence of both drug and nondrug related behavioral disturbances. In both cases, these families are much in need of preventive intervention. Since there is evidence that family therapy has served a bonafide preventive function in families of delinquents, it would seem wise to consider family therapy with families of alcoholics for its possible preventive benefits.

FAMILY AND MARITAL INTERVENTION

Working with the family of the alcoholic is the province of the family practitioner or any other provider of health care services. There are interventions with other family members short of family work by therapists trained in family and marital techniques that can be of considerable importance. Simply questioning others in the family can provide needed confirmation of an alcohol problem. A family member present at the outset of treatment can be a great help not only in clearly identifying an alcohol problem but also in effectively confronting a person with the alcohol problem. Having a spouse confirm that he or she, as well as the therapist, sees the problem as alcoholism can be a major step in overcoming the denial that both alcoholic and spouse have been living with for many years. Direct contact with family members is also the best way to detect substance abuse or other serious problems in others in the family. Undetected substance abuse in spouses, parents, or children of an alcoholic can add immeasurably to time and inefficiency of treatment.

The likelihood that spouses will attend Al Anon and children Al Ateen is greater if there is direct contact to allow for education and encouragement of others in the family. Attendance at either may have the benefit of reducing excessive reactions by spouses or children to the alcoholic's drinking, thereby reducing time wasted on fights and decreasing excuses for further drinking as well. Along a similar line, another practical way a nonfamily therapist might choose to reduce conflicts and excuses is to prescribe that Antabuse (disulfiram) be taken in front of the spouse daily. In selected couples, this has appeared to decrease fear in the spouse and speed restoration of mutual trust. Certain precautions should be taken, of course. For some couples, this latter approach would only replicate numerous previous solutions that have failed, and therefore it would be inappropriate. It is also true that, while Al Anon and Al Ateen for family members and AA for the alcoholic may increase self sufficiency for each individual, they may do so without improving relationships at all. In these situations, and when there are clear cut marital conflicts or child neglect issues, family therapy as such should be considered.

There are several approaches to family therapy which have been applied with some success in these situations. From their extensive review of the literature on marital treatment of alcoholism and their own work, Paolino and McCrady have leaned toward use of behavioral marital therapy techniques.[3] They draw particularly upon the work of Weiss, et al.[21] and of Stuart[22] on the application of conflict resolution techniques and on means of increasing the mutual rewardingness of relationships.

Berenson[23] has described approaches to family therapy for alcoholics that are taken primarily from the structural family therapy techniques of Minuchin,[24] as well as the strategic and often paradoxical approaches described by Haley[25] and by Watzlawick, Weakland, and Fisch.[26] As he indicates, these approaches are compatible with and are often combined with behavioral marital therapy techniques. He also integrates Bowen's family systems theory[27,28] with these latter approaches, either as an alternative or as part of a second phase of therapy. As was noted earlier in this chapter, young adult substance abusers seem to be surprisingly involved with their families of origin. Bowen's emphasis on the use of therapy to help the person more successfully individuate from his family of origin would seem to many in the field to go right to the heart of the issue for the alcohol or other drug abusing young adult. Nevertheless, techniques that focus more on immediate problem solving[29] may need to come first if the drinking is to cease. These include structural techniques for altering roles and coalitions and thereby shifting the structural context of the family, leaving more flexibility in roles and behaviors for the alcoholic to attempt.

Using the structural approach, there is often an essential paradox introduced, in that alcoholism is clearly defined as the number one problem and then, having done that, the focus is shifted to problems in other members of the family and within relationships. Having accomplished this, it becomes possible to achieve a redefinition of people's roles in the family. For example, the alcoholic may be seen as protecting an obese wife from depression through calling attention to his own problems, thereby placing the alcoholic's behavior into a caring context. Similarly, it may be possible to show that the spouse, whose behavior has been experienced by the alcoholic as critical and domineering, is in fact in need of and desirous of help. Children who have come to see the alcoholic parent as someone not to be taken seriously, and therefore lacking in authority over them, may find themselves surprisingly acting out the role of children in need of help turning to the more experienced and caring (alcoholic) parent. Sometimes families need to experience such redefinitions of the meaning of their family's interaction in order to dare to give up alcoholic drinking behavior. As Watzlawick, et al.[26] have indicated, often the solutions that families have come up with are in themselves the problem. Alcohol abuse or behaviors that have the effect of maintaining alcohol abuse can be seen as solutions that have become the problem. When this is the case, alternative behaviors which may be brought about by surprising or paradoxical interventions are often called for. The effects of these interventions must be accepted by all the members of the family system in which the alcoholic lives. A therapist may need family therapy techniques in order to guide family members to and help them tolerate the new and therefore unpredictable family situation.

There are a few points to be made about family therapy for alcoholism that apply without regard to type of family approach used. A very practical role for family therapy for alcoholism that is seldom written about but has much to offer is the use of family therapy in a complementary way with Alcoholics Anonymous (AA), Al Anon and Al Ateen. Davis has discussed this subject in a recent paper.[30] To summarize this paper briefly, family therapy can be used effectively to get previously recalcitrant alcoholics into AA and their spouses into Al Anon. It has also been a great help in maintaining their participation in these AA self-help groups. Family therapy and self-help groups each can reinforce the other's emphasis on taking responsibility for one's own behavior. What family therapy adds particularly to the approach of the self-help groups is direct work on relationships. Often disillusionment occurs when abstinence is newly achieved and the marital or parenting relationships are found to be no better, or sometimes even to be generating more anxiety than before. This can be anticipated, planned for, and modified through the addition of family therapy to an otherwise successful approach to change in AA.

There is much fear and resentment about psychotherapy among many of the proponents of the AA self-help groups. Many of these misgivings stem from experiences of alcoholics with individual psychotherapy, during which their problem with drinking was never explicitly addressed. The concern is that with the growth of the family therapy field, family therapy may also be offered as an alternative to the self-help groups, and that again ignorance of alcohol combined with zeal for a new therapy will lead to failure to appropriately address the alcohol problems.

When a family therapist fails to explicitly set the elimination of the drinking problem as a first priority, he is making a mistake. Altering roles or improving communication or expression of affect among family members in and of themselves is not likely to proceed well if the drinking of an alcoholic in the family continues. It is unrealistic for family therapists to assume that, if they forget about the alcohol problem and somehow deal effectively with other underlying problems, the alcoholic drinking will go away. On the other hand, when the family therapist is knowledgeable about the problems of alcohol and establishes a clear agreement with all members of the family that overcoming the drinking problem is an objective of the first priority, family therapy has much to contribute; and it can be used in conjunction with self-help groups.

Finally, here are a few practical suggestions. First, the earlier the family is brought in to see the therapist, the more likely they are to cooperate with a family approach; also, as was stated earlier, the more likely is the abuser to stay in treatment. Second, alcoholics and their families are among the most difficult of all psychotherapy patients to get into the office. Direct phone calls to each family member, especially from the eventual therapist, are often critical. Repeat calls may be necessary, but it is worth the initial effort because once a family gets involved the odds are good that they will continue. It is often critical to include in family sessions the parents of young adult alcoholics, even if they are living out of their parents' home and with a spouse. Restoration or establishment of a traditional parental-child hierarchy around the issue of the irresponsible behavior that goes along with alcohol abuse is a key step, without which the abuser's further individuation from his parents aborts and drinking is likely to resume. When the alcoholism resides in an older parent, the children should be incorporated into therapy at least temporarily. As with a spouse, children will automatically resist the changes when drinking behavior stops, unless they are helped to adapt well to the change. Finally, in family therapy for alcoholism, as in family therapy for other conditions, control in sessions must be firmly established in the therapist. An aspect of control that is critical in therapy for alcoholism is control over medication. The alcoholic is often using and abusing tranquilizers, pain medications, antidepressants or amphetamines as well. Even where the therapist is not a physician, he must be accepted by anyone else involved in providing psychoactive substances to the alcoholic or a member of his family as an authority with whom all psychoactive drug giving decisions are reviewed. Ideally, a close collaboration will evolve between the family therapist and any or all nonpsychiatric physicians. Only then does it become impossible for the alcoholic and his family to perpetuate the problems associated with an altered state of consciousness through access to prescription psychoactive drugs.

AN ETHICAL DILEMMA?

In the not-so-distant future, the alcoholism treatment field may be faced with an ethical dilemma over the question of whom to treat. Is it unethical to treat the alcoholic alone, without either involving other family members in his treatment or addressing the alcohol related problems of the significant others? Is it irresponsible to prescribe medications to an alcoholic or member of his family without first conferring with their family therapist? Clinical experience and clinical research have pointed to these questions, but they have not yet provided answers to them.

Alcoholism surely affects all members of the family of an alcoholic. Research has not proven that families can cause alcoholism in a member, but there is strong clinical evidence that family interaction can contribute to the maintenance of alcohol abuse as well as to resistance to sustaining newly achieved abstinence. The descendants of alcoholics have a greater than average risk of alcoholism themselves and perhaps of marrying alcoholics. At the same time, there is some evidence that family therapy can serve a primary prevention role, at least with the possibly related problem of delinquency.

Documented answers to our questions may be a long time in coming. In the meantime, it is likely that those in the alcoholism field with family interests increasingly will be encouraging greater collaboration between physician and nonphysician therapists working with an alcoholic and more family therapy approaches to the treatment of alcoholism.

REFERENCES

1. Vaillant, G.F. A twelve-year follow-up of New York narcotics addicts: I. The Relation of Treatment to Outcome. *Am. J. Psychiat.* 122:727–737, 1966.
2. Stanton, M.D., and Todd, T.C. Some outcome results and aspects of structural family therapy with drug addicts. Paper presented at the National Drug Abuse Conference, San Francisco, May 5–9, 1977.
3. Paolino, T.J., and McCrady, B.S. *The Alcoholic Marriage: Alternative Perspectives.* New York: Grune and Stratton, 1977.
4. Ablon, J. Family structure and behavior in alcoholism: a review of the literature, in Kissin, B. and Begleiter, H. (eds.), *The Biology of Alcoholism.* (Vol. 4). New York: Plenum Press, 1976, pp. 205–242.
5. El-Guebaly, N., and Offord, D.R. The offspring of alcoholics: a critical review. *Am. J. Psychiat.* 134:357–365, 1977.
6. Flynn, W., Davis, D.I., Foster, W., and Bast, D. The other victims of alcoholism. University Forum, Mutual Radio, WASH, August 17, 1978.
7. Cork, R.M. *The Forgotten Children: A Study of Children with Alcoholic Parents.* Toronto: Alcoholism and Drug Addiction Research Foundation, 1969.
8. Haberman, P. Childhood symptoms in children of alcoholic and comparison group patients. *J. of Marriage and Fam.* 28:152–54, 1966.
9. Goodwin, D. *Is Alcoholism Hereditary?* New York: Oxford University Press, 1976.
10. Klagsbrun, M., and Davis, D.I. Substance abuse and family interaction. *Family Process* 16:149–173, 1977.
11. Davis, D.I., Berenson, D., Steinglass, P., and Davis, S. The adaptive consequences of drinking. *Psychiatry* 37:209–215, 1974.
12. Burton, G., and Kaplan, H.M. Marriage counseling with alcoholics and their spouses II. The correlation of excessive drinking behavior with family pathology and social deterioration. *Brit. J. Addict.* 63:161–170, 1968.
13. Hore, B.D. Life events and alcoholics relapse. *Brit. J. Addict.* 66:83–88, 1971.
14. Hore, B.D. Factors in alcoholic relapse. *Brit. J. Addict.* 66:89–96, 1971.

15. Pattison, E.M., Coe. R., and Rhodes, R.J. Evaluation of alcoholism treatment: a comparison of three facilities. *Arch. Gen. Psychiat.* 20:478–488, 1969.
16. Steinglass, P. Experimenting with family treatment approaches to alcoholism, 1950–1975: a review. *Family Process* 15:97–123, 1976.
17. Janzen, C. Families in the treatment of alcoholism. *J. Stud. of Alcohol* 38:114–130, 1977.
18. Emrick, C.D. A review of psychologically oriented treatment of alcoholism. II. The relative effectiveness of different treatment approaches and the effectiveness of treatment versus no treatment. *J. Stud. of Alcohol* 36:88–108, 1975.
19. Coleman, S.B., and Davis, D.I. Family therapy and drug abuse: a national survey. *Family Process* 17:21–29, 1978.
20. Alexander J., Barton, C., Schiavo, R.S., and Parson, B.V. Systems-behavioral intervention with families of delinquents: Therapist characteristics, family behavior and outcome. *J. Consult. Clin. Psychol.* 44:656–664, 1976.
21. Weiss, R.L., Hops, H., and Patterson, G.R. A framework for conceptualizing marital conflict, a technology for altering it, some data for evaluating it, in Hamerlynch, L.A., Hardy, L.C., and Mash, E.J. (eds.), *Behavior Change: Methodology, Concepts, and Practice.* Champaign, Ill.: Research Press, 1973.
22. Stuart, R.B. Operant interpersonal treatment for marital discord. *J. Consult. and Clin. Psychol.* 33:675–682, 1969.
23. Berenson, D. Alcohol and the family system, in Guerin, P. (ed.), *Family Therapy: Theory and Practice.* New York: Gardner Press, 1976.
24. Minuchin, S. *Families and Family Therapy.* Cambridge, Mass: Harvard University, 1974.
25. Haley, J. *Uncommon Therapy: The Psychiatric Techniques of Milton H. Erickson, M.D.* New York: Ballantine Books, 1973.
26. Watzlawick, P., Weakland, J.H., and Fisch, R. *Change: Principals of problem formation and problem resolution.* New York: W.W. Norton, 1974.
27. Bowen, M. The use of family theory in clinical practice. *Compr. Psychiatry* 7:345–374, 1966.
28. Bowen, M. Alcoholism as viewed through family systems theory and family psychotherapy. *Ann. N.Y. Acad. Sciences* 233:115–22, 1974.
29. Haley, J. *Problem solving therapy: new strategies for effective family therapy.* San Francisco: Jossey-Bass, 1976.
30. Davis, D.I. Alcoholics anonymous and family therapy: or why family therapy should be seen as complementary and not as a threat to AA and Al-Anon. *J. of Marriage and Fam. Counseling.*   Oct. 1979

CHAPTER 9

Some Recent Studies of Teenage Alcoholism and Problem Drinking

REGINALD G. SMART

The past five or six years have seen a striking degree of interest in teenage drinking problems and alcoholism in North America. Much of this development has occurred because the legal drinking age has been lowered in about 25 states and all 10 Canadian provinces. This resulted in increased admission of young alcoholics to treatment facilities, increases in alcohol related traffic accidents and, of course, more drinking and heavy drinking by young people.[1] Much of the interest in youthful problem drinking has been on the part of concerned parents and government officials who have been influenced by striking media statements. For example, in 1974 the *National Observer* stated that 450,000 grade school children and teenagers in the United States were "actually alcoholics". There was a *Time* magazine editorial in April, 1974 entitled "Alcoholism: New Victims, New Treatment", which was concerned largely with increases in youthful drinking and alcohol related accidents. In fact, there are considerable difficulties in determining the trends in youthful drinking and drinking problems. There are a number of recent studies at one point in time but very few trend studies. Also there are considerable difficulties in defining exactly what is a problem and what is "teenage alcoholism". The purpose of this chapter is to review some of the recent studies of youthful drinking and drinking problems to indicate (1) the nature of the problems, (2) the characteristics of youthful problem drinkers and alcoholics, (3) treatment for young alcoholics and its outcome, and (4) some developments in preventive approaches. The present review cannot be exhaustive and readers are directed to a longer, if slightly out of date, treatment by Smart.[2]

EXTENT OF YOUTHFUL DRINKING

Several large scale studies have given recent trend information about drinking among American high school students. The oldest of these is the one conducted each year by Blackford[3] in San Mateo, California. This study was first done in 1968 and has been repeated each year. A large sample is used each year (28,000 to 35,000 students). In the 1977 study about 88% of the students were drinkers compared to only about 65.4% in 1968. This is about a 40% increase over 11 years. What is of greater interest is that the proportions of students drinking 10 or more times more than doubled in the same time period (25.4% to 54.7%). Much of the increase in drinking in Blackford's study is due to the increase in girls drinking. In this California study only alcohol and marijuana use have shown consistent increases in proportions of users over the years. Other drugs such as hallucinogens, barbiturates, etc. show fluctuations and a generally downward trend since 1971. Clearly, a major growing problem for young people in California schools has been alcohol.

The largest national study of high school students in the United States is the one conducted by Johnston and his colleagues.[4] This study unfortunately includes only seniors or students in their last year. The sample is large and carefully chosen, with approximately 18,000 students involved. The study is done every year but data have been collected only for 1975, 1976, and 1977. The trend data available do suggest an increase in the proportion of both drinkers and daily drinkers. In 1977, Johnston et al.[4] found that 92.5% of students drank alcohol and 6.1% drank daily (about half the rate of adults). This study also showed that drinking was more common among males, those living in the northern part of the country, and those living in cities rather than in rural areas.

In Ontario we have been conducting studies of youthful drinking since 1968.[5] The latest study was done in 1977 and involved a sample of 4,700 students in grades 7 to 13. We have seen a consistently increasing trend to more drinking in these studies with a large increase between 1970 and 1972. In Ontario the law was changed in 1971 to allow 18-year-olds to drink; formerly the age had been 21 years. In 1977, 82% of all students, but 95% of those aged 18 and over, drank alcohol. The rate for 18-year-olds is higher than for adults and this suggests that the next generation of adults will have even more people exposed to alcohol problems than the last. In the Ontario study we found that the highest rates of drinking and heavy drinking were among males, older students, students who have low grades in school, and those who live in the northern, more isolated areas of the province.

It should be noted that a large amount of research[6] shows conclusively that per capita alcohol consumption and problems from alcoholism such as liver cirrhosis are closely related. If more young people are drinking, and if they are drinking more often than in the past, then problems for them will also increase. The first problems will be drunkenness, alcohol-related accidents and various interpersonal problems, followed much later by physical disorders related to alcoholism.

Detailed examination of the reasons for the increase in youthful drinking is beyond the scope of this paper. It is worth noting, however, that the increase in youthful drinking followed world-wide increases in adult drinking and drinking problems,[6] and young persons are known to model their drinking on that of their parents.[5] Another reason, as mentioned, has been the lowering of drinking ages in so many parts of North America. This has led to increased drinking and drinking problems such as alcoholism and alcohol-related accidents.[1]

PROBLEM DRINKING AMONG YOUNG PEOPLE

Doubtless many people would argue that all drinking among young people represents a problem. Where parents do not wish their adolescents to drink, where they are underage, or where parents are rejecting abstainers *any drinking* may be seen as problematic. A better approach is to see adolescent drinking as part of a growth process, inevitable in most parts of North America given the high rate of adult drinking and the general acceptance of drinking in society.

How many "problems" are found depends substantially on how a "problem" is defined. If alcohol problems are restricted to alcoholism of the type usually seen in clinics and hospitals for alcoholics, then young people would have very few problems. This definition would include heavy drinking of long duration and marked by loss of control over drinking, physical dependence, withdrawal symptoms and physical complications such as liver ailments, peripheral neuritis, gastrointestinal problems, and the like. Other problems which are far more common among young drinkers include drunkenness, drinking-driving accidents, and alcohol-induced difficulties in school, family or social relationships. Many of these problems are, of course, early signs of alcoholism in later life. For some young persons the problems will increase and result in adult alcoholism. For others they are a reflection of inappropriate drinking habits which will later disappear without much serious ill effect.

Drunkenness seems to be increasing among young persons. Earlier studies done prior to 1968[7] in seven areas of the U.S.A. showed that only 11 to 17% of the students surveyed had *ever* been drunk. Only 4% reported having been drunk in the past 6 months and this is an almost insignificant proportion. However, a study by Cutler and Storm in 1973[8] showed that 40% had been drunk in the past four weeks. About 7.4% were getting drunk about once a week. A study by Smart et al.[9] in two Ontario high schools showed that 42% of the students were drunk at least once in the past month, with 5.8% being drunk 5 or more times, or about once weekly. However, only 6.7% actually passed out and 1.3% were made ill from drinking. It appears very likely that 5 to 10% of the high school students are getting drunk once a week or more. Whether this is seen as a significant problem depends on the point of view taken. Getting drunk purposely is getting to be a common recreational activity among young persons. Too much dependence on this type of recreation is likely to divert them from other more nurturing pursuits and to expose them to alcohol dependency and to alcohol-related accidents since many of them also drive cars.

Traffic accidents are a growing problem among young persons, particularly in jurisdictions which lowered their drinking ages. It has been known for some time that young persons have accidents at lower blood alcohol levels than do adults.[10] Unfortunately it is not known whether they have an especially low tolerance for alcohol because they are young or because they are inexperienced with drinking. Likely the combination of high risk-taking propensities and inexperience with both drinking and with driving is most important. Some people have suggested that learning to drink and learning to drive should not be attempted at the same time and that the legal driving age should be set at 20 or 21, long after most young people have learned to drink.

After age laws were changed, several jurisdictions found large increases in alcohol-related accidents among young people. For example, Whitehead et al.[11] in Ontario found a 339% increase in alcohol-related accidents among 18-year-olds and a 346% increase among 19-year-olds. Substantial increases were also found for 16 and 17-year-olds who technically should not have been affected by the new drinking age laws. Similar studies were done in Michigan, Vermont and Maine.[12] They showed that both single vehicle fatal crashes and night-time crashes occurred more often involving young people (under 21) after drinking ages were lowered. Comparable changes were not found in states which did not lower their drinking ages.

Other kinds of social, interpersonal and dependency problems have also been investigated among young people. Definitions of drinking problems and alcoholism are highly varied. Some definitions require the presence of a particular symptom such as intolerable craving, or physical dependence as shown by withdrawal symptoms, loss of control over drinking, or even all of these. An important and often quoted definition has been proposed by Jellinek,[13] who proposed that "alcoholism" is "any use of alcohol that causes any damage to the individual or society or both". It can be seen that no particular clinical psychological or psychiatric symptom is required. The problem word in the definition is "damage", which can be in the eye of the beholder. Surely damage would have to include physical damage, damage to social or family relationships, work potential, school performance and the like.

Most of the studies of alcoholism and problems among young people have taken this "damage" approach rather than a clinical symptoms approach. The earliest scale used to assess drinking problems among youth was developed by Straus and Bacon[14] for their studies among college students. They developed three scales—one of social complications, warning signs of problem drinking and anxiety about drinking. The social complications scale includes questions on social damage such as failure to meet obligations (missed appointments, school work), accidents or injury, formal discipline for over-drinking, losing friends, and the like). The warning signs involved problem drinking signs such as blackouts, becoming drunk alone, drinking before or instead of breakfast and participating in aggressive or destructive behaviour when drunk. In the early 1950s only 6% of the male and 1% of the female college students had drinking problems involving all of the categories.

In 1966 Globetti and Chamblin[15] used a nine point scale based on the Straus and Bacon scale. They found that 38% of the high school drinkers were "problem drinkers" with scores of 3 or more. A Canadian study using a 5 point scale found that in 1972 about 12% of the high school population or 15% of the drinkers exhibited one or more of the "problem drinking" signs.

One of the most recent studies using a modification of the Straus and Bacon scale was done in Ontario in 1975.[16] Some 1,171 students in grades 9 to 13 completed the questionnaire dealing with drinking and problem drinking and about 42% of all students reported no problem at all. About 14% reported 3 or more problems and only 2.1% 6 or more problems. This latter category should include students with very serious drinking problems although those in other categories also have problems which are far from trivial. This study found that problem drinkers were predominately males, students who drank in cars, away from home and without their parents knowing about it. These results suggest that social isolation and alienation from families are important elements in problem drinking. A great deal of the drinking of young problem drinkers occurs in situations isolated from social and parental controls.

Another study conducted in Ontario in 1977 used a 4 point scale.[1] It emphasized reactions to problems and included items on whether the student wished to drink less, whether parents felt they drank too much, if they had been arrested or warned by police or treated by a doctor or counsellor. By far the most common symptom was being arrested or warned by police. Very few had been treated or seen by any sort of counsellor. This suggests that a large proportion of youthful problem drinkers get no treatment. In all, 11.7% reported 1 or more problems but only 2.7% reported two or more. As predicted, problems were most common among older students, males, those in the higher grades of school but with a low level of success in school and those living in the northern areas of the province. The north is an area which is isolated and thinly populated. Traditionally, it has had a frontier sort of culture with strong social support for heavy drinking among men. This study together with the earlier ones suggest that in Ontario about 2 to 3% of the high school students have significant alcohol problems, probably requiring some sort of treatment or amelioration. Of course there is a much larger proportion of students with less serious problems — probably 8 to 10% of the students would be in this category.

Many youthful drinking problems appear to be more an outgrowth of inexperienced and careless drinking than of psychiatrically motivated problems. It should be expected that many will disappear with age with little need for treatment. Unfortunately, we know very little about how many problems, or what types disappear without treatment. However, one follow-up study has been made by Fillmore[17] of some of the problem drinkers seen in the original Straus and Bacon study done in 1950. This study showed that 44% of the male drinkers had one or more drinking problems in college but only 19% had a drinking problem twenty years later. Among women however, 12% were problem drinkers in college but 14% were twenty years later. This suggests that perhaps only young male drinking is likely to disappear with age. Female problem drinking appears much more likely to continue into adulthood. Of course, this is only one study and used a sample collected in the early 1950s. We know very little about how today's students will fare later with drinking problems. Also, we have no information on the persistence of drinking problems among very young adolescents. It is possible that their drinking problems could disrupt their psychosocial development to a much greater extent than for college students who are older and more mature. It is worth keeping in mind however, that at least some data show that not all youthful problem drinking is permanent.

TEENAGE ALCOHOLISM

Relative to studies of problem drinking in general populations, studies of young alcoholics are few and not very informative. Almost all studies of problem drinking involve self-report studies with large, well chosen samples of the general population. On the other hand, studies of youthful alcoholism are typically clinical or case studies of one or a few cases at most. A very few have been pre-post studies of alcoholics in treatment and some have involved follow-up as well.

In general, the appearance of alcoholism in children under the age of 14 is rare. A number of cases of liver cirrhosis have been reported in children between five and ten years of age.[18,19] The majority of these cases are from 30 to 50 years ago and it is difficult to be sure exactly how to interpret them. Almost all come from wine growing countries such as France, Brazil, Argentina and Italy. Most indicate that parents gave alcoholic beverages to their children to quiet them down or to tranquilize them at night. Unfortunately, none have involved sophisticated and modern laboratory tests of liver function. The possibility that the liver cirrhosis has been completely misdiagnosed or confused with other liver ailments such as alpha protein deficiency must be very great. In general, little by way of conclusion can be drawn from these studies.

The oldest reliable report of alcoholism among children seems to be the one by Lourie.[20] He described 20 cases of alcoholism among children between the ages of 5 and 14 seen in a Childrens' Court and Bellevue Hospital. Alcoholic drinking occurred as a means of escape, through identification with an alcoholic parent, as part of a pattern of delinquency, or in association with homosexuality.

McKay[21] made observations of the family dynamics of 20 adolescent alcoholics in the 1960s. All of the boys had alcoholic fathers. Family arguments and financial difficulties were, as expected with alcoholic parents, very common. Most of the boys were the eldest in the families and had to assume parental responsibilities at times. These children displayed hostility, impulsiveness, depression and sexual confusion.

Clinical studies by Glatt and Hills[22] indicated that young alcoholics in Britain displayed emotional deprivation early in childhood, previous exposure to heavy drinking parents, over-identification with opposite sex parent, unsatisfactory sexual adjustment and difficulties in accepting adult and parental roles (e.g. rejection of children).

The alcoholics in treatment described by Goby[23] were all 23 or under, mostly unmarried males, living with families. Most had not been treated before and few had attended AA meetings and hence were very inexperienced with treatment compared to older alcoholics. Most were abusers of other drugs such as tranquilizers, amphetamines, marihuana, and barbiturates.

The exact rate of alcoholism among young persons is difficult to determine. Jellinek estimates or other methods using liver cirrhosis deaths will be inappropriate because so few young alcoholics have liver ailments. Also, surveys of drinking problems among young people and general populations have emphasized "problems" rather than a clinically acceptable definition of alcoholism. Indeed, it is uncertain whether survey methods could ever establish the rate of alcoholics of the type seen in clinics and hospitals. Certainly a large amount of cross-validation work would be necessary to do so. Despite these difficulties there are some indications about the relative rate of treated alcoholics. Smart[2] found that by 1974 about 4% of all admissions to treatment in the alcoholism services of the A.R.F. in Ontario were aged 21 or under. At that time persons aged 15 to 21 (those at risk for admission) represented about 10% of the population of Ontario and hence young alcoholics entering treatment seem under-represented in terms of population. The study by Goby[23] found that 2.5% of all alcoholics admitted to a treatment center near Chicago were aged 23 or under.

Several studies have found evidence of increasing alcoholism among young people. The study in Ontario showed that the rate of admissions for persons under 21 was increasing until 1974. There had been no admissions of persons under 21 prior to 1965 and the rate increased dramatically for the years after 1971 (this was the year in which the drinking age was lowered). Parenthetically, it might be noted that a study in Poland in 1968[24] showed a trend to more admissions to a sobering-up station. In Scotland an increased trend was found for alcoholism admissions to mental hospitals for young persons.[25] All of these studies show increasing alcohol-related problems among young persons but surveys at two points in time have apparently not been done.

TREATMENT FOR ALCOHOLISM AMONG YOUNG PEOPLE

Despite the increased interest in youthful drinking problems, little is known of which treatments are best for them. Very few studies have been made of young persons treated in different facilities which give any indication of problems of treatment or overall recovery rates. During the past few years there has been a tendency for clinicians to believe that young alcoholics are very difficult to treat, have more symptoms, and have low recovery rates. Indeed several studies have indicated clinical impressions supporting this view. For example, Rosenberg[26] found that young alcoholics had a history of antisocial behavior, neuroticism, and anxiety and became dependent on alcohol at earlier ages than did older alcoholics. Gwinner,[27] who examined young alcoholics being treated in facilities for British Navy personnel, also found that they developed symptoms earlier than older alcoholics.

Few studies of young alcoholics in treatment have used follow-up methods with a consistent time period after treatment. Tuchmann[28] reported that alcoholics treated in Austria less often required aftercare if they were under 30 but apparently a structured follow-up was not done. Rathod[29] in England compared follow-up results for older and younger alcoholics but his study included only 8 alcoholics under 30 years of age. Of these, 7 relapsed. Similar rather depressing results were reported by Goby[23] with a follow-up varying from 11 to 25 months. Only 5 of 41 reported sobriety, with the remainder mostly using alcohol excessively.

A later study by Smart[30] examined the propositions that young alcoholics had more problems at intake and were more difficult to treat than older alcoholics. In this study 40 alcoholics aged 24 or under were compared with 40 older alcoholics of an average age of 45.1 years. The study examined drinking symptoms and demographic characteristics at intake, the type and length of treatment given to them, and overall recovery rates in terms of drinking symptoms with the Alcoholic Involvement Scale.[31] In general, the results showed that compared to older alcoholics the younger ones entered treatment with fewer resources in terms of interests and people to help them, lower social stability, poorer attitudes toward abstinence, and lower motivation for treatment. However, they did *not* have more alcoholic problems or symptoms or a higher level of alcohol consumption. The main differences seemed related to age: young alcoholics got an earlier start in their drinking careers and had fewer social supports. However, they had been treated less often and had been in the alcoholic role for a far shorter period of time. Despite the differences at intake there was no difference in recovery rates or in the type or amount of treatment received. Is it likely that young alcoholics retain some sort of resiliency because of their age which allows them to overcome their problems of low motivation for treatment? In any case, there is no good evidence for expecting that young alcoholics will do worse than older alcoholics in treatment. Probably a good deal of the pessimism about treating young alcoholics is unfounded or should really be part of the pessimism about treatment for all alcoholics.

PREVENTION

Of course, every social problem is better handled with preventive approaches than with treating affected cases. Unfortunately, few empirical studies of prevention have been attempted with young people's drinking problems. Currently, we cannot claim to know for certain how to prevent youthful drinking problems. However, a number of promising approaches can be suggested.

It seems unlikely that major changes can be made in youthful drinking without prior or concomitant changes in the society as a whole. This approach has been suggested by the Addiction Research Foundation as part of that organization's "Strategy for the Prevention of Alcohol Problems".[32] Several of the recommendations to government bear directly and others indirectly on youthful drinking and drinking problems. The recommendations in brief form include the following:

1. There should be no further liberalization of alcohol control measures and a health oriented policy to such measures should be adopted;
2. A pricing policy for alcoholic beverages should be developed which maintains a constant relationship between the price of alcohol and the consumer price index. It has been established that price increases will reduce consumption and that currently prices are too low;
3. The legal drinking age should be increased (from age 18);
4. Life style advertising of alcoholic beverages should be discouraged; and
5. There should be vigorous effort to increase public awareness of the personal hazards of heavy alcohol consumption, the economic and other consequences for society of high consumption levels and the potential public health benefits of appropriate control measures.

With regard to the latter recommendation, a recent and promising development in alcohol education should be mentioned. Research on alcohol education had traditionally been sparse and of a poor quality methodologically speaking. However, in the past year Goodstadt et al.[33] have developed a set of lesson plans for grades 8 to 10. The lesson plans were developed with the help of teachers and experts on alcohol and drugs and represent a more sophisticated approach than has been taken in the past. The plans have been tested in an experimental design in Toronto schools and have the effect of reducing drinking, intention to drink in future, and improving attitudes toward alcohol. Whether the long term use of these lessons will eventually reduce drinking problems is a matter for further research, but they hold the promise of being able to do so. More extensive testing of these lesson plans over a period of time with the same students is certainly required.

SUMMARY

The evidence available to date suggest that drinking is increasing rapidly among high school students in several areas of North America. This suggests that the next generation will have more people exposed to alcohol problems than past generations. Alcohol problems such as drunkenness, alcohol-related accidents, and pro-dromal symptoms are also increasing, especially in areas which reduced drinking ages a few years ago. The exact rate of drinking problems depends greatly upon the definition employed and how strict or conservative it is. Probably not more than 2-4% of all young persons have serious drinking problems of the type seen in clinics, although a much larger number would have less serious problems. The treatment of young alcoholics is largely unexplored. It seems likely that they have more problems at intake than older alcoholics but similar recovery rates. Real primary prevention will probably depend upon reducing alcohol consumption in society as a whole, although some promising efforts with alcohol education in schools have been made.

REFERENCES

1. Smart, R.G., and Goodstadt, M. Alcohol and drug use among Ontario students in 1977: preliminary findings, Substudy No. 889. Toronto: Addiction Research Foundation, 1977.
2. Smart, R.G. The new drinkers: drinking and drinking problems among young people. Toronto: Addiction Research Foundation, 1976.
3. Blackford, L. Surveys of student drug use: San Mateo County, San Mateo, Calif., 1978.
4. Johnston, L., et al. *Drug Use Among American High School Students, 1975-1976.* Rockville, MD.: NIDA, 1978.
5. Smart, R.G. and Fejer, D. *Changes in Drug Use in Toronto High School Students, 1968-1974.* U.N. Bulletin on Narcotics, 1975.
6. Bruun, K., et al. *Alcohol Control Policies in Public Health Perspective.* Helsinki: Finnish Foundation for Alcohol Studies, 1975.
7. Bacon, M., and Jones, M.B. *Teenage Drinking.* New York: Crowell Co., 1968.
8. Cutler, R.E., and Storm, T. *Drinking Practices in Three British Columbia Cities II. Student Survey.* Vancouver: Alcoholism Foundation of British Columbia, 1973.
9. Smart, R.G., and Gray, G. Parental and peer influences as correlates of problem drinking among high school students. In Press, *Int. J. Stud. Addict.,* 1978.

10. Borkenstein, R.F., et al. *The Role of the Drinking Driver in Traffic Accidents.* Bloomington, Indiana: Indiana University, Department of Police Administration, 1964.

11. Whitehead, P.C., et al. *Alcohol and Young Drivers: Impact and Implications of Lowering the Drinking Age, Monograph Series # 1, Ottawa: Non-Medical Use of Drugs Directorate, 1977.*

12. *Williams, A.F., et al. The Legal Minimum Drinking Age and Fatal Motor Vehicle Crashes.* Washington. Insurance Institute for Highway Safety, 1974.

13. Jellinek, E.M. *The Disease Concept of Alcoholism.* New Brunswick, N.J. College and University Press, 1960.

14. Straus, R., and Bacon, S.D. *Drinking in College.* New Haven, Conn.: Yale University Press, 1953.

15. Globetti, G., and Chamblin, F. Problem drinking among high school students in a Mississippi community. Department of Sociology and Anthropology, Mississippi State University, 1966.

16. Smart, R.G. Problem drinking among high school students in Ontario. Addiction Research Foundation, substudy No. 919, Toronto, 1977.

17. Fillmore, K.M. Drinking and problem drinking in early adulthood and middle age: an exploratory 20 year follow-up study. *Q.J. Stud. Alcohol.* 35:819–840, 1974.

18. Obarrio, J.M. Consideraciones sobre et alcoholisme en la infancia (Alcoholism among children). *Seminario Medico,* Buenos Aires 32:1096–1100, 1925.

19. Segers, A. Alcoholismo adquirido en la infancia (Acquired alcoholism in children). *Seminario Medico,* Buenos Aires 32:1238–1239, 1925.

20. Lourie, R.S. Alcoholism in children. *Am. J. Orthopsychiatry* 13:322–338, 1943.

21. McKay. J.R. Clinical observations on adolescent problem drinkers. *Q. J. Stud. Alcohol.* 22:124–134, 1961.

22. Glatt, M.M., and Hills, D.R. Alcohol abuse and alcoholism in the young. *Brit. J. Addict.* 63:183–191, 1968.

23. Goby, M.J. Follow-up study: young adult patients 1975. Alcoholism Treatment Center, Lutheran General Hospital, Park Ridge, Ill., 1977.

24. Fiszer, T., and Szezepka, K. Problemz lecznict wa alcoholikon we Wroclavia. (Problems of treatment of alcoholics in Wroclaw). *Probl. Alkzam. Wars.* 16:12–14, 1968.

25. MacCrae, A.K., at al. Alcoholism in Scotland in the 1960's. *Health Bull. of Edinburgh* 30:16–22, 1972.

26. Rosenberg, C.M. Young alcoholics. *Brit. J. Psychiat.* 115:118–188, 1969.

27. Gwinner, P.D. The young alcoholic: approaches to treatment, in Madden, J.S., et al. (eds.) *Alcoholism and Drug Dependence: A Multidisciplinary Approach.* New York: Plenum Press, 1977.

28. Tuchmann, E. Rehabilitation of alcoholics at Kalksberg (Austria). *Brit. J. Addict.* 61:59–70, 1965.

29. Rathod, N.H., et al. A two-year follow-up study of alcoholic patients. *Brit. J. Psychiat.* 112:683–692, 1966.

30. Smart, R.G. Young alcoholics in treatment: their characteristics and recovery rates at follow-up. In press, Alcoholism: Clinical and Experimental Aspects, 1978.

31. Gillies, M., et al. The alcoholic involvement scale: a method of measuring change in alcoholics. *J. Alcohol.* 10:143–147, 1975.

32. *A Strategy for the Prevention of Alcohol Problems.* Toronto: Addiction Research Foundation, 1978.

33. Goodstadt, M.S., et al. Development and Evaluation of Two Alcohol Education Programs for the Toronto Board of Education. Toronto: Addiction Research Foundation, 1978.

CHAPTER 10

Adverse Effects of Heavy Drinking During Pregnancy: Including the Fetal Alcohol Syndrome

HENRY L. ROSETT

LYN WEINER

INTRODUCTION

Although the term "fetal alcohol syndrome" was not used until 1973,[1] concern about the adverse effects of heavy drinking during pregnancy dates back to classical Greek and Roman times. In England, medical awareness of the problem increased in 1720 when Parliament lifted regulation of the distillation of alcohol unleashing the "Gin Epidemic".[2] Six years later, the Royal College of Physicians and Surgeons petitioned Parliament to reinstitute controls because of an observed increase of "weak, feeble, and distempered infants".[3]

The problem was investigated throughout the eighteenth, nineteenth, and first decades of the twentieth century. In 1899, William Sullivan, a physician at a Liverpool prison, observed that the rate of stillbirth and neonatal mortality among 600 offspring born to 120 alcoholic women, was twice as great as that of offspring born to the women's nondrinking relatives.[4] He also observed that several alcoholic women who had given birth to children with severe complications, subsequently bore healthy children when they were forced to abstain during pregnancy because of imprisonment. There also was a considerable amount of laboratory experimental research employing animal models, studying the adverse effects of alcohol on offspring. Unfortunately, many of these ideas were taken up by the temperance movement and used to illustrate the biblical admonition that sins of the parents are cast onto their children for seven generations. Between 1920 and 1930, there was a marked decrease in research activity in this area. The loss of interest probably was due to effects of prohibition and its subsequent repeal, which was accompanied by a discrediting of the temperance movement.

In 1968, Lemoine et al. described 127 offspring from 69 French families in which there was chronic alcoholism.[5] They observed retarded growth and delayed psychomotor and language development as well as a characteristic facial appearance, including a sunken nasal bridge, short upturned nose, retracted upper lip, and the like. In 1970, Ulleland et al., at the University of Washington in Seattle, observed six infants who were small for gestational age and failed to thrive.[6] Their performance was retarded on developmental tests. All of their mothers were chronic alcoholics. Subsequently, in 1973, the dysmorphologists Jones and Smith recognized a characteristic facial pattern among these infants and developed the term fetal alcohol syndrome (FAS).[1] A study group of the Research Society on Alcoholism has suggested that the diagnosis of fetal alcohol syndrome should be restricted to offspring demonstrating signs of central nervous system (CNS) dysfunction and prenatal or postnatal growth deficiency, together with the characteristic facial pattern. The central nervous system dysfunction may include mild to moderate mental retardation, poor coordination, hypotonia, irritability in infancy, and hyperactivity in childhood. Growth deficiencies include length, weight, and head circumference more than two standard deviations below the norms for the gestational age. Facial characteristics include short palpebral fissures, midfacial hypoplasia manifested by a short upturned nose, a hypoplastic philtrum, and a thin, smooth upper lip.

Clarren and Smith in 1978 reported that the Seattle group has observed 65 children demonstrating FAS.[7] Over 180 other FAS cases, including infants of most racial groups, have been reported from medical centers in different nations. Some offspring of alcoholic mothers show several characteristics of the FAS without demonstrating the complete pattern. It has been suggested that the term "possible fetal alcohol effects" (FAE) should be used for these patients.

Retrospective clinical observations were essential for description of the FAS. Prospective studies are needed in order to determine the incidence of the FAS and FAE in the population as a whole—particularly among the offspring of alcoholic women—the amount of alcohol needed to affect the fetus, and the effects of different patterns of drinking. The interaction between alcohol and the other known risk factors of pregnancy could only be investigated prospectively.

BOSTON CITY HOSPITAL STUDY

Methods

In May 1974, a prospective study was inaugurated at the Boston City Hospital (BCH) Prenatal Clinic.[8,9] Of the 1,500 women per year who deliver at BCH, 500 of them receive their prenatal care at the BCH Prenatal Clinic. At the time of registration for prenatal care, every patient was asked to volunteer for a health survey. Data was obtained on alcohol consumption as well as on cigarette smoking, drug use, nutrition, and demographic data. Since retrospective evidence suggested that heavy drinking had adverse effects on offspring, all moderate or heavy drinkers were told at the end of the interview that they had a better chance of having a healthier baby if they reduced their alcohol consumption. Heavy drinking women subsequently were seen in individual counseling scheduled to coincide with routine prenatal visits.

Heavy drinking was defined according to Cahalan's criteria for "high volume, high maximum".[10] A heavy drinker is one who reports consuming five or six drinks on some occasions and no less than 45 per month.* Rare drinkers abstained or drank less than once a month and never had five or more drinks at a time. All women who drank more than the rare drinkers but less than the heavy drinkers were classified as moderate drinkers. Among the first 962 women, approximately 10% were heavy drinkers, 40% moderate drinkers, and 50% rare drinkers.

Most mothers who receive prenatal care at Boston City Hospital are from a high-risk population. They are subjected to inner city stress, compounded by poverty and social disruption. There also is an association between heavy drinking and risk factors known to be associated with growth retardation, such as smoking, malnutrition, and the use of other drugs. Among our heavy drinking women only 17% were nonsmokers while 58% smoked a pack or more a day. Among the rare drinkers 65% were nonsmokers while only 12% smoked a pack or more a day.

Nutritional status was estimated from the patients' reply to the question,

---

* A drink is defined as the amount of beverage containing one half ounce of absolute alcohol, i.e., 12 ounces of 4% beer, 4 ounces of 12% wine, 1 ounce of 100-proof liquor, or their equivalents.

TABLE 1.–Relationship Between Infant's Clinical Status and Mother's Drinking Classification

Infant's Clinical Status	Drinking Classification at Prenatal Clinic Registration			Significant Differences of Heavy Drinkers vs. Rare and Moderate Drinkers Combined
	Rare N=152 (47%)	Moderate N=128 (40%)	Heavy N=42 (13%)	p values from chi= square test
Total number of subjects=322				
Normal	99 65%	82 64%	12 29%	<.001
*Congenital anomalies:				
major	5 3%	3 2%	5 12%	<.01
minor	8 5%	15 12%	7 17%	
*Growth abnormalities:				
†small for gestational age	14 9%	5 4%	10 24%	<.001
premature	7 5%	4 3%	7 17%	<.001
postmature	12 8%	12 9%	8 19%	NS
†head circumference below 10th percentile	11 7%	7 5%	9 21%	<.05
†weight below 10th percentile	17 11%	10 8%	11 26%	<.01
†length below 10th percentile	5 4%	4 3%	4 10%	<.01
Functional abnormalities:				
jittery	15 10%	14 11%	12 29%	<.01
hypotonic	19 13%	11 9%	7 17%	NS
poor suck	9 6%	3 2%	5 12%	NS

*Abnormalities not mutually exclusive; infants with abnormality were tested against sum of all other infants in respective drinking classification.

†Based on University of Colorado Medical Center Classification of Newborns.

"What did you have to eat yesterday?" The nutritional values of that diet were compared with the minimum daily requirements recommended by the National Research Council.[11] Among all the women registering for prenatal care at Boston City Hospital, less than 10% met minimum daily requirements for all nine categories. Most of the group was deficient in terms of the intake of vitamins, iron, and calcium. The only nutritional category on which the majority met mimimum standards was protein. This applied to the entire population. When the nutritional status of the heavy drinking women was compared with that of the moderate and rare drinkers, no significant difference was found. It should be noted, however, that this only evaluates food intake. Alcohol may also interfere with the absorption of food from the intestine, metabolism in the liver, and for some nutrients utilization at the cellular level.

While the heavy drinking women had significantly more experience with psychotropic drugs prior to pregnancy, most of them avoided opiates, psychedelic agents, amphetamines, and sedatives during pregnancy. Many had been made aware through the media that drug use during pregnancy placed their child at risk and had tried to avoid this hazard. Pregnant women on methadone maintenance were seen in a special prenatal clinic and were not included in our series.

When infants were born to mothers in our survey group, Dr. Eileen Ouellette was notified. She examined these children in the newborn nursery. At the time of the examination, she had no knowledge about the maternal history of alcohol use or other facts about the pregnancy or delivery. Since this was a pilot study, we did not know which abnormalities might be associated with heavy drinking. All minor and major anomalies were quoted. Growth abnormalities were defined as head circumference, and weight or length below the tenth percentile. Jitteriness was observed as part of a complete pediatric neurologic examination.

Results

Data on the 322 infants examined by Dr. Ouellette is shown in Table 1.[9] Among the infants born to rare and moderate drinkers, 35% of both groups had at least one abnormality. In this population the offspring of the moderate drinkers were at no greater risk than the offspring of the rare drinkers. Among the 42 infants born to heavy drinking women, however, the incidence of abnormalities was two to three times as great compared with the infants in the other two groups. Within this group of 42 heavy drinking women, there were 15 who moderated alcohol use or abstained during the third trimester. The incidence of abnormalities in their infants

TABLE 2.–Relationship Between Clinical Status of Offspring of Heavy Drinking Women and Change in Alcohol consumption Before Third Trimester

Evaluation of Newborn Total N=42	Abstinent or Reduced Drinking N=15		Continued Heavy Drinking N=27	
Normal	10	67%	2	7%
*Congenital anomalies:				
major	1	7%	4	15%
minor	0		7	26%
*Growth abnormalities:				
†small for gestational age	0		10	37%
premature	0		7	26%
postmature	4	27%	3	11%
†head circumference below 10th percentile	0		9	33%
†weight below 10th percentile	0		11	41%
†length below 10th percentile	0		4	15%
*Functional abnormalities:				
jittery	2	13%	11	41%
hypotonic	0		6	22%
poor suck	0		5	18%

*Abnormalities not mutually exclusive; infants with abnormality were tested against sum of all other infants in respective drinking classification.
†Based on University of Colorado Medical Center Classification of Newborns.

was significantly lower than among the 27 born to women who continued heavy drinking throughout pregnancy. The frequencies appear in Table 2.

We now have data on 69 newborns born to heavy drinking women. These include the 42 examined by Dr. Ouellette and an additional 27 who were born after she left Boston City Hospital, but before our current prospective study was begun. Among these 69 mothers, 25 reduced drinking or abstained during the third trimester, while 44 continued heavy drinking. The incidence of abnormalities was much greater among the offspring of women who continued heavy drinking. We are aware of the fact that there are multiple differences between those mothers who moderate their drinking during pregnancy when told it will improve their chance of having a healthy child, and those mothers who continue heavy drinking. Women who moderate are much more likely to follow other health advice and keep prenatal clinic appointments. Among the group who continued to drink heavily were eight mothers who received no prenatal care. The incidence of neonatal problems was equally frequent when women continued to drink heavily whether or not they received prenatal care.

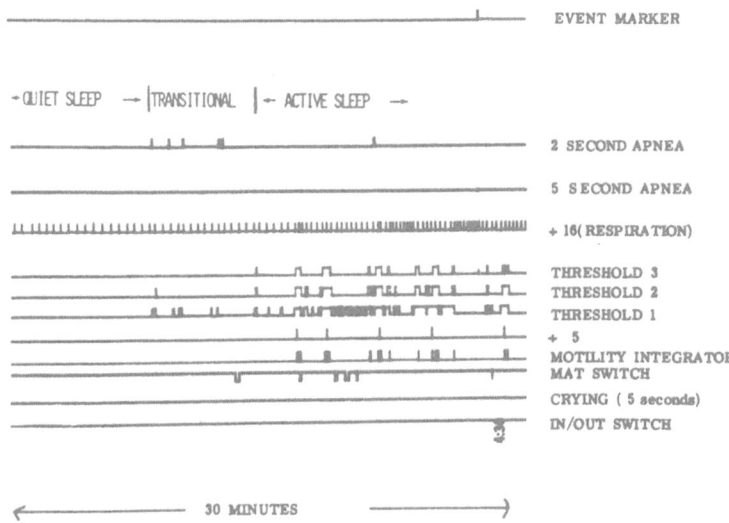

Figure 1.   Digital output of bassinet monitor labeling the 12 channels and indicating typical patterns for active, transitional and quiet substages of sleep over a 30-min. span.

We also studied effects of alcohol during pregnancy on neuro-physiologic function in terms of 24-hour sleep-awake state distribution. Dr. Louis Sander, a psychiatrist and psychoanalyst interested in the earliest days of life, has developed a bassinet monitor for this purpose.[12] During intervals between feedings, the baby rests in the monitor which looks very much like the other nursery bassinets. However, instead of the standard mattress, this one is equipped with an air mattress with multiple pressure sensors. The output from these pressure sensors is processed, digitalized, and recorded on a continuous event recorder. A standard polygraph enabled us to compare simultaneous recordings of 24-hour state regulation, with the records obtained by sleep polygraphy for shorter intervals.

Figure 1 shows a 30-minute sample of the record.[13] On the right, we have a period of active sleep, marked by irregular respirations and body movements. On the left, we can see a period of quiet sleep, during which respiration is regular and there is no body movement. There are standard criteria to define the limits of active and quiet sleep as well as the transitional phase. Other data have demonstrated a very high correlation between active sleep and quiet sleep as measured by the bassinet monitor, and quiet sleep and slow wave sleep as defined by standard polygraphy.

Figure 2 illustrates a 24-hour sleep pattern from a child born to a nondrinking mother. There are alternations between periods of active

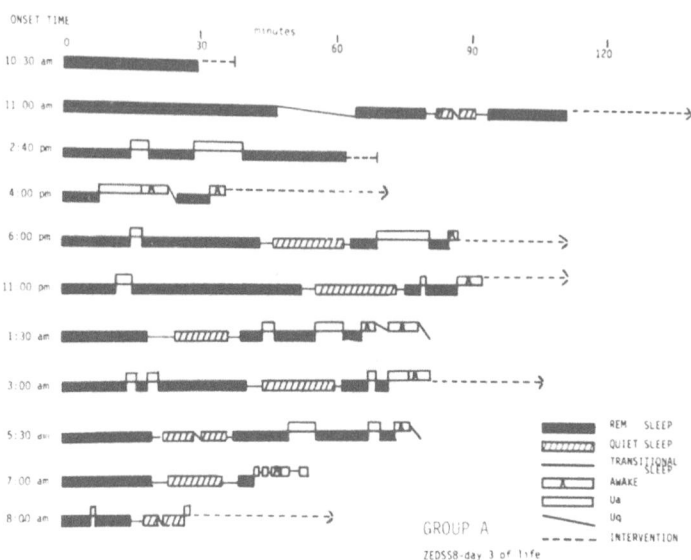

Figure 2.   The pattern of naps and distribution of sleep-awake variables in a neonate on day three of life who was exposed to heavy alcohol intake of mother during fetal life. The hour of onset of each nap is indicated vertically, and its duration in minutes horizontally. The sequence of active, quiet, and transitional, unclassified sleep states is indicated, plus awake states and interventions (time out of bassinet).

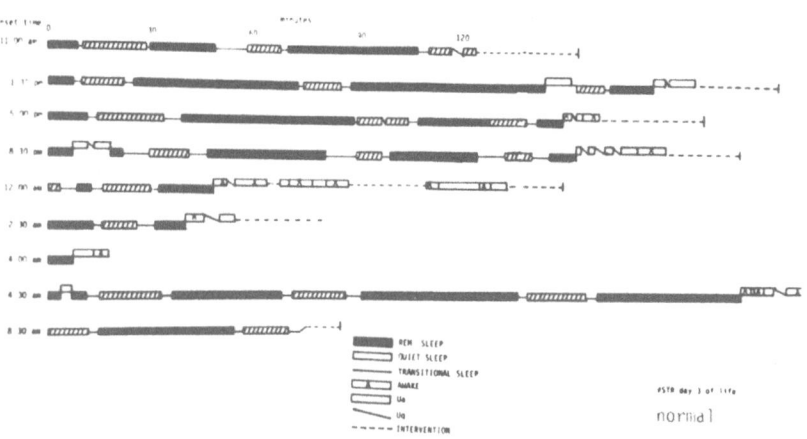

Figure 3.   The pattern of naps in a normal female infant on day three of life.

sleep and quiet, slow-wave sleep. On the third day of life, there also is the beginning of a circadian rhythm, a period during the day when the child sleeps more and another period when the child is more alert. Hopefully for the new mother, the infant will adapt to her rhythm and sleep more at night and be more alert during the day.

Figure 3 presents data from a child born to a heavy drinking mother. There is little cycling between quiet and active sleep and most quiet sleep periods are interrupted by awakening. The 24-hour pattern is irregular with no circadian rhythm. This baby would be difficult for the best mother to care for. If the mother is alcoholic and also has her own sleep problems and poor frustration tolerance, a disturbance which may begin on a neurophysiologic basis subsequently may be transformed into a disruption in mother-infant bonding and have long term behavioral consequences.[14,15]

Discussion and Conclusions

The conceptual model of the mechanism for the effects of alcohol on offspring is important in developing strategies for prevention of the fetal alcohol syndrome.[16] One model is time-specific. Alcohol is thought of as having a specific teratogenic effect at a critical vulnerable time during pregnancy analogous to the experience with thalidamide. If a time-specific effect has occurred during the first trimester, the only strategy for prevention of an abnormal child would be interruption of the pregnancy.

A second model considers the multiple effects of alcohol on biochemistry and physiology, as well as the implications for the mother-fetus system of the entire spectrum of pathophysiology of alcoholism. Alcohol can be expected to have multiple effects, depending on the variability of the blood alcohol concentration during different stages of pregnancy, as well as changes in the biological susceptibility of the mother-fetus system. During the first trimester, the effects of alcohol on the cell membrane and cell migration may affect the embryonic organization of tissue. During the second trimester, alterations in the metabolism of carbohydrates, lipids, and proteins probably affect cell growth and division. The organ systems with the most rapid growth may be most susceptible; at critical stages, this may be the central nervous system, the cardiovascular system, the urogenital system, or the musculoskeletal system. During the third trimester, rapid brain growth continues; in addition, neurophysiologic functioning begins in preparation for regulation of the infant following birth. It has been postulated that one of the functions of rapid eye movement (REM) sleep in utero is to functionally organize the central nervous system. The effects of alcohol on disruption of REM sleep in utero may be similar to the disruption of REM sleep seen in chronic alcoholic adults. Further investigation is needed to determine how long these early abnormalities in the newborn persist, and their long-term consequences.

While the initial observations of the FAS were consistent with a time-specific model, recent evidence from epidemiologic studies and animal experiments seem to be best understood in terms of the multiple effects of alcohol throughout pregnancy. In developing strategies for prevention, recognition of the multiple effects of alcohol suggests that education about the hazards of heavy drinking during pregnancy should be aimed at women who expect to become pregnant, as well as women receiving prenatal care. All professionals should be educated to obtain an adequate drinking history from all women of child-bearing age. We would recommend a separate inquiry on the use of beer, wine, and liquor. Women who report heavy drinking should be counseled and supported in their attempts to reduce alcohol use. Those who do not respond to counseling within a few weeks should be referred to more comprehensive therapeutic programs. While much remains to be learned about the specific biochemical and physiologic effects of alcohol during pregnancy, the practicing physician must make recommendations based on the best available knowledge. We believe that advising women that reduction of alcohol consumption will improve their chances of having a healthy baby is supported by a vast amount of clinical and experimental data. This should be communicated by each physician and health professional who has contact with women of child-bearing age. The interest and concern of those to whom the pregnant woman has turned for health care are powerful forces for reducing her alcohol consumption and protecting her fetus.

ACKNOWLEDGMENTS

This review is based on an earlier paper prepared under contract NIA 76-25 (P). Initial research was supported by ADAMHA Career Teacher Awards #T01DA00031 (NIDA) and PHSAA07008 (NIAAA). Further research was supported in part by NIAAA grant AA02446-01, the National Council on Alcoholism, the Massachusetts Developmental Disabilities Council, the United States Brewers Association, Inc., and both University Hospital and Boston City Hospital General Research Support Awards. We thank all our colleagues in the Maternal Health and Child Development Program and in the Boston City Hospital Department of Obstetrics and Gynecology for continued support and sharing of ideas.

REFERENCES

1. Jones, K.L., Smith, D.W., Ulleland, C.N., and Streissguth, A.P. Pattern of malformation in offspring of chronic alcoholic mothers, *Lancet* 1:1267-1271, 1973.
2. Warner, R.H., and Rosett, H.L. The effects of drinking on offspring; an historical survey of the American and British literature. *J. Stud. Alcohol.* 36:1395-1420, 1975.
3. Rosett, H.L. Effects of maternal drinking on child development: an introductory review. *Ann. N.Y. Acad. Sci.* 273:115-117, 1976.
4. Sullivan, W.C. A note on the influence of maternal inebriety on the offspring. *J. Ment. Sci.* 45:489-503, 1899.
5. Lemoine, P., Haronsseau, H., Borteyru J-P, et al. Les enfants des parents alcooliques: anomalies observées à propos de 127 cas. *Quest. Med.* 25:476-482, 1968.
6. Ulleland, C.N., Wennberg, R.P., Igo, R.P., and Smith, N.J. The offspring of alcoholic mothers. *Pediat. Res.* 4:474, 1970.
7. Clarren, S.K., and Smith, D.W. The fetal alcohol syndrome. *N. Eng. J. Med.* 298:1063-1067, 1978.
8. Ouellette, E.M., Rosett, H.L., Rosman, N.P., and Weiner, L. Adverse effects on offspring of maternal alcohol abuse during pregnancy. *N. Eng. J. Med.* 297:528-530, 1977.
9. Rosett, H.L., Ouellette, E.M., Weiner, L., and Owens, E. Therapy of heavy drinking during pregnancy. *Ob. Gyn.* 51:41-46, 1978.
10. Cahalan, D., Cisin, I.H., and Crossley, H.M. *American Drinking Practices, A National Study of Drinking Behavior and Attitudes.* New Brunswick, N.J.: Rutgers Center of Alcohol Studies, 1969.
11. *Recommended Dietary Allowances,* (8th ed.), Washington, D.C.: National Academy of Science, National Research Council, 1974.
12. Sander, L.W., Gould, J.B., Snyder, P., and Teager, H. Continuous non-intrusive bassinet monitoring of neonatal states on the sleep-awake continuum in Chase, M.H., Mitler, M.M., and Walter, P.L. (eds.), *Sleep Research,* Vol. 5. Los Angeles: Brain Information Service, University of California, 1976.
13. Sander, L.W., Snyder, P.A., Rosett, H.L., Lee, A., Gould, J.B., and Ouellette, E.M. Effects of alcohol intake during pregnancy on newborn state regulation: a progress report. *Alcoholism Clin. Exp. Res.* 1:233-241, 1977.
14. Rosett, H.L., Snyder, P., Sander, L.W., Lee, A., Cook, P., Weiner, L., and Gould, J.B. Effects of maternal drinking on neonate state regulation. *Develop Med and Child Neurol* 21(4): 464-473, 1979.
15. Rosett, H.L., and Sander, L.W. Effects of maternal drinking on neonatal morphology and state regulation, in Osofsky, J.D. (ed.), *The Handbook of Infant Development.* New York: Wiley, 1979, pp. 809-836.
16. Rosett, H.L. The effects of alcohol on the fetus and offspring, in Kalant, O.J. (ed.), *Research Advances in Alcoholism and Drug Abuse,* Vol. 5. New York: Plenum Press (In press).

CHAPTER 11

Self-Enhancing Functions of Alcohol Abuse Among Male Adolescents

HOWARD B. KAPLAN

While investigators of alcohol abuse perhaps have tended to emphasize the maleficent social and personal effects of alcohol abuse, still other observers have noted more positive functions of alcohol abuse patterns contingent upon any of a number of factors. For example, it has been concluded that "there is now available evidence for the inference that drinking behavior may function, at least in part, as an alternative mode of striving for goals otherwise unlikely to be attained or as a mode of coping with the lack of their attainment."[1] Data have been offered suggesting that alcoholism was related to a *broad* range of personal meanings and motives depending upon the sex and personality type of the subject.[2] Thus intoxication might be sought in order "to facilitate fantasy fulfillment, to enhance arbitrary interpretations of reality and to eliminate sober realizations."[3] Self-enhancing functions of alcohol abuse are suggested by the occasional reports[4] of favorable influences of experimentally induced intoxication upon the self-concepts of alcoholics and by observations of an inverse relationship between interval of sobriety and favorability of self-concept among alcoholics.[5,6] Alcohol use, depending upon the amount consumed, the setting, and personal characteristics, has been said to increase thoughts of social power (of having an impact on others for their own good) or thoughts of personalized power, that is, of winning personal victories over threatening adversaries.[7] Others have argued that intoxication permits the prealcoholic boy to satisfy his need to be dependent and at the same time to maintain his image of independence and self-reliance,[8] and Tahka[9] has concluded,

> "The effects of alcohol seem to be able to restore an emotional state comparable to that of a newly fed infant. These effects seem to be capable of giving the predisposed persons a strong and significant experience of passive gratification, characterized by pleasurable sensations of being filled with something that makes them warm, comfortable, secure and accepted."

With regard to tension-reducing functions, Williams[10] reported that alcohol does relieve tension with moderate but not severe intoxication; Stein and Bowman[11] reported that scores on an Escape-Drinking Scale (drinking to relax, to forget, to cheer up when tense and nervous) were significantly and positively correlated with amount of alcohol consumed and significantly and inversely correlated with a Behavior Rating Scale measuring social functioning among men with a primary diagnosis of alcoholism; Kalin and associates[12] observed that fear-anxiety (as assessed by TAT stimuli) was reduced by alcohol, although only in the party setting and after comparatively heavy drinking; and Pearlin and Radabaugh[13] concluded that "Intense anxiety is especially likely to result in the use of alcohol as a tranquilizer if a sense of personal efficacy is lacking and self-esteem is low."

The findings described above in general suggest that under certain (methodological and otherwise) conditions, self-enhancement will be a consequence of alcohol abuse. Although it is frequently difficult to specify such conditions (nor are they specified with any regularity by the researchers) it is often possible to hypothesize the conditions under which self-enhancing consequences will be associated with alcohol abuse. For example, that the self-enhancing/devaluing consequences of alcohol are conditional upon the contingency of evoking adverse self-devaluing responses from relevant others is suggested by several sets of findings. Nocks and Bradley[14] reported that among alcoholic patients, those who denied having a drinking problem received significantly higher scores on a measure of self-esteem than the other patients. Such denial is interpretable as reflecting continuity of relatively intact defenses that shield the subject from adverse responses by relevant others. Mindlin[15] reported that alcoholics who had reported previous therapy for alcoholism or experience with Alcoholics Anonymous (AA), relative to those who had not, manifested lowest self-esteem. Although other explanations could account for this, it is congruent with the observation that therapeutic experience might disrupt protective devices employed by the alcoholic to forestall adverse reactions to his or her alcohol abuse pattern. Such adverse reactions then might counterbalance the otherwise self-enhancing functions of alcohol treatment. That the alcoholic status of the subject might influence the beneficent/maleficent consequences of alcohol abuse is suggested by Freed's[16] conclusion, based on a review of post-1968 research on alcohol and mood. Although a good deal of variability was noted in each category, in general nonalcoholics tended to anticipate and attain elevated moods and relaxation as a consequence of drinking, while alcoholics tended to show increasing anxiety and depression with increased alcohol consumption although they expected the reverse. He further observed that "There appears to be a social factor which plays a role in determining the affective consequences of drinking."

The following report offers findings which further specify the conditions under which positive effects (particularly with regard to self-attitudes) are observed following alcohol abuse among non-institutionalized adolescent males, and, by implication, the mechanisms through which the effects are generated. The findings have the virtues of: (1) being derived within the context of a general theory of deviant behavior which permits the specification of the conditions under which effects should be observed, and (2) being generated in the course of a prospective longitudinal research design which permits the establishment of a temporal relationship between alcohol abuse patterns and subsequent changes in self-attitudes.

THEORETICAL BASIS

The theoretical basis of this study treats alcohol abuse as one among a number of deviant patterns that are more or less adaptive responses to the genesis of intrinsically distressful self-rejecting attitudes.[17,18] In brief, the theoretical model is based upon the postulate of the self-esteem motive whereby, universally and characteristically, a person is said to behave so as to maximize the experience of positive, and to minimize the experience of negative, self-attitudes. Self-attitudes refer to the person's (more or less intense) positive and negative emotional experiences upon perceiving and evaluating his own attributes and behavior.

Intense self-rejecting attitudes are said to be the end result of a history of membership group experiences in which the subject was unable to defend against, adapt to, or cope with circumstances having self-devaluing implications (that is, disvalued attributes and behaviors, and negative evaluations of the subject by valued others). By virtue of the (actual and subjective) association between past membership group experiences and the development of intensely distressful negative self-attitudes the person loses motivation to conform to, and becomes motivated to deviate from membership group patterns (those specifically associated with the genesis of negative self-attitudes and, by a process of generalization, other aspects of the membership groups' normative structures). Simultaneously, the unfulfilled self-esteem motive prompts the subject to seek alternative (that is, deviant) response patterns which offer hope of reducing the experience of negative (and increasing the experience of positive) self-attitudes. Thus, the person is motivated to seek and adopt deviant response patterns not only because of a loss of motivation to conform to the normative structure (which has an earlier association with the genesis of negative self-attitudes) but also because the deviant patterns represent the only motivationally acceptable alternatives that might effectively serve self-enhancing functions. Which of several deviant patterns is adopted, then, would be a function of the person's history of experiences influencing the visibility and subjective evaluation of the self-enhancing/self-devaluing potential of the pattern(s) in question.

Adoption of the deviant response has self-enhancing consequences if it facilitates intrapsychic or interpersonal avoidance of self-devaluing experiences associated with the predeviance membership group, serves to attack (symbolically or otherwise) the perceived basis of the person's self-rejecting attitudes (that is, representations of the normative group structure), and/or offers substitute patterns with self-enhancing potential for behavior patterns associated with the genesis of self-rejecting attitudes while permitting the person to defend against anticipated or unanticipated adverse consequences of the behavior. If self-devaluing consequences outweigh self-enhancing outcomes, the person is likely to experiment with alternative modes of deviance, since normative patterns would continue to be motivationally unacceptable.

EMPIRICAL BASIS

The data to be considered below were collected in the course of a longitudinal study of an adolescent population that was designed to test the series of hypotheses comprising the general theory of deviant behavior outlined above. Results of earlier analyses have appeared in a number of published reports.[19-29] In one of these reports[29] preliminary consideration was given to the conditions under which drinking behavior would have self-enhancing consequences. Most noteworthy among the findings was the observation that, considering only initially highly self-rejecting subjects, among males (but not among females) alcohol abuse was related to subsequent decreases in self-rejecting attitudes. This suggested that alcohol abuse in specified degrees may be a condition of conforming to a masculine role, and in more extreme degrees, may represent a deviant extrapolation from this role. Thus, alcohol used as a potentially self-enhancing deviant device by males may be more congruent with his normative roles than would be the case among females. Therefore, the male would be less likely to be the object of adverse (self-devaluing) reactions by virtue of his drinking behavior. Females, on the other hand, who adopted alcohol abuse as a self-enhancing device would be more likely to attract self-devaluing responses which would mitigate the otherwise self-enhancing consequences of the pattern. Indeed the male by displaying alcohol abuse responses (regardless of other self-enhancing consequences) might evoke approving responses from significant others, and self-approval, by virtue of conforming to culturally stereotyped masculine role expectations.

However, while alcohol abuse was observed to serve self-enhancing functions specifically among males, the data did not provide clues with regard to the mechanisms through which the self-enhancing functions were observed. Did alcohol abuse evoke punitive responses from membership groups which were the basis of the person's self-devaluation, thereby further attenuate the relationship between the subject and his membership groups and, in so doing, diminish the frequency with which the subject was exposed to self-devaluing membership group experiences? Did alcohol abuse function to increase the ability of the male subject to deny personal responsibility for self-devaluing circumstances and, thereby, diminish feelings of self-rejection? Did alcohol abuse function to reduce personal inhibitions, increase feelings of personal power, and, thereby enhance his masculine self-image and, concomitantly, his pervasive self-attitudes? It was to determine whether or not these and other processes were operative in the observed relationship between antecedent alcohol abuse and subsequent self-enhancement among adolescent males that the following analysis was undertaken. Indeed, the observation of this relationship was observed only under certain conditions. These conditional relationships suggested that the processes specified here were in fact variously operative depending upon the person's level of and change in self-rejection prior to the period of observed change in self-attitudes.

ANALYSIS

A self-administered questionnaire was presented to the seventh-grade students in half of the junior high schools in Houston Independent School District. The questionnaire was administered for the first time in the spring of 1971 and twice thereafter at annual intervals (T_1, T_2, T_3). Discussions of factors influencing sample attrition appear among the previously cited publications from this study. As noted above, only the male subjects were considered in the present analysis.

The relationships between antecedent alcohol abuse (between T_1 and T_2) and subsequent change in self-attitudes between T_2 and T_3 under specified conditions were observed separately for each of four groupings of male adolescents: (1) subjects who had relatively high levels of self-rejecting attitudes at T_1 and who maintained or increased their high levels of self-rejection between T_1 and T_2 (HH subjects); (2) subjects who had relatively high levels of self-rejection at T_1 but who decreased their levels of self-rejection between T_1 and T_2 (HL subjects); (3) subjects who had relatively low levels of self-rejection at T_1 but who increased in level of self-rejection between T_1 and T_2 (LH subjects); and, (4) subjects who were relatively low in self-rejection at T_1, and who decreased in level of self-rejection between T_1 and T_2 (LL subjects). From the theoretical perspective guiding this analysis, under specified conditions alcohol abuse was expected to have self-enhancing consequences only among the first three groups of subjects. In fact, as will be reported below, such conditional relationships were observed for these groups while for the fourth group, under several specified conditions, alcohol abuse was associated with subsequent increases in self-rejection.

Self-attitudes, conceptualized as the more or less positive (and more or less intense) affective responses to self-perceptions and self-evaluations of one's own traits and behaviors, were measured by scores on a scale composed of the following seven items. *Higher scores indicate increasing degrees of self-rejection* (parenthetical responses).

I wish I could have more respect for myself (true).
On the whole, I am satisfied with myself (false).
I feel I do not have much to be proud of (true).
I'm inclined to feel I'm a failure (true).
I take a positive attitude toward myself (false).
At times I think I'm no good at all (true).
I certainly feel useless at times (true).

The derivation of the scale, validity and reliability issues, and scoring procedures are variously discussed in the other reports from the more inclusive study. Initial *level* of self-rejection was determined by division of the distribution of the T_1 scores into two intervals: low and high. Level of *change in self-rejection* T_1–T_2 was categorized as "low" if there was an arithmetic decrease in self-rejection from T_1 to T_2. *Change in self-rejection* T_2-T_3 was measured by a residual gain score which removed "from the post-test score, and hence from the gain, the portion that could have been predicted linearly from the pretest status ... The residualized score is primarily a way of singling out individuals who changed more or less than expected."[30]

The decision to use a "base-free" measure of self-attitude change was necessary since the adoption of deviant response patterns is associated with or preceded by increases in self-rejection. Since the purpose of the analysis was to test the hypothesis that alcohol abuse has self-enhancing consequences, it was necessary to rule out alternative explanations that might result from the relatively higher self-derogation scores at T_2 among the alcohol-abuse subjects by using a "base-free" measure of change.

More negative residual gain scores indicate greater than expected decreases in self-derogation while more positive scores indicate greater than expected increases in self-rejection from T_2 to T_3.

Alcohol abuse subjects were defined as those who reported at the second test administration (T_2) that they used wine, beer, or liquor more than two times during the preceding week. Subjects who denied such use at T_2 were said to be "non-alcohol-abusers." The issues relating to the deviant nature of this behavior by the (then) eighth-grader is considered in an earlier publication.[29]

The theoretical conditions (reflected by scale responses at T_2) under which a relationship between alcohol abuse and subsequent decrease in self-rejection might be expected will be considered below in conjunction with the presentation of the results. The distribution of scores reflecting each of the conditional variables were divided into "high" and "low" categories thus permitting the following format for analysis of the data. For each of the four groupings of adolescent males delineated above, for the subjects variously manifesting high and low values on the conditional variables, alcohol-abusing subjects are compared with nonalcohol-abusing subjects with regard to mean residual gain scores between T_2 and T_3 on the measure of self-rejection. Significance of difference between means was determined by t-test (one-tailed) assuming unequal variances.[31]

RESULTS

In view of limitations of space only the statistically significant ($p < .05$) findings will be presented and textual rather than tabular presentation will be employed. The findings will be grouped according to categories of subjects formed by cross-tabulation of T_1 self-rejection categories and the T_1–T_2 raw change in self-rejection categories.

Among subjects who were high in self-rejection at T_1 and who either maintained or increased that high level of self-rejection between T_1 and T_2, the self-enhancing consequences of alcohol abuse were contingent upon one particular variable—perceived self-enhancing potential of the normative environment. This four-item scale (By the time I am 25 I will probably be married; I like our society pretty much the way it is; By the time I am 30 I will probably have a good job and a good future ahead of me; My parents always expected a lot of me) reflects the subject's identification of the normative environment with future personal gratification. Among subjects who scored high on this variable, alcohol abuse patterns were significantly associated with subsequent decreases in self-rejection. For the subjects scoring low on this measure no differences were observed between abusers and non-abusers with regard to subsequent decreases in self-rejecting attitudes. Nor were such differences observed for those in the high or low categories on this variable among subjects in the remaining three groupings (HL, LH, LL).

Among HH subjects, then, why should high scores on this variable have been a specific condition for self-enhancing consequences of alcohol abuse? Since subjects were high in self-rejection at T_1 and were unable to reduce their level of self-rejection at T_1–T_2 it must be assumed that the normative environment served as a continuing source of self-devaluing circumstances. Self-rejection could thus be reduced only by seeking alternative self-enhancing patterns which at the same time might diminish the significance of the normative environment as a basis for self-attitudes. For subjects who perceived their future gratification as tied to the normative environment and apparently did not perceive alternative routes to self-enhancement, however, such mechanisms were not available. For these subjects, if reduction in self-rejecting attitudes were to be achieved, it would be necessary to intervene in the process and attenuate the relationship between the person and his membership groups.

For these subjects alcohol abuse is interpreted as just such an intervening circumstance. Alcohol abuse and concomitant deviant patterns will evoke negative responses from others, reduce the expectation of future gratification from the normative environment, and intensify the subjective association between normative patterns and the genesis of self-rejecting attitudes. As a consequence the person will withdraw from the normative environment, question the worthiness of the normative structure, and search for alternative deviant routes to self-enhancement. In so doing he will reduce the experience of self-devaluing circumstances (in the past associated with the genesis of self-rejecting attitudes), reduce the affective significance of rejecting others in his membership groups, and in fact find alternative routes to self-enhancement.

Although these findings will not be described in detail here, it may be observed that the preceding interpretation is consistent with other findings observed in the present study, notably the association of alcohol abuse patterns on the one hand with subsequent increases in perception of rejection by family and school, contra-normative attitudes and identification with a deviant subculture on the other. Alcohol abuse was also associated with subsequent decreases in affective identification with the normative structure.

In short, among subjects experiencing continuing highly self-rejecting attitudes, those subjects who perceive their future gratifications as tied to the normative environment are likely to benefit with regard to subsequent reduction of self-rejecting attitudes from alcohol abuse patterns, presumably through the effects of these patterns on the attenuation of the relationship between the self-rejecting subject and the normative environment which was the basis of the subject's pervasive self-rejection.

Among *subjects who were high in self-rejection at* T_1 and who decreased in self-rejection between T_1 and T_2, the self-enhancing consequences of alcohol abuse were also contingent upon one particular variable. In this instance the variable was the need to avoid judgment of personal responsibility for self-devaluing circumstances. The subject's need in this regard was measured in terms of the number of affirmative responses to the following items:

Are most of your friends older than you?
Do you often lose track of what you were thinking?
Do you tell lies often?
Do you try to avoid situations in which you have to compete with others?
It's mostly luck if one succeeds or fails.
I would like to travel with a circus or carnival.
If someone insulted me I would probably avoid talking to him in the future.
When I do something wrong, it's almost like it's someone else who is doing it, not me.

Often I feel that I don't have enough control over the direction my life is taking.
I don't care much about other people's feelings.
People often talk about me behind my back.

The avoidance of self-judgments of personal responsibility for wrongdoing or failure might be accomplished through the disavowal of personal, as opposed to external, control over one's behavior and outcomes, emotional detachment that precludes the experience of self-blame, interpersonal avoidance of situations characterized by risks of self-devaluation, and/or denial of reality.

This measure appears to encompass the two patterns of protective attitudes identified by Washburn.[32] The "Self-Other Distortion" pattern was said to involve the defenses of projection, displacement of hostility, substitution, and conversion. The "Reality-Rejection" pattern included suppression, regression, withdrawal, and negativism. Washburn reported a correlation of $r=.28$ between measures of these two patterns for a grouping of 100 high school students, thus suggesting a common underlying factor (here interpreted as avoidance of judgments of personal responsibility).

Among subjects who scored *low* on this variable, alcohol abuse patterns were significantly associated with subsequent decreases in self-rejection. For the subjects scoring high on this measure no differences were observed between abusers and nonabusers with regard to subsequent decreases in self-rejecting attitudes. Nor were such differences observed for those in the high or low categories on this variable among subjects in the remaining three groupings (HH, LH, LL).

Among the HL subjects, then, why should low scores on this variable have been specific condition from self-enhancing consequences of alcohol abuse? In answer to this question, a number of issues must be considered. First, the diminution of self-rejection (T_1-T_2) among initially (T_1) self-rejecting subjects (the defining characteristics of this grouping of subjects) may indicate the effectiveness of adaptive patterns and/or the reduction of environmental stress. Insofar as these characteristics reflect (at least in part) the effectiveness of adaptive patterns, then the interaction between characteristic adaptive behavior and alcohol abuse becomes a critical consideration in the interpretation of the conditional relationship under consideration. High levels on this variable are interpretable as reflecting the use of intrinsically ineffective patterns and/or patterns that evoke negative responses that mitigate what would otherwise be effective responses to self-devaluation. In the present study (data to be reported elsewhere) it was observed that high scores on this measure were related to subsequent increases in self-rejection. Alcohol abuse might serve to exacerbate the use of these patterns. This conjecture is not unwarranted in view of the frequent observation among alcoholic populations between externality (reflected in a number of items on the measure under consideration) on the one hand and helplessness, depression, isolation, and general clinical pathology on the other hand.[33]

However, among subjects who are not characteristically high on this measure, the use of alcohol might permit episodic adoption of these self-other-distorting, reality-reflecting patterns in less pathological form (e.g., denial, intellectualization, repression), that is, toward the other end of the scale, in response to self-devaluing circumstances which would permit short-term avoidance of the self-devaluing implications of discrete events (by distorting and/or denying the reality that would be the basis of self-blame).

Among subjects who were low in *self-rejection at* T_1 but who increased in self-rejection between T_1 and T_2, the self-enhancing consequences of alcohol abuse were contingent upon three variables: subjective perception of being rejected by peers; aggressive responses to self-devaluing circumstances; and, perceived inconsistency of parental rules. Perceived peer rejection was indicated by affirmative responses to the following four items:

More often than not I feel put down by the kids at school.
I am not very good at the kinds of things the kids at school think are important.
The kids at school are usually not very interested in what I say or do.
Most of the kids at school do not like me very much.

A tendency toward aggressiveness was indicated by the parenthetical responses to the following items. The opposite responses (low scores) would indicate more passive/less aggressive responses.

If someone insulted me I would probably hit him (true).
If someone insulted me I would probably insult him back (true).
If someone insulted me I would probably try to understand why he did it (false).
If someone insulted me I would probably forgive him (false).
If someone insulted me I would probably think about ways I could get even (true).
If someone insulted me I would probably feel very angry but not do anything about it (false).

Inconsistency of parental rules was indicated by the parenthetical responses to the following items. A low score on the other hand would reflect the subjective perception of a firm and consistent parental code of behavior for the child.

My parents pretty much let me do what I want to do (true).
Sometimes my parents will punish me for doing something that at another time they didn't mind me doing (true).
Very often I do not know whether my parents would approve of what I am doing (true).
My parents pretty much agree about how I should be raised (false).
My experiences outside my home make me wonder whether my parents' ideas are right or not (true).
I was often punished unfairly as a child (true).
My parents believe that children should be raised according to firm rules (false).
My parents love me less when I am bad than when I am good (false).

Among the male adolescent subjects who scored low on each of these variables, alcohol abuse patterns were significantly associated with subsequent decreases in self-rejection. For the subjects scoring high on these measures no differences were observed between alcohol abusers and nonabusers with regard to subsequent decreases in self-rejecting attitudes. Nor were such differences observed for those in high or low categories on these variables among subjects in the remaining three groupings (HH, HL, LL).

The fact that the self-enhancing consequences of alcohol abuse were observed where the subject was not characteristically aggressive in response to self-devaluing circumstances, where the adolescent male perceived a firm and consistent parental code of conduct, and where the boy was not alienated from his peer group suggests that the self-enhancing consequences of alcohol abuse were effected through the interrelated mechanisms of release of inhibitions, increased sense of power, and demonstration of perceived masculine virtues in a peer context. The first mechanism is consistent with Tahka's[9] report that among the premorbid personality characteristics of alcoholics were inhibitions of aggressive and sexual impulses. The second mechanism is consistent with McClelland's[7] argument that the effect of alcohol is to increase power fantasies, perhaps through physiological mechanisms by providing a quick source of energy and by stimulation of adrenalin secretion with its mobilizing effects. He further notes that in *supportive* settings (the peer group would certainly be perceived as such) larger amounts of alcohol often lead to an increase in thoughts of personal power which, in younger men and appropriate settings, are frequently expressed in terms of sexual and aggressive conquests. The third mechanism is consistent with the observation of McCord and McCord[8] who considered the relationship between alcohol use to the attempt to suppress intensified dependency needs among prealcoholic boys. They noted that insofar as the intoxicated state was correlated with feelings of warmth, comfort, and omnipotence, the boy could simultaneously satisfy his strong need to be dependent and maintain his image of independence and self-reliance. In this last connection they observed that "The hard drinker in American society is pictured as tough, extroverted and manly—exactly the masculine virtues the alcoholic strives to incorporate into his own self-image."

The fact that these conditional relationships were observed only for the subjects who were relatively low on self-rejection at T_1 but increased their level of self-rejection between T_1 and T_2 further suggests that these mechanisms operate only where the threats to self-esteem are situational rather than characteristic and environmentally pervasive.

According to the present theory, alcohol abuse was said to be adopted in response to feelings of self-rejection and functioned more or less effectively under specifiable circumstances to reduce such feelings. Thus, it was not anticipated that among *adolescent males who were low on self-rejection at* T_1 and who decreased in self-rejection between T_1 and T_2 conditions would be noted whereby these subjects would manifest a decrease in self-rejection subsequent to the reports of alcohol abuse; and, therefore, it was not surprising when, in fact, no decreases in self-rejection were observed. On the contrary, a number of conditions were noted under which increases in self-rejection were observed. Since the focus of the present study is on the positive consequences of alcohol abuse the data specifying these conditional effects will not be described in detail. It may be noted, however, that where the adolescent male does not manifest problems with regard to self-rejection (that is, among LL boys), alcohol abuse is likely to result in an increase in self-rejection where its consequences are not compatible with the boy's normal modes of adapting to stress, where the behavior represents a contra-normative response, where the person is negatively sanctioned by the family, and where the person views his future gratifications as tied to the normative order. In this connection it may also be noted that among female subjects only LL female adolescents displayed reductions in self-rejection under some conditions following reports of alcohol abuse, and these conditions were those suggesting that alcohol "abuse" was an acceptable pattern and unlikely to be associated with self- or other-administered negative sanctions. These findings are consistent with the observation by Jessor and his associates[1] that males reported a greater intake of alcohol and more numerous drinking-related complications than female college students and with the report by Waller and Lorch[34] that men faced a greater number of social complications as a result of their alcohol abuse.

CONCLUSION

It is apparent then, whatever adverse consequences alcohol abuse may have for other subjects, among adolescent males characterized by pervasive and/or situationally induced ephemeral self-rejecting attitudes this pattern may have the subjectively desirable consequence of reducing self-rejecting attitudes. Depending upon whether the occasions for self-rejection are pervasive and related to a high level of self-rejection (HH), variably experienced against the background of a high level of self-rejection (HL), or variably experienced by relatively self-accepting subjects (LH), the self-enhancing consequences of alcohol abuse may be accomplished through alternative mechanisms. Analysis of the conditions under which self-enhancing consequences of alcohol abuse by adolescent males are observed suggested that such consequences may be effected variously by attenuation of the subject's affective relationship with the normative environment which served as the basis of his self-rejection, disinhibition of the expression of uncharacteristic self-other distorting/reality-rejecting self-protective patterns, and increased sense of power (in part gained from rule violation and in part, perhaps, from physiological sensations) accompanied by the gratifications received from being better able to approximate the idealized adolescent masculine role.

The findings reported above, whatever intrinsic value they may have, are perhaps more significant insofar as they suggest the need to continue investigation of the *positive* functions of alcohol abuse and the method by which this may be accomplished—through the specification of the conditions under which these subjective gratifications occur.

REFERENCES

1. Jessor, R., Carman, R.S., and Grossman, P.H. Expectations for need satisfaction and patterns of alcohol use in college, in Maddox, G. (ed.), *The Domesticated Drug: Drinking among Collegians.* New Haven, Conn.: College and University Press, 1970, pp. 321–342.
2. Mogar, R.E., Wilson, W.M., and Helm, S.T. Personality subtypes of male and female alcoholic patients. *Int. J. Addict.* 5:99–113, 1970.
3. McGuire, M.T., Stein, S. Mendelson, J.H. Comparative psychosocial studies of alcoholic and non-alcoholic subjects undergoing experimentally induced ethanol intoxication. *Psychosom. Med.* 28:13–26, 1966.

4. Berg, N.L. Effects of alcohol intoxication on self-concept: studies of alcoholics and controls in laboratory conditions. *Q. J. Stud. Alcohol.* 32:442–453, 1971.
5. White, W.F., and Gaier, E.L. Assessment of body image and self-concept among alcoholics with different intervals of sobriety. *J. Clin. Psychol.* 374–377, 1965.
6. White, W.F., and Porter, T.L. Self concept reports among hospitalized alcoholics during early periods of sobriety. *J. Coun. Psycho.* 13:352–355, 1966.
7. McClelland, D.C. Examining the research basis for alternative explanations of alcoholism, in *The Drinking Man.* McClelland, D.C., Davis, W.N., Kalin, R., and Wanner, E. (eds.) New York: The Free Press, 1972, pp. 276–315.
8. McCord, W., and McCord, J. *Origins of Alcoholism.* Stanford, Calif.: Stanford University Press, 1960.
9. Tahka, V. *The Alcoholic Personality.* Helsinki: Finnish Foundation for Alcohol Studies, 13, 1966.
10. Williams, A.F. Social drinking, anxiety, and depression. *J. Per. Soc. Psychol.* 3:689, 1966.
11. Stein, L.I., and Bowman, R.S. Reasons for drinking: relationship to social functioning and drinking behavior, in Seixas, F.A. (ed.), *Currents in Alcoholism,* vol. II. New York: Grune and Stratton, 1977, pp. 479–485.
12. Kalin, R., McClelland, D.C., and Kahn, M. The effects of male social drinking on fantasy. *J. Per. Soc. Psychol.* 1:441, 1965.
13. Pearlin, L.I., and Radabaugh, C.W. Economic strains and the coping functions of alcohol. *Am. J. Sociol.* 82:652–663, 1976.
14. Nocks, J.J., and Bradley, D. Self-esteem in an alcoholic population. *Dis. Nerv. Syst.* 30:611–617, 1969.
15. Mindlin, D.F. Attitudes toward alcoholism and toward self: differences between three alcoholic groups. *Q. J. Stud. Alcohol.* 25:136–141, 1964.
16. Freed, E.X. Alcohol and mood: an updated review. *Int. J. Addict.* 13:173–200, 1978.
17. Kaplan, H.B. *Self-Attitudes and Deviant Behavior.* Pacific Palisades, Calif.: Goodyear, 1975.
18. Kaplan, H.B. Toward a general theory of psychosocial deviance: the case of aggressive behavior. *Soc. Sci. Med.* 6:593–617, 1972.
19. Kaplan, H.B. Increase in self-rejection as an antecedent of deviant responses. *J. Youth. Adol.* 4:281–292, 1975.
20. Kaplan, H.B. Sequelae of self-derogation: predicting from a general theory of deviant behavior. *Youth Soc.* 7:171–197, 1975.
21. Kaplan, H.B. The self-esteem motive and change in self-attitudes. *J. Nerv. Ment. Dis.* 161:265–275, 1975.
22. Kaplan, H.B. Antecedents of negative self-attitudes: membership group devaluation and defenselessness. *Soc. Psychiat.* 11:15–25, 1976.
23. Kaplan, H.B. Self-attitudes and deviant response. *Soc. Forces* 54:788–801, 1976.
24. Kaplan, H.B. Self-attitude change and deviant behavior. *Soc. Psychiat.* 11:59–67, 1976.
25. Kaplan, H.B. Antecedents of deviant responses: predicting from a general theory of deviant behavior. *J. Youth. Adol.* 6:89–101, 1977.
26. Kaplan, H.B. Increase in self-rejection and continuing/discontinued deviant response. *J. Youth Adol.* 6:77–87, 1977.
27. Kaplan, H.B. Social class, self-derogation and deviant response. *Soc. Psychiat.* 13:19–28, 1978.
28. Kaplan, H.B. Deviant behavior and self-enhancement in adolescence. *J. Youth Adol.* 7:253–277, 1978.
29. Kaplan, H.B., and Pokorny, A.D. Alcohol use and self-enhancement among adolescents: a conditional relationship, in Seixas, F. (ed.), *Currents in Alcoholism,* vol. IV. New York: Grune and Stratton, 1978, pp. 51–75.

30. Cronbach, L.J., and Furby, L. (1970). How should we measure "change"— Or should we? *Psychol. Bull.* 74:68–80.
31. Welch, B.L. The generalization of "student's" problems when several different population variances are involved. *Biometrika* 34:28–35, 1947.
32. Washburn, W.C. Patterns of protective attitudes in relation to differences in self-evaluation and anxiety level among high school students. *Calif. J. Educ. Res.* 13:84–94, 1962.
33. Rohsenow, D.J. and O'Leary, M.R. Locus of control research on alcoholic populations: a review, II. relationship to other measures. *Int. J. Addict.* 13:213–226, 1978.
34. Waller, S., and Lorch, B.D. Social and psychological characteristics of alcoholics: a male-female comparison. *Int. J. Addict.* 13:201–212, 1978.

CHAPTER 12

Phenomenology and Treatment of Alcoholism in the Elderly

MARC A. SCHUCKIT

INTRODUCTION

My goal is to help physicians better identify the older alcoholic, understand their probable clinical course and offer the most efficient therapeutic interventions. The literature on this topic is sparse, perhaps reflecting the diminished level of social and police problems experienced by older alcoholics coupled with the fact that the rate of alcoholism in the elderly is not any higher than in the general population. Thus, much of the information offered here is a common sense application of knowledge of problems of the elderly to knowledge of alcoholism to arrive at the best estimate of the problems of the older alcoholic. I present relevant references where appropriate and encourage the reader to go back to the original material to form his own conclusions.

In the course of this paper I will introduce some basic background information on problems of the elderly in our society, note why alcoholism is of major importance in this group, and discuss some alcohol related problems as they affect some alcoholic older individuals. The remainder of the paper will center on alcoholism itself, offering the definition, giving the epidemiology of this problem in the elderly, relating the usual clinical course, and discussing treatment. My primary focus is on clinical problems with the hopes that you will be able to apply many of the lessons here to your daily practice.

THE ELDERLY: A VULNERABLE POPULATION

Becoming elderly is an individual process which depends not only on chronological age but a variety of social factors. The arbitrary statistical cut off for the "geriatric" group is usually age 65, and it is important to know that this is no longer a small population in America. The number of elderly have increased 7 fold from the 3.1 million aged 65 and older in 1900, while the general population has only increased 2.5 fold.[1] Older persons now represent 10% of the population with the projection of an increase to at least 13% by the 1990s.[1] Noting the necessity of older people to seek medical care, these individuals now represent a significant proportion of daily clinical practice and the figures cited above indicate that they will become more and more prevalent.

There are many stresses involved in growing old in a youth oriented culture. Most of these can be summarized as feelings of loss of stability and of self-worth. The problems may be generated by the difficulty in obtaining employment and a subsequent decreased income, resulting in a lowered level of mobility and a lack of money for daily necessities and enjoyable activities, and a lowered level of responsibilities with the resultant feeling that the elderly person is no longer recognized or valued. While these stresses may have nothing to do with the development of alcoholism per se (a direct cause and effect relationship is difficult to prove as so many individuals with these factors do not develop serious alcohol misuse), they are important aspects of a patient's life to be considered when treating any disorder.[23]

A major stress, and one that affects drinking in nonalcoholics as well as alcoholics, is the lowering of physical reserve which occurs with advancing age.[2] All body systems tend to lose resiliency with the result that wounds and fractures take longer to heal the older one becomes and vital body organs are stressed to the limit with daily living alone. Thus, any type of stress including a change in environment, an infection, an electrolyte imbalance caused by vomiting, etc. can cause failure of these organs. This vulnerability to stresses and bodily insults extends to alcohol, which can cause temporary failure of the cardiovascular, hepatic, or central nervous systems in older people at levels easily tolerated in a 35 or 40 year old.

These difficulties are exacerbated by changes in metabolism of medications and toxins which occur with advancing age.[4] As the lean body mass decreases and adipose tissue increases there is a tendency toward greater distribution of all fat soluble substances with a resulting decreased rate of elimination. In addition, with increasing age there is probably a decreasing amount of liver tissue available and there is some evidence that mitochondria are less efficient in their metabolic role.[4] The result is that, at least theoretically, older individuals might be expected to attain a higher and/or more persistent blood alcohol level when given the same amount of alcohol per body weight as a younger person.

Another relevant organ system which probably changes with age is the central nervous system (CNS).[4] Older individuals demonstrate an increased reaction time and a tendency to show levels of confusion during stress, infection or other bodily insults, or when taking CNS depressing drugs. They might be expected to demonstrate lowered levels of cognition and perhaps a frank organic brain syndrome (OBS) (i.e. confusion and disorientation) with low doses of alcohol. A related phenomenon, important for those with decreased lung functioning (e.g. chronic obstructive lung disease), could be the effect of alcohol through its CNS depressing activities on the drive to breathe.

Alcohol also adversely affects the cardiovascular system.[1] An individual demonstrating decreased cardiac functioning for any reason will show a decreased cardiac output and an increased heart work load with levels of alcohol as low as one drink.[5] Those individuals complaining of angina will note that when they drink they can work harder before the cardiac pain begins, but the electrocardiogram demonstrates ischemic changes at lower work levels which are not being perceived by the patient.[6] In addition, alcohol adversely affects the cardiovascular system through increasing the blood pressure, increasing the free fatty acids, and as a direct cardiac muscle toxin.[6-9] The result is that older patients with heart disease should probably not drink, even if they are not alcoholic.

As one grows older, the number of prescribed and over-the-counter medications imbibed increases.[8] Alcohol interacts adversely with many of these drugs, a problem especially significant for other CNS depressants as their actions are likely to be potentiated by ethanol.[3,4] Through its effect on the liver, alcohol may also increase the rate of metabolism of *some* drugs but interfere with the degradation of others.

It is, thus, apparent that one cannot discuss alcohol problems in the elderly by limiting the notation to older alcoholics alone. Elderly individuals with a variety of medical problems including diabetes, heart disease, liver disease and CNS degeneration do not tolerate alcohol well. It is also wise to advise older individuals on medication to avoid drinking. While an adverse drug-alcohol interaction might be well tolerated in a 35-year-old, the decrease in reserves in vital organ systems can make such a stress potentially life threatening on the elderly person.

ALCOHOLISM IN THE ELDERLY

Some Definitions

No clinical diagnostic system is perfect. The reasons for applying a label vary and include attempts at describing an individual's condition at one point in time, a desire to indicate a probable cause of the problem and an attempt to establish the likely prognosis and response to treatment.[10,11] In clinical psychiatry and in alcoholism I prefer to use a diagnosis as a guide for my future plans for the individual.

The diagnosis of alcoholism has been approached from a variety of standpoints. If one wishes to use relatively objective criteria, however, the most useful label utilizes the history of serious alcohol problems.[1,12,13] Thus, an alcoholic is an individual who has demonstrated any one or more serious problems including a marital separation or divorce because of alcohol, been fired or laid off from a job because of drinking, experienced multiple arrests because of drinking, or has developed physical evidence that alcohol has harmed his/her health. Others who show persistent alcohol related problems, but not to the level described above, would be labeled as probable alcoholics, thus indicating that they would probably run the course of this disorder but also noting a level of uncertainty regarding prognosis.

This life problem definition of alcoholism outlines a group with a relatively homogeneous prognosis and response to treatment when applied to younger individuals. As of yet, there are no longitudinal studies of alcoholism in the elderly, but, remembering that the criteria for alcoholism might not have the same degree of relevancy when applied to older populations, this approach is the best clinical label available.

One further common sense step is required. After determining whether an individual fulfills a life problem definition of alcoholism, it is worthwhile to further evaluate whether the alcohol problems occurred independent of any major preexisting psychiatric disorder.[12,13] An individual who demonstrated alcohol-related difficulties but *only* in the midst of a severe depression would be labeled as having primary affective disorder and secondary alcoholism, while a second individual with serious alcohol problems who shows a basically normal mood state except while drinking would be labeled as having primary alcoholism with a secondary affective disorder. The primary affective disorder patient demonstrating secondary alcoholism tends to run the course of his primary illness, inferring (although not proving) that the major treatment mode might best be aimed to the affective disorder and not the alcoholism itself.

In summary, my bias is to use a diagnostic label to indicate prognosis and response to treatment. Within this context, the diagnostic criteria most clearly related to prognosis and treatment while being stated in the most objective terms center on the occurrence of any one of a number of serious life problems related to alcohol. Those persons who have alcohol related pathology but not to the point of fulfilling the research criteria for alcoholism would be labeled probable alcoholics. One further step required to adequately indicate prognosis is the division of alcoholics into those with a pre-existing psychiatric disorder, such as affective disorder, and those who have no such history and are primary alcoholics. Most of the material related below will deal with the primary alcoholic, probably making up 70% to 80% of groups of alcoholics in treatment.[12,13]

Epidemiology

There are no hard data on the rate of alcoholism in any age group.[14] All attempts at establishing such numbers have inherent biases with the result that studies done in public hospitals may have different results from those done in inpatient settings in the private sector and these in turn might differ from outpatient clinic data which would also be distinguished from surveys of alcoholism in the general population.[14] The best estimate would indicate that the lifetime risk for ever showing alcoholism (not the number of individuals alcoholic at any one point in time) is between 5% and 10% for men with figures for women probably resting between 3% and 5%. The greatest prevalence of more minor and transient alcohol related problems which are *not closely associated* with alcoholism[15] is probably in the 18- to 24-year-old range while the greatest prevalence of alcoholism itself is probably in the 35 to 55 age range.[14]

As difficult as it is to establish the rate of alcoholism in the general population, problems are even greater in the elderly. Older people are less likely to work and thus less likely to lose jobs related to alcohol, they are less likely to be apprehended and officially charged by the police, they are more likely to be widowed and thus not in danger of losing their marriage because of their drinking, and, perhaps related to the "shame" of having an alcoholic father or grandfather, they are less likely to be brought in for treatment.[2,16] Once entering a treatment sphere, because they do not fit the prototype of the alcoholic, the proper diagnosis is more likely to be missed, a problem exacerbated by the tendency of older people to receive treatment from a variety of programs without anyone coordinating the care.[17]

The overall rate of alcohol problems in populations of the elderly ranges from 2% to 10% with a number of subpopulations at elevated risk.[1]

As might be expected, higher rates of serious alcohol-related pathology are noted in widowers, those who are single, and individuals demonstrating difficulty with the police.[18] Because alcohol causes such serious pathology in most body systems, the rates of alcoholism in elderly individuals in nursing homes, psychiatric facilities and general medical or surgical wards are probably in excess of 20%,[19-22] figures in the same general range as those reported for younger populations.[23] It is probable that about 10% of alcoholics in treatment are age 60 or older.[17]

It is thus obvious that alcohol problems do occur in elderly individuals and greatly impact on the treatment offered by any practitioner in a clinical setting. When one considers the adverse effects alcohol has on existing medical pathology, the adverse drug interactions which can ensue when alcohol is added to any medication, and the high rate of alcoholism in elderly populations entering treatment in medical and psychiatric settings, it is in the best interest of the practitioner to query each patient about alcohol related life problems.

The Clinical Course of Alcoholism in the Elderly

The generalizations given in this section relate to primary alcoholics,— those who demonstrate no pre-existing major psychiatric disorders. When older alcoholics are compared to elderly nonalcoholics, the former relate higher rates of suicide attempts and are more likely to show signs of mental deterioration including an OBS.[19] Alcoholics, compared to other elderly individuals, are more likely to be living alone, less likely to be married, and less likely to be living at their present address for five or more years.[19] Most of the generalizations made for the older alcoholics appear to apply equally well for alcoholic men and women.[24]

When older alcoholics are compared with younger alcohol abusing patients, the former demonstrate more life stability, showing less difficulty with early school and job performance, lower rates of drug and alcohol related difficulties in early life and less interpersonal problems. It appears as if many of the older alcoholics have been more stable in early life and then, for unknown reasons, in later years develop alcohol problems.[1,19]

The psychiatric problems seen in older alcoholics are very similar to those demonstrated in younger alcoholic populations. Serious depression of proportions almost equal to that of primary affective disorder are often noted *during* active drinking bouts but tend to clear within 2 to 7 days on their own with proper detoxification and probably do not necessitate prescription of antidepressants or lithium.[13] Another common problem in older alcoholics, the development of confusion, might appear at low blood alcohol levels or after relatively short periods of heavy drinking, and tend to persist longer than would be seen in younger alcoholics. While there is little data available on this, an alcohol induced OBS in an elderly person might be more prone to run a chronic course. Similarly, problems of paranoia and hallucinosis, while seen in all alcoholics, might be at a higher rate in older individuals.[16] This information on psychopathology is a combination of some clinical experience, the literature as it relates to psychiatric manifestations in younger alcoholics, and some common sense applications of what such problems might mean in a geriatric sample. They do point out, however, how alcoholism must be considered as part of the differential diagnosis for almost any psychiatric syndrome in older individuals.

There are still clinically relevant subgroups within the primary alcoholic group. One relevant distinction is based on the age of first occurrence of alcohol related problems.[19]

The importance of the age of onset of alcoholism was addressed in a series of medical and surgical patients admitted to the San Diego Veterans Administration Medical Center.[19] A random sample of men admitted to selected nonpsychiatric wards were asked to participate by taking part in an interview, having their medical records reviewed, and giving permission for an interview with a spouse or additional resource person. Thus, it was possible to establish that 15% to 20% of these individuals had at some point in their life fulfilled the criteria for alcoholism with the group breaking down into equal subgroups of those who had their first alcohol problem prior to the age of 40 and those who did not demonstrate alcoholism until after that age. These two groups of individuals, the alcoholic demonstrating the more typical age of onset and the late onset alcoholic, were very different.

The "normal" onset alcoholic reported the same high rate of social (police and job) problems as would be expected in any group of alcoholics, experienced alcohol related serious life difficulties over a span of 10 to 15 years, and had been "dry" or "almost dry" for an average of about 10 years prior to interview—they were alcoholics who were no longer drinking at the time of entering the study. The remaining individuals, those with a later age of onset of alcohol related pathology, experienced much lower levels of social problems but elevated rates of medical disorders and marital disruptions related to their drinking. Almost all of these individuals were actively drinking at the time of interview.

Whether the person demonstrated a "normal" or late onset of alcoholism, if they were actively drinking, they showed a number of unique characteristics compared to the literature on the younger alcoholic. In most studies, the average practicing elderly alcoholic drinks between 5 and 7 days a week with an average intake of 4 drinks per day, a rate lower than might be expected for younger alcoholics. He or she also reports a mean of 2 or 3 alcohol-related life problems, also slightly lower than that seen for most younger populations. Drinking history is paralleled by smoking, as alcoholics appear to be less likely to abstain from smoking while actively drinking but seem to be better able to give up their tobacco when they become abstinent from ethanol.[1,19]

In summary, the clinical course of alcoholism in older individuals does not appear to differ greatly from that in younger people. About half of the older alcoholics began their alcohol abuse at a younger age and survived past age 65, usually by acquiring abstinence sometime in their late fifties or early sixties. The actively drinking older alcoholic tends to have a later age of onset for alcohol misuse and demonstrates a lowered level of social pathology but has increased medical disorders. Alcoholics can present a variety of psychopathological pictures ranging from obvious alcoholism, to depression, to psychosis and this problem must be considered as part of a differential diagnosis of any psychiatric picture in older populations. Once alcohol problems begin, the older alcoholic usually does not drink every day and consumes levels of alcohol which might not be considered pathological in younger populations. This last finding is not surprising in light of the differences in body composition, metabolism of drugs, and increased medical pathology seen with advancing age.

Treatment of Alcoholism in Older Populations

The actively drinking older alcoholic is likely to present a less obvious picture of social and interpersonal pathology than the younger alcoholic. The health care practitioner, reluctant to see a grandfatherly or grandmotherly figure as an alcoholic, may overlook the diagnosis, even when it is obvious.[1] The result can be a group of stop-gap measures aimed at treating individual symptoms without the treatment personnel understanding the total picture. As the patient's condition deteriorates, the practitioner is likely to add more levels of intervention, including medications which result in decreasing functioning.

There is little data indicating what the optimal treatment is for the older alcoholic. I know of no controlled studies which would demonstrate that one type of therapy is better than any other. However, there are some common sense modifications one might make in the usual alcohol treatment program until adequate data develops.[25,26] These can be developed for all stages of treatment ranging from detoxification, to rehabilitation, to outpatient follow-up.

Detoxification

Some alcoholics enter treatment solely because of medical or psychological problems caused by continued heavy drinking and do not desire rehabilitation, while others want help in stopping to drink but present an intoxicated state. In either instance the patient must be carefully withdrawn from their CNS depressant using the basic approach outlined by Sellers and Kalant with some proposed modifications for older individuals.[27]

First, the serious physical pathology associated with alcoholism and the decreased physical reserves of the elderly make an adequate medical evaluation of even greater importance in older individuals than in the usual alcoholic. A thorough physical examination including a good neurological evaluation and adequate blood screens are mandatory. Any abnormalities must be carefully followed up as they might potentially lead to great complications during treatment.

Once this is accomplished, the alcoholic must be offered rest, nutrition, and vitamin supplementation. While multiple vitamins will frequently suffice, the decrease in body reserves for thiamine and the role this important vitamin plays in adequate heart functioning (such as Beri-beri or heart disease) and neurologic functioning (for example Wernicke-Korsakoff's disease) make specific thiamine supplementation in the range of 100 mg IM for one to three days advisable.

If the individual is truly addicted to the CNS depressant, alcohol, the smoothest withdrawal with the least chance for the development of the serious sequela of an OBS, hallucinations, or convulsions rests with the careful administration of another CNS depressant to alleviate symptoms. This is based on the fact that abstinence symptoms develop because the addictive drug was stopped too quickly. I prefer to use the benzodiazepines such as chlordiazepoxide as they tend to decrease respirations and cardiac functioning less than most other CNS depressants.[28] Because older people tend to metabolize drugs more slowly and demonstrate more CNS sensitivity to depressant drugs with a possible resulting OBS, benzodiazepines must be administered very carefully to older individuals with careful monitoring of vital signs and the level of alertness before the final drug level is decided. Thus, while the average younger alcoholic going through withdrawal might require 150 mg of chlordiazepoxide on the first day (which is then decreased by 20% of the original day's dose each subsequent day), the older alcoholic might conceivably require only 25 or 50 mg the first day. While no convincing data can be given on this point, I would carefully monitor any doses of chlordiazepoxide, withholding the medication if the patient develops a major drop in blood pressure or a decreased level of alertness.

The Usual Rehabilitation Program

As has been discussed in detail elsewhere, rehabilitation of the alcoholic basically involves taking advantage of the patient's initial level of motivation and attempting to maximize the chances of achieving abstinence. This usually is carried out through a short inpatient stay (often two weeks or less) during which the patient receives education about alcohol, counseling regarding day to day life problems which is usually given by nondegreed paraprofessionals, supervision by a physician, an introduction to Alcoholics Anonymous, and, in some settings, various forms of aversive conditioning.[25,26,29]

There is no reason to believe that the elderly should receive any radical departure from this usual program, but common sense dictates the possible benefit of creating group discussions and Alcoholics Anonymous meetings for the older alcoholic to meet with other older alcoholics. This follows the assumption that the day-to-day life stresses and needs for counseling may be quite different in the seventh decade of life than for the 40-year-old individual.

In a similar light, in dealing with the older alcoholic one might have to recognize interactions with the children as much as with the spouse. It is also important to recognize that while vocational rehabilitation might have less relevance to older alcoholics, opening their eyes to various types of volunteer work and older age activities in their community might be important. Of course, the older alcoholic's tendency towards physical disorders would require adequate supervision by a physician who will hopefully attempt to coordinate all medical care for that individual. The older alcoholic also has greater potential need for social service help in guaranteeing an adequate income for his living situation and food.

The Older Alcoholic in a Nursing Home

Alcoholics evidencing either a severe physical disorder or a persistent organic brain syndrome are often placed in nursing homes. The staff of such facilities have limited experience with alcoholics and usually hold the erroneous opinion that alcoholics are hopeless skid-row bums who cause trouble. As a result, the staff often seeks to avoid having alcoholics placed in their facilities and may try to have them transferred as soon as possible following admission. This is extremely unfortunate, as there are rarely any adequate long-term treatment facilities for alcoholics with mental or physical deterioration. The result is a great deal of strain between the patient, programs interested in the treatment of alcoholism, and nursing home staff.

There is no easy answer for this unfortunate situation. In a perfect world, specific facilities for the older impaired alcoholic might be developed, but limitations in public funding make this unlikely. Thus, a common sense approach is to attempt to educate nursing home staff about alcoholism and its treatment, working with them in establishing programs aimed at controlling the patient's access to alcohol while in the nursing home, and offering nursing home staff a high level of back-up from alcoholic treatment facilities and Alcoholics Anonymous. The result, while not perfect, is all one usually has to offer in a clinical setting.

SOME FINAL THOUGHTS

Alcohol is a potent drug adversely affecting many older individuals who drink despite their medical problems or present medications. In addition, the rate of alcoholism in older individuals is approximately the same as the general population. These two factors result in high levels of physical and mental pathology which impact on health care delivery systems.

I have presented an introduction to alcohol related pathology in the nonalcoholic geriatric patient and an overview of the diagnosis, usual clinical course, and treatment of the older alcoholic. This is not a hopeless disorder as, based on data in younger populations, probably more than one-third of the individuals with alcoholism reach and sustain abstinence. It is also important to note that the older alcoholic is likely to drink with some level of moderation even without treatment.

There are no magic cures for this problem and, unfortunately, there is little data to indicate what specific therapies should be offered the geriatric alcohol abuser. However, I have related a number of common sense modifications of usual treatment approaches which have helped me in dealing with the elderly alcoholic and which hopefully can be of use in clinical practice.

REFERENCES

1. Eisdorfer, C., and Schuckit, M.A. Drug and alcohol misuse in the elderly. Alcohol and Drug Abuse Institute Technical Report No. 77-32, University of Washington, Oct. 1977.

178   SCHUCKIT

2. Schuckit, M.A., and Pastor, P.A. The elderly as a unique population: alcoholism. *Alcoholism: Clin. Exper. Res.* 2:31–38, 1978.
3. Schuckit, M.A. Geriatric alcoholism and drug abuse. *The Gerontologist* 17:168–174, 1977.
4. Raskind, M., and Eisdorfer, C. Psychopharmacology of the aged, in Simpson, L.L. (ed.), *Drug Treatment of Mental Disorders.* New York: Raven Press, 1976, pp. 237–266.
5. Gould, L., Zahir, M., and Demartino, A. Cardiac effects of a cocktail. *J. Am. Med. Assoc.* 218:1799–1802, 1971.
6. Horowitz, L.D. Alcohol and heart disease. *J. Am. Med. Assoc.* 239:959–960, 1975.
7. Klatsky, A.L. Friedman, G.D., Siegelaub, A.B., et al. Alcohol consumption and blood pressure. *N. Engl. J. Med.* 1194–1200, 1977.
8. McDonald, C.D., Burch, G.E., and Walsh, J.J. Alcohol cardiomyopathy managed with prolonged bed rest. *Ann. Intern. Med.* 74:681–691, 1971.
9. Mendelson, J.H., and Mello, N.K. Alcohol-induced hyperlipidemia and beta lipoproteins. *Science* 180:1372–1374, 1973.
10. Guze, S.B. The need for toughmindedness in psychiatric thinking. *S. Med. J.* 63:662–671, 1970.
11. Woodruff, R.A. Goodwin, D.W., and Guze, S.B. *Psychiatric Diagnosis.* New York: Oxford University Press, 1974.
12. Schuckit, M.A. Alcoholism and sociopathy—diagnostic confusion. *J. Stud. On Alcohol* 34:157–164, 1973.
13. Schuckit, M.A. Alcoholism and affective disorder: diagnostic confusion, in Goodwin, D.W. (ed.), *Alcoholism and Depression,* Jamaica, N.Y.: Spectrum Publications, Inc. (In press).
14. Haglund, R.M.J., and Schuckit, M.A. The epidemiology of alcoholism. In Estes, N. and Heinemann, E. (eds.), *Alcoholism: Development, Consequences & Interventions.* St Louis: C.V. Mosby Co., 1977.
15. Fillmore, K.M. Drinking and problem drinking in early adulthood and middle age. *Q. J. Stud. Alcohol.* 35:819–840, 1974.
16. Schuckit, M.A., and Pastor, P.A. Alcohol-related psychopathology in the aged, in Kaplan, O.J. (ed.), *Psychopathology in the Aging.* New York: Academic Press (In press).
17. Rosin, A.J., and Glatt, M.M. Alcohol excess in the elderly. *Q. J. Stud. Alcohol.* 32:53–59, 1971.
18. Bailey, M.B. Haberman, P.W., and Alksne, H. The epidemiology of alcoholism in an urban residental area. *Q. J. Stud. Alcohol.* 26:19–40, 1965.
19. Schuckit, M.A., and Miller P.L. Alcoholism in elderly men: a survey of a general medical ward. *Ann. N.Y. Acad. Sci.* 273:558–571, 1976.
20. Graux, P. Alcoholism of the elderly. *Rev. Alcsme.* 15:46–48, 1969.
21. Gaitz, C.M., and Baer, P.E. Characteristics of elderly patients with alcoholism. *Arch. Gen. Psychiat.* 24:829–836, 1971.
22. Daniel, R. A five-year study of 693 psychogeriatric admissions in Queensland. *Geriatrics* 27:132–155, 1972.
23. Moore, R.A. The prevalence of alcoholism in a community general hospital. *Am. J. Psych.* 128:638–639, 1971.
24. Schuckit, M.A. Morrissey, E.R., and O'Leary, M.R. Alcohol problems in elderly men and women. *Addict. Dis.* 3:405–416, 1978.
25. Schuckit, M.A. Treatment of alcoholism in office and outpatient settings, in Mendelson, J.H., and Mello, N.K. (eds.) *Diagnosis and Treatment of Alcoholism.* New York: McGraw-Hill Co., 1979.
26. Schuckit, M.A. Inpatient and residential approaches to the treatment of alcoholism, in Mendelson, J.H., and Mello, N.K. (eds.), *Diagnosis and Treatment of Alcoholism.* New York: McGraw-Hill Co. 1979.

27. Sellers, E.M., and Kalant, H. Medical intelligence—alcohol intoxication and withdrawal. *N. Engl. J. Med.* 2:757–762, 1976.
28. Greenblatt, D.J., and Shader, R.I. *Benzodiazepenes in Clinical Practice.* New York: Raven Press, 1974.
29. Elkins, R.L. Aversion therapy for alcoholism: chemical, electrical, or verbal imaginary? *Int. J. Addict.* 10:157–209, 1975.

CHAPTER 13

Differential Treatment of Alcoholism

E. MANSELL PATTISON

The field of alcoholism is still beset by controversy over the effectiveness of treatment. We continue to hear ideological statements of pessimism such as "we really know little about how to treat alcoholism", or ideological statements of optimism such as "we know that alcoholism is a treatable disease". Ideologies do not advance our understanding of alcoholism treatment.

In 1966, I proposed that we adopt the general epidemiological model of medicine for the investigation of alcoholism treatment, which requires the analysis of multiple treatment variables.[1] This model poses the following multi-question of alcoholism treatment:

What alcoholism syndromes, at which stages of development, and in what kind of patients, respond under what conditions, in what short and long range ways, to what measures, administered by whom?

In the ensuing decade we have acquired a substantial body of research toward answering this question.[2] Therefore, in this chapter I shall address the advances we have made in differential treatment, by which I mean matching different alcoholism syndromes in alcoholic subpopulations with congruent facilities, treatment methods, and treatment personnel.

THE CONCEPT OF ALCOHOLISM AS A SYNDROME

A major hindrance to the development of selective treatment of alcoholism has been the "unitary" concept of alcoholism. That is, there is one discrete disease entity which can properly be defined as the disease of alcoholism. Logically, if there is one specific disease, then we should properly seek one specific treatment.

This simplistic concept of alcoholism has proved inadequate. For example, the objective assessment of alcoholism by scaling tests reveals a multidimensional profile, rather than a measurable unitary entity.[3] Numerous studies of the psychological and social characteristics of alcoholics reveal no consistent unitary pattern,[4] and the characteristics of alcoholics themselves appear less predictive of outcome than variations in treatment programs.[5]

There is now a general consensus that there are multiple types of alcoholics or alcoholism problems which require a spectrum of treatment programs appropriate to the type of alcoholism problem.[6] This is commonly called a "multivariate" concept of alcoholism to reflect the variation in alcoholic persons, alcoholism problems, and alcoholism treatments.[7,8]

When Jellinek[9] proposed the disease concept of alcoholism, he used the term "concept" quite deliberately to indicate a wide panoply of patterns of alcohol abuse and misuse. In fact, he reserved the use of the term "disease" for only one type of alcoholic pattern—the gamma alcoholic. This type he considered to be an alcohol addiction, which merited definition as a disease. His other four types of alcohol abuse were considered to be alcohol problems. Unfortunately, the conventional wisdom of the field soon wrenched the Jellinek formulation out of context to produce the unitary concept of alcoholism.[10]

Roughly, the unitary concept proposes:

There is a unitary phenomenon called alcoholism, in which all persons so afflicted are substantially the same, who experience a similar progressive deterioration, who will respond to a singular treatment, resulting in one specific outcome—abstinence.

This unitary concept has been implemented by multiple isolated treatment personnel, each preferring a singular treatment, to achieve one simple outcome.[11]

Although major scientific advances have been made in both our understanding of the alcoholism syndrome and our treatment methods, there has been significant reluctance to abandon the unitary approach to alcoholism in clinical practice.[12]

At this point, the question of whether alcoholism is to be considered a disease is not at debate. Rather the issue is whether alcoholism is a unitary disease or a multivariate *syndrome*. A syndrome can be defined as:

A group or set of concurrent symptoms which together can be considered a disease.

To consider alcoholism as a disease does not necessarily require a unitary set of symptoms, nor necessarily a uniform clinical course. For a syndrome is a concatenation of symptoms that can be usefully aggregated to describe a clinical problem. To formulate alcoholism as a syndrome does not do violence to the clinical utility of defining alcoholism as a disease. On the other hand, it may be distinctly inaccurate and clinically misleading to ignore the multivariate nature of the alcoholism syndrome.[13]

Let us first consider the Jellinek proposition that there are five distinct sub-types of alcoholism, one of which, the addictive gamma alcoholic, is distinctly different from the others. Since 1960 there has been extensive research on a wide variety of alcoholic populations, which has rather conclusively demonstrated that there are no distinct categories of alcoholics. Certainly, the five sub-types proposed by Jellinek have not been validated. Rather there are pattern clusters. That is, certain sets of symptoms, behaviors, and disabilities tend to cluster out on factor-analytic studies. Thus, one can generate sub-types of alcoholics. But these sub-types are composed of complex personality, social, and drinking variables, not simple drinking categories such as Jellinek proposed. Further, this research has not validated the Jellinek concept of the gamma addictive alcoholic. Rather, degrees of severity of alcohol use are complexly intertwined with other psychosocial variables. Thus, the "true" gamma addictive alcoholic has proved nonexistent.[14-18] The syndrome of alcoholism has one constant feature: *a significant life problem associated with the use of alcohol.* Beyond that, we find a wide variation in pre-existent and consequent variables associated with a given person's alcohol problem.

Second, let us consider the extent to which the clinical course of the alcoholism syndrome can be considered unitary. Jellinek proposed that there were distinct clinical phases leading to alcohol addiction. He postulated a sequence of 43 specific symptoms of alcoholism, with three symptoms—blackouts, loss of control, and prolonged intoxication (binges)—serving as phase markers to identify the onset of each major phase—the prodromal phase, the crucial phase, and the chronic phase, respectively. Jellinek, however, cautioned that:

Not all symptoms ... occur necessarily in the same sequence.

The Jellinek model suffers from multiple methodological problems. His notion of a unitary phase sequence was derived from his interpretation of an open-ended questionnaire distributed only to AA members via their in-house newsletter, *The Grapevine*.[19] Of those questionnaires returned, only 98 (6.13%) were adequate for analysis. Thus, the sample consisted of a small group of persons willing to respond to an open-ended questionnaire, who were self-identified as recovered alcoholics from one organization. Among the inadequacies of this method is the fact that the sampling methodology is highly biased and the returns are nonrepresentative of the sample. Second, as Seiden[20] has pointed out, members of AA are nonrepresentative of the alcoholic population in general. The technique used retrospective reconstruction and self-report. It is likely that the ideology of AA greatly influenced the nature of the reconstructed symptom development. Third, the questions were open-ended, and the data were coded by Jellinek in a post-hoc manner. Thus, pre-existing assumptions or biases may have influenced the analysis of the data. Finally, several more refined research studies have failed to confirm Jellinek's analysis. A re-analysis of the Jellinek data by Park[21] using new statistical techniques revealed that the original Jellinek data did not support a phase sequence of symptoms. Orford[22] assessed a large sample of alcoholics in England, and found a large variation in ordering of symptoms, unrelated to Jellinek's postulates. Similarly, in his own data from Finland, Park[21] found:

If there be three phases in the development of alcohol addiction ... a sizeable proportion of experiences do not occur in the phases to which they are assigned ... the presumed manifestations of alcoholism do not necessarily develop in the order given by Jellinek.

Finally, although a specific set of sequential symptoms cannot be substantiated, can we concur with the unitary concept that in the alcoholism syndrome there is a relatively common progressive course of deterioration? Could we consider characteristic early, middle, and late stages of alcoholism common to all?

The vast majority of observations on this issue have come from clinicians working within circumscribed clinical populations and without comparative or longitudinal data. Thus, this clinical data is subject to the distortions of a severely disabled population, retrospective analysis, and lack of generalizability to larger populations of alcohol users.

In contrast, in large scale national and regional epidemological surveys of drinking practices, which have followed individuals over time with varying degrees of drinking problems, it has been shown: (1) that people move in and out of symptomatic drinking, (2) that severity of drinking problems may remain constant and non-progressive, and (3) that remissions and progressions significantly vary with time, place, and circumstance.[23-26]

In a study of problem drinking over only a four year span, Clark and Cahalan[27] found that there was a substantial turnover in the number of persons who moved into or out of the problem drinking population. Thus, entry into the category of problem drinker does not necessarily imply an inexorable progression toward middle and late stages of the alcoholism syndrome. The abuse of alcohol does not necessarily, in itself, move from one stage to another. As Chandler, et al,[28] conclude:

It may be useful to call alcoholism a disease, but the notion is simplistic in the extreme if it ignores the probably vital influence of social circumstances and personality in patterning the consequences of abnormal drinking.

In still another fashion, the development or cessation of drinking problems may be related to stages of life and life circumstances, rather than to the use of alcohol per se. For example, Fillmore[29] followed up a group of college students who then had drinking problems. After twenty years, she found that 68% of the males and 67% of the females had become nonproblem drinkers, while 10% of those who had been abstainers in college now were problem drinkers. Similarly, Goodwin, et al.[30] followed a group of 451 Army men in Vietnam subsequent to their return to civilian life. They found that most of those with drinking problems in Vietnam discontinued their abusive use of alcohol and had no subsequent problems associated with alcohol. Hyman[31] conducted a fifteen year follow-up and found the majority of young severe drinkers had become moderate drinkers or abstainers.

A different pattern is described by Blum and Levine[32] for "reactive" alcoholics. In contrast to the "progressive" pattern in which the person moves from early to middle to late stages of alcoholism in mid-life, they have found that "reactive" alcoholics develop a significant alcohol syndrome only in mid-life associated with acute life stress and inability to cope effectively at this point in the life cycle.

And then there is the pattern of alcoholism problems emerging only toward the end of the life cycle among the aged. In this case there may have been a life history of nonproblematic drinking. However, the stresses of retirement and aging may precipitate significant alcoholism problems among the aged.[33,34,35]

All of this data does not indicate that there is no progression of severity in the alcoholism syndrome. Orford and Hawker[36] found that there is a small number of clusters of events that can be seen as a clinical sequence—first, the onset of psychological dependence; second, tremor, morning drinking, and amnesia; third, aspects of alcoholic psychosis. They conclude:

> There is a characteristic ordering of new events or symptoms in the development of alcoholism, but we would argue strongly that the extensions of this notion to include a wide range of events encompassing psychophysiological, social, and treatment events is not feasible and has served only to obscure a number of more basic and relatively circumscribed processes.

If we observe the alcoholism syndrome throughout a continuing clinical course, we may separate that clinical course into early, middle, and late stages.[37] The point is that the alcoholism syndrome is not necessarily an invidious "disease". Rather significant symptoms associated with alcohol use will vary with each person in accord with his/her own life history. Garitano and Ronall[38] suggest that we can view the alcoholism syndrome as the particular expression of the use of alcohol embedded in the "life style" of a given person.

In summary, the alcoholism syndrome is just that—a syndrome. There is a general set of symptoms associated with early, middle, and late stages of the syndrome. Yet, there is such variability in the syndrome, that we must assess each individual in terms of the particular array of symptoms, disabilities, and potential for change that characterize the alcoholism syndrome for each individual.

It is the failure to properly define and address alcoholism as a syndrome that then gives rise to simplistic approaches to alcoholism treatment as a personal "monopoly" in a competitive monolithic array of treatment entrepreneurs. Babow[39] comments:

> Particular treatment modalities or treatment programs ... are praised as 'the only effective way' by their enthusiasts and denigrated by advocates of competing models.

The result is lack of professional and public accountability, and anti-scientific bias against the accumulation of evidence for efficacy or the development of new methodologies, and the failure to develop collaboration, coordination, or cooperation among treatment resources. Babow concludes:

A vicious circle thus operates in which a program policy of rigid ideology tried to shut off anyone or anything that does not fit.

The problem is illustrated in a study of alcoholism treatment personnel by Einstein, et al.[40] They report that treatment personnel focus on only one aspect of the alcoholism syndrome and then pursue one personal line of rehabilitation. They conclude:

Is it reasonable to expect that effective treatment and/or prevention of a condition as complex as alcoholism can be achieved by such a simplistic approach?

Similarly, Hadley and Hadley[41] studied the social climate of ten different alcoholism treatment programs. Not only were the attitudes and social behavior different in each program, but within each program the individual staff held individual philosophies and treatment approaches at variance with each other and their common program. In a factor analytic study of dimensions of change in alcoholic rehabilitation, Pemper[42] isolates six sociopsychological variables, but found that treatment focused on only one variable—personal maladjustment.

An alternative approach to treatment which has become popular is the eclectic, laissez-faire multiple treatment philosophy of "a little bit of everything for everybody". In a methodological review of treatment programs, Costello[43,44] found that such "multiple indiscriminate" programs had the lowest rehabilitation rates, the highest dropouts, and largest number of overt treatment failures.

In contrast, the approach to alcoholism as a syndrome has stimulated the development of what many of us term the "multivariate-multimodal" model of alcoholism.[7,45-51] In brief, the multivariate-multimodal model recognizes that there are multiple variables that produce multiple syndromes, which require multiple modes of treatment based on differential treatment selection.

There are several clinical implications of this model that must be briefly discussed.

First, this model states that there is a series of factors involved in alcoholism treatment. Our goal is to *match* a particular patient with the appropriate treatment facility, in which he will be matched with the appropriate personnel, who in turn will match treatment interventions to the needs of the person.

This is a large order, and in fact most reviewers of treatment methods report that no large-scale clear indicators for selective treatment matching

can be determined from the data.[44,52-56] In view of the widespread
indiscriminate utilization of treatment methods, such a conclusion from
global reviews is not surprising.[57,58]

On the other hand, small scale discrete research projects have
demonstrated the utility of developing a match of patient facility-
therapist-method. For example, Pattison, et al.[59-61] have shown that
different types of alcoholics present themselves at different facilities,
receive distinctly different treatments, and achieve different treatment
outcomes. This data suggests that some covert "matching" already occurs.
Similar findings in other research projects have demonstrated some
predictors for matching.[62,63] Perhaps the clearest illustration of the
potential value of the "matching" concept is provided by McLachlan,[64]
who reported:

> When the patient was matched to both therapy and after-care
> environments, 77 percent were recovered; when matched to either
> the after-care or therapy environment alone, 61 and 65 percent were
> recovered; when mismatched to both therapy and after-care only 39
> percent recovered.

Second, the model states that there are multiple factors in the outcome
of rehabilitation. That is, abstinence itself is not an adequate criterion of
successful rehabilitation. In fact, the alcoholism syndrome is comprised of
multiple disabilities, some of which may predate the development of
alcoholism, some of which may be a consequence of the alcoholism.[65] In
either case, a focus on drinking behavior per se is likely to be misleading.
For then the clinician may overlook life variables that perpetuate the
alcoholism, or even if the drinking behavior is changed there may remain
unattended major disabilities in the life of the alcoholic that preclude
successful rehabilitation. As Rohan[66] concludes:

> The results show that the label alcoholic subsumes great quantitative
> diversity and that the present dichotomy of normal vs. abnormal
> drinker, or social drinker vs. alcoholic should be replaced with a
> concept of continuum. The adverse effects of drinking are not
> linearly dependent on the quantity of drinking but depend on many
> other factors as well.

One simple way of looking at these factors is in terms of "Life Health",
which is the total adaptation of the person. We can divide this into five
parts: "Drinking Health", "Emotional Health", "Interpersonal Health",

"Vocational Health", and "Physical Health". So in a given alcoholism syndrome the person may have disability of varying severity in each area of life health. The successful outcome of treatment would be assessed in terms of relative improvement in each area of life health where disability exists.

It must be emphasized that the relationship between Drinking Health and the other areas of life health is not a simple cause and effect. Changes in Drinking Health do not necessarily relate to areas of improvement in other life health areas. Conversely, there may be improvement in the other four life health areas, not closely related to improvement in the Drinking Health area.[2,67] This is illustrated by Bowman, et al.[68] who found that changes in drinking only accounted for 50% of the variance in treatment outcome.

This means that the clinician must construct treatment goals and implement treatment methods relevant to each area of impairment. And the success of treatment must be assessed in terms of multiple outcome variables. For example, Lowe and Thomas[69] evaluated successful outcome in three areas. In their alcoholic population at follow-up, 70% had achieved vocational rehabilitation, 62% psychosocial behavioral rehabilitation, and 34% abstinence. Thus, we see that successful rehabilitation is not a unitary phenomenon. It is probably rare that there is either total failure or total success. There are different degrees of rehabilitation in different lives.

Third, the model is multimodal. We can pose two questions about methods of treatment. First, is there data to support a specific treatment method for specific alcoholics? Second, is there data to support the use of multiple treatment methods with the same person? Unfortunately, the data is equivocal, but there are some plausible conclusions.

To address the first question, we must separate specific and nonspecific factors in treatment. Treatment methods may differ in philosophies and techniques, but the differences may be clinically unimportant. The fact of involvement in treatment, of interested treatment staff, of mobilization of resources, all of a *nonspecific* nature, may be the most critical factors. Baekeland, et al.[70] support this conclusion.

If differences in improvement rates indeed depend more on the kinds of treatment being used—and this did seem to us to be the case—an obvious question arises: since the treatments studied have all been applied somewhat indiscriminately to rather heterogeneous populations but nonetheless seem to help many patients, why are they as effective as they are? In other words, what do they have in common and how do they work?

It is surprising that much alcoholism treatment is rather effective despite the little attention given to selection of treatment. It is reasonable to anticipate that more careful attention to treatment selection will not provide exact answers, but it may well *improve* the effectiveness, efficiency, and precision of the treatment methods available to us.

In regard to the second question of multiple treatments, we must distinguish between selected interventions that are coordinated and focused on areas of impairment versus an indiscriminate pot-pourri of treatments that have no logical relationship to each other or to the clinical status of the patients. Some evidence is presented in the report by Costello.[43,44] He finds that the best treatment programs do offer multiple treatment methods that are clearly organized, carefully defined, and systematically conducted, whereas the poorest treatment programs have little organization or definition and merely present multiple indiscriminately conducted therapies.

Thus, it appears that the issue of selection of treatment methods is not a single treatment method versus multiple treatment methods. Rather, the best options appear to lie in *focusing on a group of treatments relevant to a set of specific disabilities, with some range of viable alternatives within that group of treatments.*

VARIATIONS IN ALCOHOLIC POPULATIONS

There is now general agreement that there is no such person as "the" alcoholic. On the other hand, certain general typologies may be generated that are clinically useful.

Early attempts to define the "alcoholic personality" have failed. Blane[71] considers the concept of a personality structure *unique* to alcoholics and *to only* alcoholics a straw man. Or as Keller[72] put it: "Alcoholics are different in so many ways that it makes no difference."

It is important to differentiate between attempts to define a uniformity among all alcoholics—which has failed—versus attempts to define a number of personality factors which might predict individual vulnerability to develop alcoholism or to predict response to treatment. Recent research has demonstrated such great diversity in personality structure that one cannot find specific personality attributes, traits, or mechanisms that would predict alcoholism.[16,66] Likewise, personality variables alone are not reliable predictors for treatment.[73-76] Thus, the use of psychological tests to predict or select treatment has not been successful.[77,78]

Another way of looking at alcoholic populations is in terms of the populations who constitute the clientele of specific treatment facilities. Pattison, et al.[60] reported on clientele at three different alcoholism treatment facilities. They found that the successful cases at each facility were substantially different from each other, constituting unique subpopulations. Each facility subpopulation improved, but improved in different patterns. Subsequently, Pattison, et al.[61] studied the populations presenting before treatment at four different treatment facilities. They found that the subpopulations were not just the result of treatment, but were distinct pre-existent subpopulations who entered each facility. Other researchers have published confirmatory studies that indicate that different alcoholism treatment facilities tend to attract populations distinctive to that type of facility.[62,79-85]

Finally, within facilities there is variation. Here we must consider individual differences in perceived needs,[86] as well as motivations and attitudes toward different treatment methods and personnel.[87,89]

In conclusion, there is no unitary population of alcoholics. Yet combinations of psychological, social and cultural variables together describe relatively distinct clinical subgroups. In his recent review of population variables as predictors of treatment, Ogborne[90] concludes that we may have underestimated the potential value of creating useful clinical typologies of alcoholics that may aid selection of treatment.

VARIATION IN TREATMENT FACILITIES

There has been relative neglect of systematic study of alcoholism treatment facilities. Bromet, et al.[91] have pioneered in evaluating the "social climate" of different treatment facilities. They found that different treatment facilities which have the same overall goal of alcoholism rehabilitation have major variations in ideology, operation, and climate.

Are there common characteristics among treatment facilities that relate to effective function? The best indicators come from a comprehensive review by Costello[43,44] of comparative treatment methods. He found that the most effective treatment programs had the following characteristics: (1) Had a well organized treatment philosophy that was implemented in consistent and logical fashion; (2) Had inpatient resources for medical care and for nonmedical rehabilitation; (3) Had an aggressive post-discharge follow-up; (4) Provided involvement and assistance for the significant people in the life of the alcoholic, or what might be termed collateral counseling and participation; (5) Had aggressive outreach with community agencies to both bring alcoholics into the program through community contacts and effect transition back into community resources; (6) Had adjunctive use of Antabuse available; and (7) Provided behaviorally oriented interventions in addition to purely verbal therapies.

In short, effective treatment facilities are *systems of treatment,* that have coherent organization, aggressive intake and follow-up procedures, and provide a wide spectrum of carefully constructed treatment options.

There is great variation between even these successful alcoholism facilities. Each type of facility is likely to recruit a particular sub-type of alcoholic from the community. In addition, the same type of facility may vary from community to community. Therefore, it is necessary that each facility use selection procedures as follows:

1. Identify the subpopulation of alcoholics that it actually serves or desires to serve.
2. Identify the treatment needs of that specific population.
3. Evaluate and organize their treatment programs to match the needs of their specific clientele.
4. Develop appropriate collaboration between their facility and other facilities in the community.

VARIATION IN TREATMENT METHODS

Recently, Bromet, et al.[92] have published large scale studies which indicate that treatment method and selection are more important to successful outcome than previously realized. Thus, there is evidence to support more careful differentiation between treatment methods.

Further, selection of treatment must be in accord with the *specific phase of treatment.* Thus, we need to consider emergency treatments, initial intake treatment methods, the selection of ongoing treatments, and termination and follow-up methods of treatment. Thus, rather than ask "what is the treatment of alcoholism?" we might better ask: "Which treatments are most appropriate to what phase of a longitudinal rehabilitation process?"

Next is the *target* of treatment. We may consider treatment that will impact on five areas of health of the alcoholic person: drinking behavior per se, emotional/psychological function, interpersonal relations, vocational function, and physical health. Each area will likely require different target interventions. Just providing vocational rehabilitation is no more sensible than just providing medical care, etc. We do *not* treat "alcoholism", but rather we need to treat specific areas of life dysfunction.

Finally, there is the problem of "over-treatment". By this, I mean a shotgun approach of a little bit of everything. It is *not* true that if a little bit of treatment is good, a lot of treatment is better. Nor is it true that all therapies help, so mixing lots of therapies together can do no harm. Such a shotgun approach may merely confuse the patient. More importantly, neither patients nor therapists may develop solid commitments to a treatment approach, or no one person may assume responsibility to carefully monitor and guide a patient toward a successful therapeutic experience, but rather let the patient drift among many therapists and programs. As we have noted, such unsystematic treatment programs have poor results.

In conclusion, multiple treatment methods do have a place, and indeed the need for multiple treatment is stressed here. However, we need to define "multiple treatments" as the appropriate selection of treatment methods in accord with the phase of rehabilitation, selecting target areas where disability exists and treatment intervention is likely to be useful, and matching treatment methods with the patient's own participation in selection according to personal proclivity. It does *not* mean exposing the patient to everything in the hope that something will "take".

VARIATIONS IN TREATMENT PERSONNEL

Treatment may be significantly effected by the selection of the treatment personnel. This is an area devoid of much systematic attention, much less empirical data. Only recently has concerted attention been focused on the peculiar and particular manpower problems in the field of alcoholism.[93,94]

First, the field of alcoholism services has been ignored by health professionals in general, and mental health professionals in particular. Repeated surveys of professional agencies and professional attitudes indicate that there is a general negativistic attitude toward alcoholics, that generic service agencies ignore or screen out alcoholics, much less make measured efforts to make their services available to them, and that professionals both avoid choosing services to alcoholics as a professional option and avoid those who seek services in their agencies.

The result has been a curious and perhaps tragic vacuum. For the major bulk of alcoholism services manpower has come from the ranks of volunteers and paraprofessional personnel. Until at least 1950, the vast bulk of alcoholism programs and services were nonprofessional in nature. As Cahn[95] has documented, what professional alcoholism services were developed tended to be staffed by second class professional staff, with second class funding, resulting in second class professional programs operating in the back-waters of the main stream of professional developments.

Second, the training of mental health professionals has rarely included much preparation in the field of alcoholism.[96] Hence, professional recruitment has been difficult. Perhaps most professional recruits have been those who have been alcoholic themselves, achieved sobriety, and then sought professional training to return to the field of their personal experiences. The influence of this type of professional has not been critically evaluated.

One response to this professional vacuum has been the development of specialized professional training programs for alcoholism counselors. These range from new careers training of recovered alcoholics to B.A. and M.A. level academic curricula. Although such programs are personally successful, we must question their overall national value if they continue apart from a more general manpower development program. Such specialized alcoholism personnel have little lateral mobility into other human services jobs, they have little vertical mobility except on an idiosyncratic basis within a specific program, and they have ambiguous professional status and sanction at this time. On the other hand, where professional training programs do interdigitate with more general manpower training and manpower personnel series, they do offer a highly potent specialized manpower development track for personnel directed toward alcoholism services.[97]

Third, a major problem in the development of manpower, from a professional point of view, is the fragmented professional orientation towards alcoholism. Some medical professionals view alcoholism solely as a biological problem; some psychiatric professionals view alcoholism solely as a neurotic emotional problem; some psychological professionals view alcoholism solely as a conditioned behavioral problem, etc. In sum, there is no widely accepted professional frame of reference within which professional training can be developed. Hence, we have partisan professionalism rather than scientific professionals. Until a more adequate professional conceptual base for manpower preparation is developed, we may expect difficulties in the recruitment and training of adequate manpower.

A further complication in the manpower field is the split between the layman and professional approaches to alcoholism treatment. Kalb and Propper[11] describe the differences in terms of the cognitive style and commitments of the two manpower groups. According to them, the professionals use an analytical-objective-inductive cognitive style, whereas the lay personnel use an intuitive-subjective-deductive style. They point out that lay personnel often have a strong personal commitment to a personalized treatment style, whereas the professional is likely to lack intense personal commitment and look at treatment methods as a scientific problem. The result, say Kalb and Propper, is a conflict of power and ideology between two manpower pools in the field.

It is important to match personnel to programs, so that the skills, values, and ideologies of the staff match the values, ideology, and programmatic goals of the facility. Where this does not occur, staff are likely to provide services not congruent with program goals.[18] Our staff attitudes may be shaped by external factors that bias treatment services. For example, Smart, et al.[98] studied a large alcoholism program in which careful treatment recommendations were made at diagnostic intake based upon individual need assessment. Yet they found that the actual treatment received was based on social class biases of the staff, which ignored the actual treatment needs of the individual alcoholics.

With a comprehensive treatment program, then, I recommend that careful attention be given to matching treatment personnel in terms of their specific skills and values with individual alcoholic clients who need those specific treatment skills and share similar values.[49,70] Then we are likely to develop collaborative and mutually committed therapeutic relationships.

SELECTION OF TREATMENT IN PHASE SEQUENCES

Up to this point, we have only considered differential treatment in terms of variations in the different syndromes, populations, facilities, treatments, and personnel. Now we must turn our attention to selection of treatment throughout the phase sequence of treatment.

Selection of treatment is not one single event, but a *series of decision points* throughout the *entire community system* of alcoholism treatment. Thus, selection of treatment is *longitudinal* as well as cross-sectional.

Table 1 represents the rehabilitation process as a flow chart, in which alcoholic clients enter the alcoholism treatment system through multiple ports of entry. From this point onward we can identify seven phases of treatment, each of which involves selective treatment decisions. Ultimately, the alcoholic client will exit from the treatment system back into multiple ongoing involvement in community relationships.

As illustrated, Phase A. (Identification) and Phase B. (Triage) involve TYPE 1. treatment decisions, which are DEFINITIONAL. That is, the decisions involve defining persons with alcohol problems, defining the nature of the problems, defining the appropriate resources for referral. These decision points are located in multiple agencies throughout the community, and may include churches, hospitals, social welfare agencies, business and industry, legal agencies, mental health services, etc. These decisions are the most generalized.

TABLE 1.–Phase Sequences of Treatment

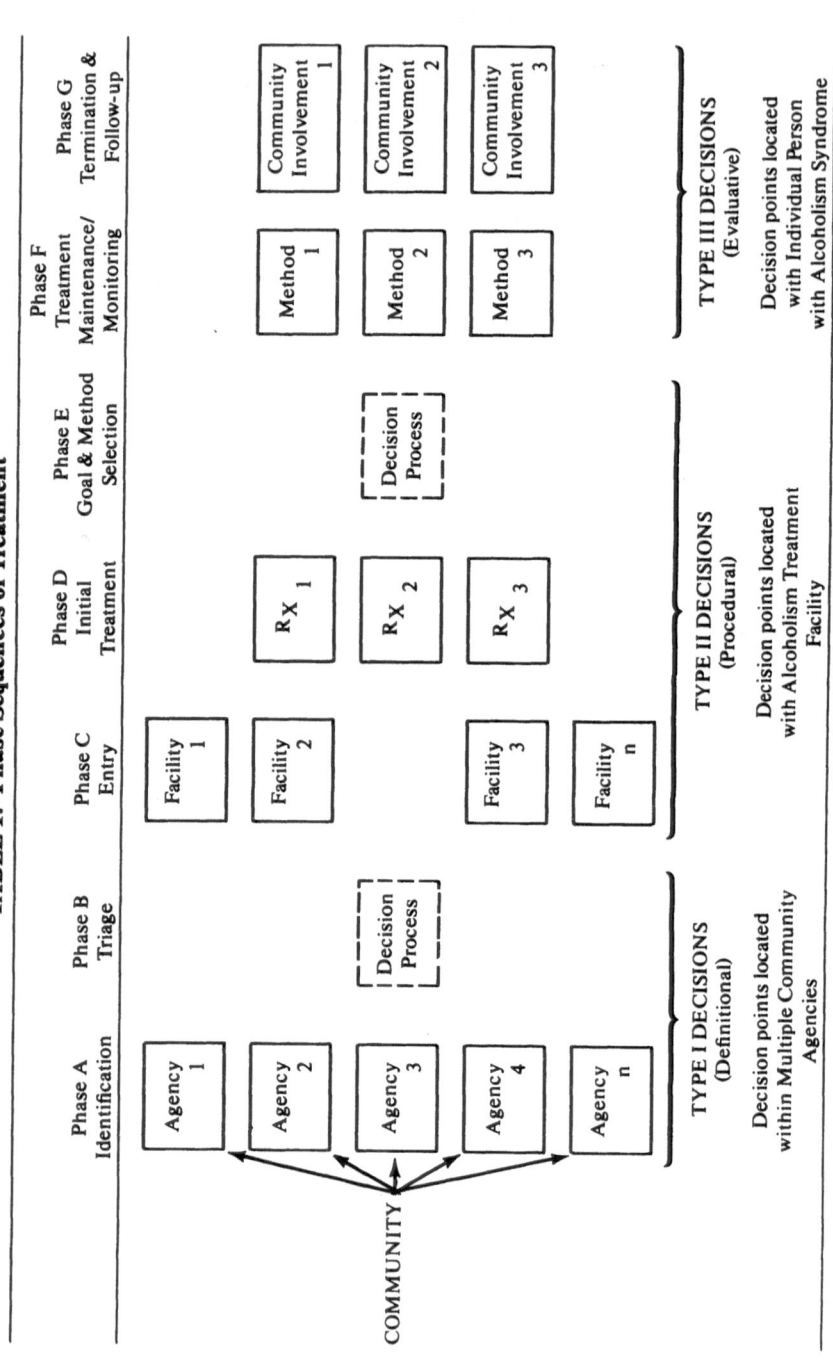

Phase A Identification	Phase B Triage	Phase C Entry	Phase D Initial Treatment	Phase E Goal & Method Selection	Phase F Treatment Maintenance/ Monitoring	Phase G Termination & Follow-up
Agency 1		Facility 1				
Agency 2		Facility 2	RX 1		Method 1	Community Involvement 1
Agency 3	Decision Process		RX 2	Decision Process	Method 2	Community Involvement 2
Agency 4		Facility 3	RX 3		Method 3	Community Involvement 3
Agency n		Facility n				

COMMUNITY

TYPE I DECISIONS (Definitional)

Decision points located within Multiple Community Agencies

TYPE II DECISIONS (Procedural)

Decision points located with Alcoholism Treatment Facility

TYPE III DECISIONS (Evaluative)

Decision points located with Individual Person with Alcoholism Syndrome

The next three phases, Phase C. (Entry), Phase D. (Initial Treatment), Phase E. (Goals and Method Selection) involve TYPE II. treatment decisions, which are PROCEDURAL. That is, the decisions revolve around methods to involve the alcoholic initially in the treatment process and then conduct appropriate individual assessment as to which particular treatment goals and methods should be provided from among the options available within the treatment programs. These decision points are located within each treatment facility, and the decisions are intermediate in specificity.

The final two phases, Phase F. (Treatment Maintenance/Monitoring), and Phase G. (Termination and Follow-up) involve TYPE III. treatment decisions, which are EVALUATIVE. That is, these decisions involve regular review of the client's progress toward stated treatment goals, appropriate utilization of specific treatment methods, assessment of individual progress toward termination, and specific individual plans for re-involvement in community life. These decision points are, therefore, located within each individual; while the decisions are the most specific of all.

Thus, we see that the rehabilitation process as a system involves multiple levels of decision-making, which range from the community to the individual. Different types of decisions are involved in each phase of the rehabilitation process, while the decisions become increasingly specific throughout the rehabilitation process. It is obvious that highly specific decisions in the early phases are just as inappropriate as highly global and generalized decisions are inappropriate in the later stages of rehabilitation. Optimally, decisions about treatment should be made within the framework of the overall process of rehabilitation. In this manner, we can clearly define *what types of treatment decisions need to be made in each phase.*

GUIDELINES FOR TREATMENT SELECTION

In this abbreviated chapter I have only been able to touch upon some of the major principles of treatment selection. Elsewhere, I have documented and presented the empirical data in detail that serve as the basis for the following summary of the "state of the art" in treatment selection.[99,100]

Facility Principles

One, each clinical facility should examine its own population clientele, to determine what type of alcoholic subpopulation it predominantly serves.

Two, each facility should determine which treatment methods it can best offer that are relevant to the population it serves.

Three, the facility should discard treatment methods that are irrelevant to its population, and discard treatment methods that it cannot effectively deliver.

Four, clientele should be *pre-screened* so that only those alcoholics are accepted into a program to whom realistically relevant services can be given.

Five, a facility should provide effective *referral* and *transfer* mechanisms for the inappropriate clientele, so that those alcoholics are successfully placed in a program suited for them elsewhere.

Six, a facility should provide a *group* of alternative treatment approaches so that the alcoholic client may select the treatment approach most suited to his personal preference.

Seven, the alcoholic client should be actively engaged in the process of *mutual selection* of treatment methods and selection of treatment goals.

Eight, a treatment program should provide *continuity of care* through each phase of rehabilitation; or if necessary, provide careful transfer of the alcoholic from phase to phase to different facilities. Programs that deal with only one phase of alcoholism rehabilitation without specific linkages are likely to be ineffective.

Nine, a facility should provide ancillary services, directly or in careful collaboration with other community agencies. These include provision of shelter, food, clothes, welfare support, legal aid, and vocational rehabilitation.

Ten, inpatient alcoholism programs are likely to be ineffective if they do not provide for continuing outpatient care after discharge.

Eleven, short-term inpatient programs of less than 3–4 weeks are likely to not engage alcoholics in a rehabilitative process, whereas lengthy programs of over 6 weeks are likely to foster withdrawal from self-sufficiency and create dependency upon the institution.

Twelve, programs that offer indiscriminate treatment, without specific individualized treatment plans, or offer only a general domicile milieu are likely to be ineffective, whereas carefully organized, logical treatment programs, with specific individual plans are likely to be more effective.

Population Principles

One, simple psychological and social data are likely to provide better indicators for treatment selection than any available complex tests and measurements.

Two, a history of prior successful social and psychological adaptation is positively correlated with treatment success, regardless of the treatment.

Three, clients who are currently functioning well in psychological, social, vocational and physical areas of life, but who are nevertheless drinking in an abusive pattern, may likely not accept psychological treatment, but may be good candidates for aversive conditioning hospital programs, or alcoholism hospital programs that stress the medical and disease aspects of alcoholism.

Four, clients who are functioning reasonably well in psychological, social, vocational, and physical areas of life, but in addition, experience some self-defined emotional distress, are likely to accept various forms of psychotherapy, and are probable good candidates for broad-spectrum behavioral approaches.

Five, clients who have a past history of reasonable life function, but are seriously impaired at present in their ability to be self-sustaining, may likely need vocational assistance, short to medium term living facilities, and careful attention to the restoration of family and community relationships.

Six, clients who have always been seriously impaired in life, such as the prototype skid-row alcoholic, will need supportive types of care over a long period of time. Intensive psychotherapy, aversive-conditioning, disulfiram, tranquilizers and antidepressants, and behavior modification approaches, all are probably inappropriate here.

Treatment Method Principles

One, Alcoholics Anonymous (AA) appears to be a limited resource, that should not be used indiscriminately. Alcoholics who are guilt-prone, desire group affiliations in life, have a prior history of positive social relations, and who tend to develop dependent relations are likely to affiliate with AA.[101,102]

Two, the use of disulfiram (Antabuse®) seems best suited for those who have a stable social and vocational history, are personally motivated to refrain from drinking after some years of problem drinking, and who are able to establish and maintain a positive on-going relationship with the treatment staff who dispense the drug. Major elements of depression seem a contraindication, as well as evidence of impulsivity. The more careful, controlled, obsessive compulsive person is a better treatment risk.

Three, broad-spectrum behavioral treatment methods, and marital/

family psychotherapeutic methods appear to offer the best potential for long-term intensive treatment methods. These methods seem best suited for persons who are relatively functional despite their alcohol abuse, or who have prior good function, with a potential to reestablish their prior level of life adaptation. Methods that link the patient with his community life appear most promising.

Four, drug maintenance may be feasible where the patient is socially stable, but is psychologically more dependent and positively oriented toward authority figures.

Five, where there has been severe impairment of ability to function, and a major loss of social, family, job, and community ties, the treatment of choice seems to be reality-based retraining for life. Reeducation, vocational training, structured living settings, specified social responsibilities, supervised use of time, energy, and money, etc. all appear paramount.

Six, the management of acute detoxification problems remains a major issue that challenges us. Available data indicate that many detoxification problems can be handled on an outpatient basis. On the other hand, many of the people seen for detoxification are not medical problems, but present the problem of social vagrants and public intoxication.

Treatment Goal Principles

One, when the individual alcoholic is first seen, the first task is to engage in a personal contact and establish a working agreement to participate in a rehabilitation program.

Two, only *after* engagement should a careful preliminary evaluation be made, which should include the suitability of the client for this program.

Three, evaluation should include an assessment of the degree of impairment in terms of major areas of life function—which I have for convenience termed drinking health, psychological health, social health, vocational health, and physical health.

Four, evaluation should determine degree of impairment, the stage in the person's life and alcoholism career, and what the *potential* is for change in this area.

Five, evaluation should then lead to a client-worker mutual decision and treatment plan for each area of impairment, where change is *desired* and *possible*.

Six, the treatment plan should include both specific *goals* and specific *methods* to achieve these goals, for each area of life where change is planned.

Seven, the client and worker should develop specific times for *review* of treatment progress, so that there is ongoing feedback to both the alcoholic client and the treatment staff as to areas of specific progress toward goals, of areas where plans need revision or more specific attention given. The result is a specific plan that can be monitored and revised in the light of actual clinical progress by the alcoholic client.

SUMMARY

Ten years ago the notion of differential treatment selection in the field of alcoholism had just emerged as a potential approach to treatment. In the past decade, we have substantially clarified the meaning of differential treatment, which has gained wide acceptance in the field. This multivariate-multimodal model of alcoholism treatment is now widely used in both research and in clinical programs. Although our concepts are much more clear than our data, this is a substantial progress, and the directions for more precise research on treatment can be set forth.

REFERENCES

1. Pattison, E.M. A critique of alcoholism treatment concepts with special reference to abstinence. *Q. J. Stud. Alcohol.* 27:49–71, 1966.
2. Pattison, E.M. Ten years of change in alcoholism treatment and delivery systems. *Am. J. Psychiat.* 134:261–266, 1977.
3. Miller, W.R. Alcoholism scales and objective assessment methods: a review. *Psychol. Bull.* 83:649–674, 1976.
4. Gibbs, L., and Flanagan, J. Prognostic indicators of alcoholism treatment outcome. *Int. J. Addict.* 12:1097–1141, 1977.
5. Smart, R.G., and Gray, G. Multiple predictors of dropout from alcoholism treatment. *Arch. Gen. Psychiat.* 35:363–367, 1978.
6. Costello, R.M., Biever, P., and Baillargen, J.G. Alcoholism treatment programming: historical trends and modern approaches. *Alcoholism: Clin. Exp. Res.* 4:311–318, 1978.
7. Kissin, B. Theory and practice in the treatment of alcoholism, in Kissin, B., and Begleiter, H. (eds.), *The Biology of Alcoholism. Vol. 5 Treatment and Rehabilitation of the Chronic Alcoholic.* New York: Plenum Press, 1977, pp. 1–51.
8. Replogle, W.H., and Haim, J.F. Multivariate approach to profiling alcoholic typologies. *Multivariate Exp. Clin. Res.* 3:157–164, 1977.
9. Jellinek, E.M. *The Disease Concept of Alcoholism.* Highland Park, N.J.: Hillhouse Press, 1960.
10. Robinson, D. The alcohologists addiction—some implications of having lost control over the disease concept of alcoholism. *Q. J. Stud. Alcohol.* 33:1028–1042, 1972.
11. Kalb, M., and Propper, M.S. The future of alcohology: craft or science? *Am. J. Psychiat.* 133:641–645, 1976.

12. Verden, P., and Shatterley, D. Alcoholism research and resistance in understanding the compulsive drinker. *Ment. Hyg.* 55:331–336, 1971.
13. Robinson, D. *From Drinking to Alcoholism: A Sociological Commentary.* New York: Wiley, 1976.
14. Horn, J.L., and Wanberg, K.W. Symptom patterns related to excessive use of alcohol. *Q. J. Stud. Alcohol.* 30:35–58, 1969.
15. Horn, J.L., and Wanberg, K.W. Dimensions of perception of background and current situation of alcoholic patients. *Q. J. Stud. Alcohol.* 31:633–658, 1970.
16. Horn, J.L., Wanberg, K.W., and Adams, B. Diagnosis of alcoholism: factors of drinking, background, and current conditions in alcoholics. *Q. J. Stud. Alcohol.* 35:147–175, 1974.
17. Hurwitz, J.I., and Lelos, D. A multilevel interpersonal profile of employed alcoholics. *Q. J. Stud. Alcohol.* 29:64–76, 1968.
18. Mogar, R.E., Helm, S.T., Snedeker, M.R., Snedeker, M.H., and Wilson, W.M. Staff attitudes toward the alcoholic. *Arch. Gen. Psychiat.* 21:449–454, 1969.
19. Jellinek, E.M. Phases of alcohol addiction. *Q. J. Stud. Alcohol.* 13:673–684, 1952.
20. Seiden, R.H. The use of alcoholics anonymous members in research on alcoholism. *Q. J. Stud. Alcohol.* 21:506–509, 1960.
21. Park, P. Developmental ordering of experiences in alcoholics. *Q. J. Stud. Alcohol.* 34:473–488, 1973.
22. Orford, J.A. Notes on ordering of onset of symptoms in alcohol dependence. *Psychol. Med.* 4:281–288, 1974.
23. Cahalan, D. *Problem Drinkers: A National Survey.* San Francisco: Jossey-Bass, 1970.
24. Cahalan, D., and Room, R. *Problem Drinking Among American Men.* New Brunswick, N.J.: Rutgers, 1974.
25. Cahalan, D., Cisin, I.H., and Crossley, H.M. *American Drinking Practices: A National Survey of Behavior and Attitudes.* New Brunswick, N.J.: Rutgers, 1969.
26. Mulford, H.A., and Miller, D.E. Drinking in Iowa. IV. Preoccupation with alcohol, and definitions of alcoholism, heavy drinking, and trouble due to drinking. *Q. J. Stud. Alcohol.* 21:279–291, 1960.
27. Clark, W.B., and Cahalan, D. Changes in problem drinking over a 4 year span. *Addict. Beh.* 1:251–259, 1976.
28. Chandler, J., Hensman, C., and Edwards, G. Determinants of what happens to alcoholics. *Q. J. Stud. Alcohol.* 32:349–363, 1971.
29. Fillmore, K.M. Relationships between specific drinking problems in early adulthood and middle age: an exploratory 20-year follow-up study. *J. Stud. Alcohol.* 36:887–907, 1975.
30. Goodwin, D.W., David, D.H., and Robins, L.N. Drinking amid abundant illicit drugs: the Vietnam case. *Arch. Gen. Psychiat.* 32:230–233, 1975.
31. Hyman, M.M. Alcoholics fifteen years later. *Ann N.Y. Acad. Med.* 273:613–623, 1976.
32. Blum, J., and Levine, J. Maturity, depression, and life events in middle-aged alcoholics. *Addict. Beh.* 1:37–45, 1975.
33. Gaitz, C.M., and Baer, P.E. Characteristics of elderly patients with alcoholism. *Arch. Gen. Psychiat.* 24:372–378, 1971.
34. Schuckit, M.A. Geriatric alcoholism and drug abuse. *The Gerontologist* 17:168–174, 1977.
35. Simon, A., Epstein, L.J., and Reynolds, L. Alcoholism in the geriatrically mentally ill. *Geriatrics* 23:125–131, 1968.
36. Orford, J.A., and Hawker, A. Investigation of an alcoholism rehabilitative half-way house. 2. Complex questions of client motivation. *Brit. J. Addict.* 69:315–323, 1974.
37. Mulford, H.A. Stages in the alcoholic process: toward a cumulative, nonsequential

index. *J. Stud. on Alcohol.* 38:563–583, 1977.
38. Garitano, W.A., and Ronall, R.E. Concepts of life style in the treatment of alcoholism. *Int. J. Addict.* 9:585–592, 1974.
39. Babow, I. The treatment monopoly in alcoholism and drug dependence: social critique. *J. Drug Issues* 5:120–128, 1975.
40. Einstein, S., Wolfson, E., and Gecht, P. What matters in treatment: relevant variables in alcoholism. *Int. J. Addict.* 5:54–67, 1970.
41. Hadley, P.A., and Hadley, R.G. Treatment practices and philosophies in rehabilitation facilities for alcoholics. *Proc. Am. Psychol. Assoc.* 80:729–780, 1972.
42. Pemper, K. Dimensions of change in the improving alcoholic. *Int. J. Addict.* 11:641–649, 1976.
43. Costello, R.M. Alcoholism treatment and evaluation: I. In search of methods. *Int. J. Addict.* 10:251–275, 1975.
44. Costello, R.M. Alcoholism treatment evaluation: II. Collation of two year follow-up studies. *Int. J. Addict.* 10:857–868, 1975.
45. Pattison, E.M. A critique of abstinence criteria in the treatment of alcoholism. *Int. J. Soc. Psychiat.* 14:260–267, 1968.
46. Pattison, E.M. Rehabilitation of the chronic alcoholic, in Kissin, B. and Begleiter, H. (eds.), *The Biology of Alcoholism. Vol. 3 Clinical Pathology.* New York: Plenum Press, 1974, pp. 587–658.
47. Pattison, E.M. Non-abstinent drinking goals in the treatment of alcoholism: a clinical typology. *Arch. Gen. Psychiat.* 33:923–930, 1976.
48. *Differential Treatment of Drug and Alcohol Abuses.* Edited by Davis, C.S., and Schmidt, M.R. Palm Springs, Calif.: ETC Publ. 1977.
49. Larkin, E.J. *The Treatment of Alcoholism: Theory, Practice, and Evaluation.* Toronto: Addiction Research Foundation, 1974.
50. Ruggels, W.B., Armor, D.J., and Polich, J.M. *A Follow-up Study of Clients at Selected Alcoholism Treatment Centers Funded by NIAA.* Menlo Park, Calif.: Stanford Research Institute, 1975.
51. Williams, P.J.A., Letemendia, F.J.J., and Arroyave, F. A categorization of the assessment of programs and outcomes in the treatment of alcoholism. *Brit. J. Psychiat.* 122:649–654, 1973.
52. Armor, D.J., Johnson, P., Polich, S., and Stanbul, H. *Trends in U.S. Adult Drinking Practices.* Santa Monica, Calif.: Rand Corporation, 1977.
53. Baekeland, F. Evaluation of treatment methods in chronic alcoholism, in Kissin, B., and Begleiter, H. (eds.), *The Biology of Alcoholism. Vol. 5 Treatment and Rehabilitation of the Chronic Alcoholic.* New York: Plenum Press, 1977, pp. 385–440.
54. Baekeland, F., Lundwall, L.K., and Kissin, B. Methods for the treatment of chronic alcoholism: a critical appraisal, In Israel, Y. (ed.), *Research Advance in Alcohol and Drug Problems.* New York: Wiley, 1975, pp. 247–328.
55. Emrick, C.D. A review of psychologically oriented treatment of alcoholism: II. The relative effectiveness of different treatment approaches and the effectiveness of treatment versus no-treatment. *J. Stud. Alcohol.* 36:88–108, 1975.
56. Emrick, C.D. A review of psychologically oriented treatment for alcoholism: I. The use and interrelationships of outcome criteria and drinking behavior following treatment. *Q. J. Stud. Alcohol.* 35:534–549, 1974.
57. Crawford, J.J., and Chalopsky, A.B. The reported evaluation of alcoholism treatment (1968-1971): a methodological review. *Addict. Beh.* 2:63–74, 1977.
58. Swint, J.M., and Nelson, W.B. Prospective evaluation of alcoholism rehabilitation efforts. *J. Stud. Alcohol.* 38:1386–1404, 1977.

59. Pattison, E.M. Non-abstinent drinking goals in the treatment of alcoholism, in Gibbins, R. (ed.), *Research Advances in Alcohol and Drug Problems.* New York: Wiley, 1976, pp. 401–455.

60. Pattison, E.M., Coe, R., and Rhodes, R.A. Evaluation of alcoholism treatment: comparison of three facilities. *Arch. Gen. Psychiat.* 20:478–488, 1969.

61. Pattison, E.M., Coe, R., and Doerr, H.O. Population variation among alcoholism treatment facilities. *Int. J. Addict.* 8:199–229, 1973.

62. Kern, J.C., Schmelter, W., and Fanelli, M. A comparison of the alcoholism treatment populations: implications for treatment. *J. Stud. Alcohol.* 39:785–792, 1978.

63. Trice, H.M., Roman, P.M., and Belasco, J.A. Selection for treatment: a predictive evaluation of an alcoholic treatment regimen. *Int. J. Addict.* 4:303–317, 1969.

64. McLachlan, J.F.C. Therapy strategies, personality orientation, and recovery from alcoholism. *Canad. Psychiat. Assoc. J.* 19:25–30, 1974.

65. Belasco, J.A. The criterion question revisited. *Brit. J. Addict.* 66:39–44, 1971.

66. Rohan, W.P. Quantitative dimensions of alcohol use for hospitalized problem drinkers. *Dis. Nerv. Sys.* 37:154–159, 1976.

67. Pattison, E.M. A conceptual approach to alcoholism treatment goals. *Addict. Beh.* 1:177–192, 1976.

68. Bowman, R.S., Stein, L.I., and Newton, J.R. Measurement and interpretation of drinking behavior. *J. Stud. on Alcohol.* 36:1154–1172, 1975.

69. Lowe, W.C., and Thomas S.D. Assessing alcoholism treatment effectiveness: a comparison of three evaluative measures. *Q. J. Stud. Alcohol.* 37:883–889, 1976.

70. Baekeland, F., and Lundwall, L.K. Dropping out of treatment: a critical review. *Psychol. Bull.* 82:738–783, 1975.

71. Blane, H.T. *The Personality of the Alcoholic: Guises of Dependency.* New York: Harper and Row, 1968.

72. Keller, M. The oddities of alcoholics. *Q. J. Stud. Alcohol.* 33:1147–1148, 1972.

73. Donovan, D.M., Hague, W.H., and O'Leary, M.R. Perceptual differentiation and defense mechanisms in alcoholics. *J. Clin. Psychol.* 31:356–359, 1975.

74. Gellens, H.K., Gottheil, E., and Alterman, A.I. Drinking outcomes of specific alcoholic sub-groups. *J. Stud. Alcohol.* 37:986–989, 1976.

75. Hague, W.H., Donovan, D.M., and O'Leary, M.R. Personality characteristics related to treatment decisions among inpatient alcoholics: a non-relationship. *J. Clin. Psychol.* 32:476–479, 1976.

76. O'Leary, M.R., Donovan, D.M., and Hague, W.H. Relationship between locus of control and defensive style among alcoholics. *J. Clin. Psychol.* 31:360–363, 1975.

77. Jacobson, G.R. *The Alcoholisms: Detection, Diagnosis, and Assessment.* New York: Human Sciences Press, 1976.

78. Neuringer, C., and Goldstein, B. The use of psychological tests for the study of the identification, prediction, and treatment of alcoholism, in Goldstein, J., and Neuringer, C. (eds.), *Empirical Studies of Alcoholism.* Cambridge, Mass.: Ballinger, 1976, pp. 7–30.

79. Delahaye, S. An analysis of clients using alcoholism agencies within one community service, in Madden, J.S., Walker, R., and Kenyon, W.H. (eds.), *Alcoholism and Drug Dependence.* New York: Plenum Press, 1977, pp. 335–350.

80. Edwards, G., Kyle, E., and Nocholls, P. Alcoholics admitted to four hospitals in England. *Q. J. Stud. Alcohol.* 35:499–522, 1974.

81. English, G.E., and Curtin, M.E. Personality differences in patients at three alcoholism treatment agencies. *J. Stud. Alcohol.* 36:52–61, 1975.

82. Moos, R.H., Mehren, B., and Moos, B.S. Evaluation of a Salvation Army Alcoholism Treatment Program. *J. Stud. Alcohol.* 39:1217–1225, 1978.

83. Orford, J.A., Hawker, A., and Nicholls, P. An investigation of an alcoholism rehabilitative halfway house. I. Types of clients and modes of discharge. *Brit. J. Addict.* 69:213–224, 1974.

84. Orford, J.A., Hawker, A., and Nicholls, P. An investigation of an alcoholism rehabilitative halfway house. IV. Attractions of the halfway house for residents. *Brit. J. Addict.* 70:179–186, 1975.

85. Tomsovic, M. Hospitalized alcoholic patients. A two-year study of medical, social and psychological characteristics. *Hosp. & Comm. Psychiat.* 19:197–204, 1968.

86. Hart, L. Rehabilitation need patterns of men alcoholics. *J. Stud. Alcohol.* 38:494–511, 1977.

87. Kammeier, M.L., Lucero, R.J., and Anderson, D.J. Events of crucial importance during alcoholism treatment as reported by patients: a preliminary study. *Q. J. Stud. Alcohol.* 34:1172–1189, 1973.

88. Pisani, V.D. Assessing inpatient attitudes toward an alcoholism treatment center. *Q. J. Stud. Alcohol.* 30:640–644, 1969.

89. Price, R.H., Curlee-Salisbury, J. Patient-treatment interactions among alcoholics. *J. Stud. Alcohol.* 36:659–669, 1975.

90. Ogborne, A.C. Patient characteristics as predictors of treatment outcome for alcohol and drug abuse, in Israel, Y. (ed.), *Research Advances in Alcohol and Drug Problems*. New York: Plenum Press, 1978, pp. 177–223.

91. Bromet, E., Moos, R.H., and Bliss, F. The social climate of alcoholism treatment programs. *Arch. Gen. Psychiat.* 33:910–916, 1976.

92. Bromet, E., Moos, R.H., Bliss, R., and Wuthman, C. The post-treatment functioning of alcoholic patients: its relation to program participation. *J. Consult. Clin. Psychol* (In press).

93. Blacker, E. Training for professionals and non-professionals in alcoholism, in Kissin, B., and Begleiter, H. (eds.), *The Biology of Alcoholism. Vol. 5 Treatment and Rehabilitation of the Chronic Alcoholic.* New York: Plenum Press, 1977, pp. 567–592.

94. Blume, S. Role of the recovered alcoholic in the treatment of alcoholism, in Kissin, B., and Begleiter, H. (eds.), *The Biology of Alcoholism. Vol. 5 Treatment and Rehabilitation of the Chronic Alcoholic.* New York: Plenum Press, 1977, pp. 545–563.

95. Cahn, S. *The Treatment of Alcoholics: An Evaluation Study.* New York: Oxford University Press, 1970.

96. Einstein, S., and Wolfson, E. Alcoholism curricula: how professionals are trained. *Int. J. Addict.* 5:295–307, 1970.

97. Staub, G.E., and Kent, L.M. *The Para-Professional in the Treatment of Alcoholism.* Edited by Staub, G.W., and Kent, L.M. Springfield, Ill.: Charles C. Thomas, 1973.

98. Smart, R.G., Schmidt, W., and Moss, M.K. Social class as a determinant of the type and duration of therapy received by alcoholics. *Int. J. Addict.* 3:543–556, 1969.

99. Pattison, E.M., Sobell, M.B., and Sobell, L.C. *Emerging Concepts of Alcohol Dependence.* New York: Springer, 1977.

100. Pattison, E.M. *Selection of Treatment for Alcoholics.* Piscataway, N.J.: Rutgers University Press, 1979.

101. Edwards, G., Hensman, C., Hawker, A., and Williamson, V. Alcoholics Anonymous: the anatomy of a self-help group. *Soc. Psychiat.* 1:195–204, 1967.

102. Edwards, G., Gisher, M.Y., Hawker, A., and Hensman, C. Clients of alcoholism information centers. *Brit. Med. J.* 4:346–349, 1967.

CHAPTER 14

Lithium Treatment of Alcoholism

MARTIN H. KEELER

INTRODUCTION

Most alcohol dependent patients either do not accept or do not respond to treatment. This generates a demand for new treatment methods. The usual cycle for a treatment is introduction, reports of success usually with unselected patients, general use with unselected patients, reports of failure, and general abandonment but continued use by a small number of treatment facilities. Aversive conditioning, apomorphine in subemetic doses, disulfiram to an extent, and perhaps tricyclic antidepressants and benzodiazepines have gone through this cycle. Lithium is entering the cycle. The cycle works well as a means of avoiding the large scale continuing use of a treatment for inappropriate patients. Unfortunately it works equally well at preventing the identification of patients who would benefit from the treatment. An analogy is useful. A new antibiotic is not tested by comparing it to existing antibiotics or placebo to the broad class of patients who have any infectious disease, but treatments for alcoholism are evaluated by applying them to all alcoholic patients. There is more possibility that specific indications for the use of lithium as a treatment for alcoholism will be missed than that such treatment will be extensively misapplied.

The need to obtain blood samples at regular intervals and monitor serum values of lithium has restrained the extensive prescription of lithium to alcoholics. This was the situation despite the belief that lithium, if properly controlled, caused fewer and less serious unwanted effects than did tricyclic antidepressants or benzodiazepines. Recent studies indicate that long term lithium use is often associated with interstitial fibrosis of the renal distal convoluted tubules and with decreased urinary concentrating ability that does not always reverse itself when lithium treatment is discontinued.[1,2] If lithium protects a patient from killing himself, undoing his life's accomplishments during a manic episode, living in an intolerable up and down mood state, or even drastic psychological, physical, or social damage, calculated risk of renal toxicity can be justified. Lithium, however, can no longer be described on the basis that it does no harm so it does not make much difference if it does no good. The chronic toxicity of lithium probably excedes that of tricyclic antidepressants, benzodiazepines, and disulfiram.

PRESENT USE OF LITHIUM

Lithium is the treatment of choice for manic episodes.[3] It is the treatment of choice for decreasing the frequency and severity of episodes of mood disorders among patients with bipolar affective disorders.[4] Lithium and tricyclic drugs are equal as protection against depression among such patients but lithium is more effective than tricyclic drugs as a means of preventing manic episodes. It is an effective treatment for depression that occurs as part of bipolar affective disorder. Both lithium and tricyclic drugs are equally effective and more effective than placebo as means of preventing depressive episodes among patients with unipolar recurrent depressive disorder.[5] Lithium has been reported to decrease aggression.[6] Part of this may be related to lithium preventing the irritable or paranoid-destructive variant of hypomania or mania. It is often forgotten and almost as often rediscovered that mania can manifest itself by irritability and aggression as well as by elation and grandiosity.

RATIONALES FOR THE USE OF LITHIUM TO TREAT ALCOHOLISM

Mood disturbance precipitates or aggravates drinking

An obvious reason to use lithium to treat alcoholism is the assumption that episodes of mood disorder precipitate or aggravate drinking. Lithium can decrease the frequency and severity of such episodes and so would decrease drinking. It might be argued that patients with bipolar or unipolar affective disorder would receive lithium whether or not they were alcoholic or lithium would not be utilized as a treatment for alcoholism. Not all patients with unipolar or bipolar affective disorders receive lithium because of the risks and difficulties of such treatment. If lithium also relieved alcoholism among patients with alcoholism and a recurrent mood disorder this would be reason to administer it to more such patients.

An associated question is whether an appreciable number of alcoholics have unipolar or bipolar affective disorder. Such disorder must be diagnosed using strict criteria. A manic depression or a manic episode should be observed. If less strict criteria are used most alcoholics can be diagnosed as depressed. Rates as high as 71%[8], 75%[9], and 98%[10] have been reported on this basis. Most such depression responds equally to tricyclic antidepressants and placebo and as such does not indicate unipolar or bipolar disorder. In the study in which 71% of patients would be diagnosed as depressed by loose standards only 8.6% could be diagnosed as having depression of the type justifying pharmacological treatment.

There is evidence that unipolar recurrent depressive illness is present at a higher rate among alcoholics than among the general population.[11,12] One study has demonstrated a rate of occurrence of both diagnosis that excedes chance alone. Studies involving patient diagnoses are difficult to evaluate.

If depression is detected after alcoholism and both reported the inevitable inclusion of some alcohol precipitated transient depression will increase the rate of coincidence. If any depression occurring in an alcoholic is considered secondary to alcoholism, patients with genuine unipolar or bipolar disorder may be excluded when excessive drinking accompanies and masks an initial episode of mood disorder. There are genetic studies[13] which definitely demonstrate a linkage between alcoholism and unipolar depressive disorder.

One such study demonstrates an increased incidence of depression among the female relatives of male alcoholics. This indicates linkage and also suggests that there is a condition which manifests itself by depression in women and by alcoholism in men.

The more rigorous studies indicate no increased rate of bipolar affective disorder among alcoholics.[14,15] Studies involving patient diagnoses would miss such a coincidence even if it were present because any affective episode or disorder diagnosed after alcoholism would be considered secondary and not diagnosed as bipolar or unipolar disorder. In one study based on interviewing 507 relatives of alcoholic probands only two had experienced a manic episode, but 78 had had a depressive episode. It is possible that alcoholism and bipolar illness may occur together with increased frequency among hospitalized alcoholics on the basis that the two conditions together are likely to precipitate hospitalization.

Lithium blocks desired reactions to alcohol

The use of lithium as a treatment for alcoholism derives from the concept that it might decrease desired reaction or cause unpleasant reactions from drinking. There is evidence that some desired effects of alcohol are triggered by the release of catechol amines after drinking.[16] Some studies of the interaction of central adrenergic symptoms and drinking indicate that lithium and alcohol have opposite effects on the release of central adrenergic transmitters.[17] Several studies indicate that lithium decreases the voluntary consumption of alcohol by rats.[18,19] These studies do not state the blood levels of alcohol at which this effect occurs so extrapolation to human subjects is difficult but such studies do provide impetus to study the interaction of lithium and alcohol in human subjects.

There is an anecdotal report that lithium decreases alcohol "highs".[20] Judd and his colleagues[21] conducted a controlled study of lithium effect on a response to alcohol employing non-alcoholic subjects. Lithium serum levels varied from .7 to 1.3 mEq/liter and blood alcohol levels from .7 to 1.53mEq/liter. Lithium neither blocked nor decreased desired responses to alcohol. The same group conducted an essentially similar study of lithium and pentobarbital. This study indicated that subjects who received lithium had lower values for positive subjective sensation both before and after receiving pentobarbital than did those who received placebo and then pentobarbital.[22] The authors concluded that lithium did not decrease pentobarbital's effects but these started from a lower baseline. This lithium dysphoria or lack of euphoria might cause difficulties in patients' compliance with taking lithium.

It has been reported that patients receiving lithium report decreased response to amphetamine.[23] In a well controlled study, lithium did decrease amphetamine caused activation and euphoria. The subjects were severely depressed. The decrease of positive response to amphetamine by severely depressed patients cannot be equated to a decrease in positive response to alcohol by non-depressed patients.

There is a theoretical basis for lithium antagonizing alcohol induced euphoria. Lithium decreased alcohol consumption by rats. Studies fail to demonstrate that lithium decreased desired effects of alcohol in human subjects. If lithium does decrease such effects this might lead to the use of an increased amount of alcohol to overcome this partial blockade rather than decreased use. It is possible that lithium might cause unpleasant reactions to alcohol. If so there might be as much difficulty in persuading patients to take lithium as there is in persuading them to take disulfiram. Added to these considerations is the fact that lithium produces unpleasant effects which would further decrease patient compliance with taking the drug.

Lithium may decrease withdrawal reactions after alcohol use

There is evidence from animal and human studies that lithium may decrease certain aspects of withdrawal from alcohol. One theory of the cause of alcoholism is that alcoholics have experienced extremely unpleasant withdrawal reactions and once they have started drinking are afraid, consciously or unconsciously, to stop lest these unpleasant reactions recur.[24] By attenuating such reactions, lithium would permit them to stop drinking. Benzodiazepines also decrease withdrawal reactions after alcohol use.[25,26] There is no comparative study of lithium and benzodiazepines in this respect but it is likely that the benzodiazepines are more effective. Benzodiazepines have some dependency-inducing potential and most have additive or synergistic effects with alcohol, but the renal toxicity problems associated with chronic use of lithium excede the chronic toxicity of benzodiazepines. Benzodiazepines have not proven to be an effective treatment for alcoholism despite their attentuation of alcohol withdrawal symptoms so it would have to be established that lithium does have such action.

Lithium may produce a taste aversion to alcohol

Lithium has been reported to cause a taste aversion to alcohol in animals. The only reports of lithium taste aversion in human subjects refer to butterfat and certain vegetables and do not mention alcohol.[27,28] No systematic studies have been reported. Complaints of lithium-induced changes in taste are not common. There is no good reason to suspect that lithium causes appreciable taste aversion to alcohol in human subjects.

CLINICAL STUDIES OF THE USE OF LITHIUM TO TREAT ALCOHOLISM

Kline, Wren, Cooper, Varga, and Canal[29] treated alcoholics with lithium or placebo for 48 weeks using double blind procedures. Their patients were reported as depressed at the onset and having neither unipolar nor bipolar affective disorder. Thirty of seventy-three (41%) completed the study. The only criteria for alcoholism was hospitalization resulting from excessive drinking. Of those who completed the study 4 of 16 who received lithium and 9 of 14 who received placebo were rehospitalized during the study. This difference is significant at p<.05. Lithium and placebo had equal influence on depression as determined by the Zung Self-Rating Depression Scale.

Merry, Reynolds, Bailey, and Cooper[30] administered either lithium or placebo for six weeks to 71 patients, half of whom, equally distributed in the lithium and placebo groups, were depressed as determined by clinical interview and the Beck Inventory. Most of the patients probably had neither unipolar nor bipolar affective disorder. Thirty-eight (53%) equally distributed between the lithium and placebo groups completed the study. Outcome in terms of alcoholism was determined by asking patients how many days they drank at all and how many days they had been incapacitated by drinking. There were no differences, during the six weeks studied, in the nondepressed group between those who received lithium and those who received placebo. The depressed patients who received lithium reported significantly fewer days of drinking and significantly fewer days of incapacitation caused by drinking than did the depressed patients who received placebo. There were no significant differences between lithium and placebo effect on depression.

Kline, Bennet, Calobrisi, Cooper, Neidengaard and Snyder[31] described a double-blind study with 172 patients neither selected for nor excluding nor testing for initial depression. The study lasted one year and 17% of those who started the study completed it. The only outcome criteria was presence or absence of hospitalization for alcohol withdrawal. Those who completed the study who received lithium did significantly better than those who completed the study and received placebo.

Young and Keeler[32] described the treatment, using lithium, of fifteen patients with bipolar affective disorder and histories of excessive drinking. Treatment was initiated immediately after recovery from an observed manic episode and continued for six months. Eight patients had neither disabling alcoholism nor affective symptoms during this period but five of these patients also required tricyclic drugs or disulfiram. Seven patients had some alcohol caused disability and two of these also had exacerbation of affective disorder.

It is possible to derive some hypothesis from these reports despite the differences in subjects and the methodologies employed:

1. The usual outcome criteria for alcoholism should be applied. Outcome should be evaluated for at least one year and measures of daily use as well as of incapacitation are required.

2. Patients with bipolar illness should be studied separately. Their responses appear to differ from those of other patients.
3. Patients with unipolar recurrent depressive illness should be studied as such. It is probable that some such patients were included in both Kline's studies and in Merry's study but the numbers are uncertain.
4. Most patients will continue to take neither lithium nor a placebo but those who continue to take lithium do better in terms of alcoholism. An explanation for this may be the methodologies used screen out a group whose alcoholism improves with lithium treatment. It must be repeated that this has been demonstrated only in one study which lasted only six weeks and in two studies in which rehospitalization was the only outcome measure.

DISCUSSION

The use of lithium as a treatment for alcoholism requires administration on a chronic basis. Such use thus depends on risk-benefit factors. The initial use of lithium as a treatment for alcoholism was based on the assumption of negligible toxicity. Present knowledge of lithium induced renal interstitial fibrosis and irreversible loss of urinary concentrating ability changes the situation. Lithium is still a relatively safe treatment but the real and predictable risks require a definite benefit that cannot be attained by other treatment.

Lithium is good treatment for patients with bipolar affective disorder. An accompanying history of disabling alcoholism gives increased reason to utilize lithium for such patients. It is superior to tricyclic drugs or placebo in decreasing the frequency and severity of bouts of mania. Hypomania and mania may aggravate or precipitate excessive drinking.

Lithium is a treatment for patients with unipolar recurrent depressive disorder and excessive drinking. It is equal to tricyclic drugs and more effective than placebo in decreasing the frequency and severity of depressive episodes among such patients. If effect against alcoholism is mediated only by antidepressant effect, the greater safety of the tricyclic drugs would make them preferable to lithium as a treatment for patients with unipolar affective disorder and alcoholism until controlled studies demonstrate otherwise. The early reports of the ineffectiveness of tricyclic drugs as a treatment for alcoholism in unselected patients did not demonstrate that such treatment was ineffective for patients with unipolar recurrent affective disorder and alcoholism.

There is no clear evidence from clinical trends that lithium is an effective treatment for alcoholism when depression is not present and one study reports that it is ineffective in this circumstance. The only controlled study of lithium effect on reaction to alcohol indicates that lithium neither blocks nor diminishes desired reactions to alcohol.

Even if lithium did have a slight blocking effect this might be overcome by increased drinking. There is also the problem that lithium causes mild dysphoric effects and some impairment of cognitive function which would make patients unwilling to take it. When all of these are added to the known toxicity of lithium, the conclusion is reached that the lithium treatment of alcoholism not existing in patients with recurrent affective disorders is a matter for clinical investigation rather than clinical practice.

It is impossible to overlook the reports that lithium is reported as having useful effect as a treatment for alcoholism among some patients not identified as having unipolar or bipolar disorders. This was more apt to occur if the patients are depressed. It occurred in the patients who took lithium on a long-term basis, which most patients will not do. One hypothesis is that alcoholic patients have undiagnosed unipolar or bipolar affective disease. It is difficult to tell hypomania with alcoholism from a severe bout of drinking. Alcoholism so often precipitates depression that it is possible to miss the relatively few instances in which depression precipitates alcoholism. Some diagnostic practice considers all affective disorder that occurs subsequent to the diagnosis of alcoholism to be secondary. It is thus possible that there are a considerable number of alcoholics who have undiagnosed bipolar or unipolar affective disorder and who would benefit by lithium treatment. It is necessary, in this regard, to repeat that those with unipolar disorder might benefit by treatment with the less toxic tricyclic antidepressants.

It lithium treatment is of some help to as many as 5% of alcoholics this should not be overlooked. If the evaluations of lithium as a treatment for alcoholism prompts a re-examination of the use of tricyclic drugs as a treatment of alcoholism this too is important.

REFERENCES

1. Hestbech, J., Hansen, H.E., Amdisen, A., et al. Chronic renal lesions following long-term treatment with lithium. *Kidney Int.* 12:205–213, 1977.
2. Burrows, G.D., Davis, B., Kincaid-Smith, P. Unique tubular lesions after lithium. *Lancet* 1:1310, 1978.
3. Prien, R.F., Caffrey, E.M., and Klett, C.J. Comparison of lithium and chlorpromazine in the treatment of mania. *Arch. Gen. Psychiat.* 26:146–153, 1972.
4. Davis, J.M. Maintenance therapy in psychiatry II: affective disorders. *Am. J. Psychiat.* 133:1–13, 1976.

5. Baastrup, P.C., Poulsen, J.C., Schou, M., et al. Prophylactic lithium: Double blind discontinuation in manic depressive and recurrent depressive disorders. *Lancet* 2, 326–329, 1970.
6. Sheard, M.H., Marini, J.L., Bridges, C.I., et al. The long term use of lithium in aggressive prisoners. *Compr. Psychiat.* 14:311–317, 1973.
7. Murphy, D.L., Beigel, A. Depression, elation, and lithium carbonate responses in manic patient subgroups. *Arch. Gen. Psychiat.* 31:647–648, 1974.
8. Keeler, M.H., Taylor, C.I., and Miller, W. Diagnostic criteria for depression among alcoholics. *Currents in Alcoholism* 4, 1968.
9. Weingold, H.P., Lachin, J.M., Bill, A.H., et al. Depression as a symptom of alcoholism. *J. Am. Psychology* 33:195–197, 1968.
10. Shaw, J.A., Donley, P., Morgan, W., et al. Treatment of depression in alcoholism. *Am. J. Psychiat.* 132:641–644, 1975.
11. Winokur, G., Reich, T., Rimmer, J., et al. Alcoholism III: Diagnosis and familial psychiatric illness in 159 alcoholic probands. *Arch. Gen. Psychiat.* 23:104–111, 1970.
12. Winokur, G., and Clayton, P. Family history studies: IV. Comparison of male and female alcoholics. *Q. J. Stud. Alcohol.* 29:885–891, 1968.
13. Winokur, G., Rimmer, J., Reich, T. Alcoholism IV: Is there more than one type of alcoholism? *Brit. J. Psychiat.* 118:525–31, 1971.
14. Woodruff, R.A., Guze, S.B., Clayton, P.J., et al. Alcoholism and depression. *Arch. Gen. Psychiat.* 28:97–100, 1973.
15. James, N., Chapman, C.J. A genetic study of bipolar affective disorder. *Brit. J. Psychiat.* 125:496–499, 1974.
16. Truitt, E.B., and Wash, M.J. Role of acetaldehyde in the actions of ethanol, in Kissen, B.J., and Begleiter, H. (eds.), *The Biology of Alcoholism, Vol I: Biochemistry,* Chap. 5. New York: Plenum Press, 1971.
17. Schou, M. Pharmacology and toxicology of lithium. *Ann. Rev. Pharmacol.* 16:231–243, 1976.
18. Ho, A.K.S., and Tsai, C.S. Lithium and ethanol preference. *J. Pharm. Pharmac.* 27:58–60, 1975.
19. Ho, A.K.S., and Tsai, C.S. Effects of lithium on alcohol preference and withdrawal. *Ann. N.Y. Acad. Sci.* 371–377, 1976.
20. Flemenbaum, A. Affective disorders and chemical dependence: lithium for alcohol and drug addiction. *Dis. Nerv. Syst.* 35:281, 1974.
21. Judd, L.L., Hubbard, B., Huey, L.Y., at al. Lithium carbonate and ethanol induced "highs" in normal subjects. *Arch. Gen. Psychiat.* 34:463–467, 1977.
22. Judd, L.L., Hubbard, R., and Attewell, P.A. The effects of lithium carbonate upon subjective state changes induced by sodium pentobarbital. *Psychopharmacology Communications* 1(6), 631–639, 1975.
23. Flemenbaum, A. Does lithium block the effects of amphetamines: a report of three cases. *Am. J. Psychiat.* 820:7, 1974.
24. McCloud, L.D. The "craving" for alcohol: symposium. *Q. J. Stud. Alcohol.* 16:34–66, 1955.
25. Sellers, E.M., Cooper, S.D., Sen, A.K., et al. Lithium treatment of alcoholic withdrawal. *Clin. Pharm. Ther.* 15(2):212, 1974.
26. Woodruff, R.A., Guze, S.B., Clayton, P.J., et al. Alcoholism and depression. *Arch. Gen. Psychiat.* 28:97–100, 1973.
27. Duffield, J.E. Side effects of lithium carbonate. *Brit. Med. J.* 1:491, 1973.
28. Himmelhoch, J.M., and Hanin, I. Side effects of lithium carbonate. *Brit. Med. J.* 4:233, 1974.

29. Kline, N.S., Wren, J.C., Cooper, T.B., et al. Evaluation of lithium therapy in chronic and periodic alcoholism. *Am. J. Med. Sci.* 268:15–22, 1964.
30. Merry, J., Reynolds, C.M., and Barley, J. Prophylactic treatment of alcoholism by lithium. *Lancet* 2:481–482, 1976.
31. Kline, N.S., Bennett, J., Calobrisi, A. et al. Lithium in the treatment of chronic alcoholism (Unpublished).
32. Young, L.D., and Keeler, M.H. Sobering data on lithium in alcoholism (letter). *Lancet* 1:144, 1977.

CHAPTER 15

Countertransference in the Treatment of the Alcoholic Patient

DAVID W. KRUEGER

INTRODUCTION

Medical professionals frequently misdiagnose and mismanage the alcoholic patient due to the professional's own attitudes and countertransferences as well as a lack of understanding of the syndrome of alcoholism. A study of 800 medical professionals revealed that 15 of every 20 were bothered by some emotional impact of alcoholism which rendered them unable to deal effectively with this problem.[1] Reasons for the above finding included training, unresolved alcoholism in the medical professional's family, negative experiences with previous alcoholic patients, and a rigid personality structure precluding emotional empathy.[1] Often a vague and largely unrecognized cynicism, discomfort, or sense of hopelessness may exist regarding the alcoholic patient and/or his family.[1] More effective treatment of alcoholism requires that these underlying aspects of subtle attitudes, countertransferences, and expectations be recognized, differentiated, and subjected to scrutiny and new evidence.

The study and understanding of countertransference phenomenon should have much wider berth than analytically based therapy; this chapter considers a broader range of applicability and necessity for recognition in treatments, including supportive and pharmacologic.

Alcoholics constitute a difficult patient population. Patients who abuse drugs, including alcohol, are more likely than nonabusing patients to be critical and defiant, to alienate others, and to resist cooperation when in treatment.[2] The countertransference potential of this behavior on most therapists is readily apparent. Because of the ego-syntonic element of drinking behavior these patients may evoke reactions in the therapist ranging from direct reactions to the drinking behavior, to the alienating characteristics which are provoking, to more subtle reactions which are far from obvious counterreactions to the patient's character pathology.

Countertransference in the treatment of alcoholic patients is seldom mentioned in the literature, perhaps due partly to the association of countertransference feelings with shame or guilt in the therapist. Countertransference may imply to many therapists a contraindicated set of reactions to the patient which should be taboo and thus be avoided in a phobic manner. It is viewed as a professional sin rather than as a guide to deeper understanding.

A more complete understanding of the patient is the result of freely working attention and emotional sensitivity in the therapist to perceive empathetically and identify emotional movement and unconscious fantasies.[3] The emotional sensitivity of the therapist includes the *necessity* for countertransference and its awareness for a thorough therapeutic endeavor.[4]

The use of the term countertransference varies from the conception of an inclusive definition of all feelings and attitudes of the therapist toward his patient[5] to more specific use in which countertransference is seen as the unconscious reaction of the therapist to specific transference phenomenon in the patient. Implicit in this latter position is the use of countertransference as the *counterpart* in the therapist to the transference in the patient.[6] In this paper the term countertransference will correspond with the latter usage, specifically as a transference parallel in the therapist which is a counterpart to the transference reaction in the patient. Countertransference is, in this sense, analogous to the function of controls in a scientific study, emphasizing the counterpart and parallel processes of patient transference/therapist countertransference. This more limited usage affords more specificity of response in the understanding of certain issues in the patients which, when their component parts are recognized in the therapist, may provide additional therapeutic understanding and leverage in addition to the content and process communication of the patient. It likewise bestows the possibility of leading to a misunderstanding of inappropriate response toward the patient if it remains unconscious in the therapist. Countertransference as the complement to transference gives precision to the concept, and divides the interrelated concepts of countertransference, the real relationship, the working alliance, and transference reactions on the part of the therapist toward the patient.[7]

Obviously not *all* responses of the therapist to the patient are countertransferential in origin, but only those which are responses to the transference reaction of the patient in the therapeutic situation.[8]
The important question then is whether the countertransference has been *recognized, understood,* and *utilized* by the therapist. The utilization of countertransference has much wider application than analytic therapy alone, as this paper considers the utilization in a broader scope of therapeutic approaches, including supportive treatment. Obviously only a very limited number of alcoholic patients may have analytic therapy prescribed.

Countertransference is constantly present in therapeutic work as a normal phenomenon[9] and has been called a necessary prerequisite for therapeutic work and thoroughness in understanding the patient.[4,10] Countertransference reactions may point to specific contents, mechanisms, anxieties, or other characteristics which may elucidate the patient's psychological events.[11]

There may be relatively little problem with objectivity by the therapist as long as the material and fantasies from the patient are about external events which do not directly involve the therapist. However, the therapist becomes more prone to countertransference when he becomes the object of attack or of fantasy.[12]

While the broad span of psychopathologies underlying alcoholism are complex,[13,14] we are specifically concerned here with the more common issues in the patient-physician relationship which produce certain *predictable countertransference reactions* in working with the alcoholic patient which can be therapeutic or antitherapeutic depending on their recognition, understanding, and implementation.

ATTITUDES, TRANSFERENCES TO THE PATIENT, AND INADEQUATE INFORMATION VS. COUNTERTRANSFERENCE

Attitudes

The differentiation of the therapist's response ranges from a diagnosis of (1) countertransference reactions to the alcoholic patient, (2) transference reactions to the alcoholic patient with a preset or predetermined set of attitudes, expectations, and feelings, and (3) lack of information and education regarding the treatment of the alcoholic.

The initial distinction between a therapist's basic attitudes toward the alcoholic should be made. An extensive survey showed inconsistent attitudes and behavior in rejecting the disease concept in alcoholism.

While advocating psychiatric treatment, treatment benefits were considered to be extremely limited. Therapists were as well very reluctant to participate themselves in rendering this treatment.[15] Another survey of physician's attitudes and approaches toward the treatment of alcoholism reports that 35% of physicians studied stated that they *avoided* alcoholics as patients.[16] This study established the existence of significant negative emotional attitudes toward alcoholism as well as some degree of ignorance regarding treatment programs. The conclusion reached was that these negative attitudes were of sufficient magnitude to interfere both with the identification of the alcoholic and subsequent therapy of the alcoholic. Physicians tend not to diagnose alcoholism in patients who have definite and serious problems with alcohol if the patient is married, voluntarily comes for help, has a medical problem which should be focused on by the physician, is employed, or has health insurance.[17,18] The therapist's attitude that the alcoholic is untreatable and therefore hopeless may be accusingly rationalized as "lack of motivation" or "lack of will-power" on the patient's part.

Recognition of the therapist's basic attitudes toward alcoholism is important to recognize, and some therapists may have such deep-seated and fixed resentments that their treating of alcoholism would be precluded and a referral indicated. The recognition of an attitude that the alcoholic patient is hopeless, is simply not accepting responsibilities, is not exerting sufficient will-power, or is just self-inflicting this behavior for some secondary gratification are clues which should be rigorously scrutinized by the therapist within himself.

It is also well-known that therapists' and physicians' attitudes often vary little from those of the general public regarding alcoholism and treatability, as well as the impugned judgment regarding alcoholism and the alcoholic.[18] These preset and predetermined attitudes of the therapist, thus technically the transference of the therapist onto an alcoholic patient (rather than the specific counter-part reactions to a patient's transference) should be distinguished.

Transferences to the Patient

Responses, attitudes, and expectations which are both characterological kinds of problems, perhaps even the same form, are not characteristics of countertransference, but they may be characteristics of "transferences" in the therapist, including unresolved aspects of the therapist's own unconscious.[4] This lack of specificity to a certain patient, communication, or dynamic meaning makes the response not only unhelpful but detrimental to treatment as well. Thus, deficiencies or defects in the therapist's experience, knowledge, perceptions of patient communication, and transferences to the patient may be incorrectly labeled "countertransference".[4]

The distinction should be made between the therapist's transference reactions to his patients, derived from unconscious unresolved conflicts which generate distorted and inappropriate responses, and the more specific "counter" reaction to the patient's transference, appropriately called countertransference. Both strong countertransference reactions and transference difficulties unrecognized within the therapist interfere with the working alliance with the patient, and both disturb the therapist's capacity for empathy, but the therapist's transferences to the patient imply a more pervasive and unworkable problem, specifically one which does not yield information about the particular counterpart reaction in the patient at a specific time. The kinds of deep and abiding counterproductive biases and attitudes, disguised perhaps as "experience", speaks incisively to the early working alliance with an alcoholic patient.

Inadequate Information

Countertransference reactions must also be distinguished from inadequate information and incorrect understanding of the patient's material. Frustration and anger at patients may be created by insufficient information combined with unrealistic or omnipotent expectations of permanent abstinence. Both therapist and patient may share reactions of failure, hopelessness, guilt, and anger at the failure of this abstinence as the sole criterion for successful treatment. This basic failure to recognize the chronicity of alcoholism is thus a mixture of educational and dynamic misunderstanding.[15] There has been recommendation for getting physicians and therapists into a learning situation which would allow them to become aware of the lack of knowledge about alcoholism, about antitherapeutic attitudes toward alcoholics, and even about the extent of their own drinking problems.[1]

Countertransferences in Treatment

Countertransference phenomena are by definition as multiple and varied as the counterpart transference phenomenon arising from the patient, and as the various personalities of the individual therapists and patients. Both phenomena may change from patient to patient and even

from day to day within the same patient. The evidence of countertransference may occur in various forms, but some of the more common
manifestations include stereotyped feelings or behavior, feelings or
responses of love or hate, erotic preoccupations, persistence of affects (i.e.,
anxiety, depression) after the therapeutic hour, feeling argumentative with
the patient, dreams about the patient, feeling the patient must get better
for the doctor, being afraid of losing the patient, difficulty in detecting
certain material and drowsiness or boredom within the hour.[4,6] There are,
however, some transference reactions which seem particular to the
treatment of alcoholic patients and appear with some consistency. We will
consider these responses individually.

Denial

Denial may be the major defense mechanism operative in the
personality of the alcoholic, particularly in the denial of the nature, extent,
and effects of drinking behavior. A common countertransference reaction
is the therapist's own unconscious denial colluding with that of the
patient, especially if the patient is well-to-do, intelligent, and married.[18]

Acceptance of the patient's denial and rationalization, consciously or
unconsciously, reflects countertransference feelings regarding the avoidance of confrontation of this denial and of the critical necessity of
intervention to disrupt the life-threatening illness of alcoholism. The
aspect of helpessness in dealing with problems, especially drinking, on the
part of the patient may be the result of attributing difficulties or projecting
blame to some external component of the patient's world. This denial of
responsibility may become reflected in the therapist's attitudes or
unconscious expectations, resulting in pessimistic expectations of change,
as well as the minimization of the extent or impact of drinking.

The denial may be exemplified by the therapy of a patient who, while
being extremely well-to-do and successful in her own right, was in analytic
therapy originally for problems other than alcoholism. During the course
of therapy as her denial softened, the patient talked increasingly of the
major role and significance of alcohol in her pathology. As the therapist
continued to focus on the dynamic underpinnings and meaning of related
aspects of her pathology, the patient one day brought a fifth of bourbon,
pulled it out of her purse, and set it on the corner of the therapist's desk.
She stated, "I wanted to show you this so that both of us wouldn't
continue to deny my drinking."

A related problem has been the demonstration that physicians in the
United States have high rates of alcoholism themselves.[19] There has been

substantiation for the supposedly facetious statement defining an alcoholic as anyone who drinks more than his physician, as there is a denial of the diagnosis of alcoholism demonstrated in those patients who actually do report less drinking than the physician, yet have objective alcoholism.[19] The denial by the patient of the extent of his alcoholism offers a convenient hitchhiking vehicle for the countertransference denial in the physician or therapist.

Anger, Guilt, Withdrawal

A consistently seen psychodynamic characteristic of alcoholic patients is an entanglement of passive-dependent wishes, a concomitant need to control a need-fulfilling object, and manifestation of anger when this need is thwarted.[20,21] The consensus regarding therapeutic approach is an attempt to meet this need constructively.[22] Certain alcoholic patients may lack the integrated ego function to soothe or calm themselves and thus insulate against over-stimulation.[23] This inability to internally supply tension-reducing gratification results in turning to an external method: alcohol and/or the therapist.

The dynamic picture of the personality excessively indulging in alcohol extends from frustration when demands are not met to hostile acts for which he feels guilty and punishes himself masochistically. As re-assurance there is an excessive demand for affection and indulgence.[24] The rage at parents who initially frustrated gratification is later displaced onto alcohol and/or the therapist to achieve both gratification and revenge, resulting in the need for punishment to alleviate guilt when sober.[25] The patient who may be convinced of his badness, that he deserves the guilt and concomitant punishment he experiences, concludes that he will be rejected because of this badness if he seeks help. This may indeed be the case if the physician acts out this expectation by turning the patient away or becoming angry at the patient for drinking.

The potential exists for regressive and at times archaic relationships with the therapist. The boundaries of self and other may be blurred at times. The therapist is needed at these regressive moments to help the patient calm himself, much as the mother has initially provided support for self-comforting activities, rather than resort to the maladaptive use of alcohol.

The patient's environment may be characterized by its tendency to fulfill his unconscious aims and expectations, by which, for example, a person who feels unloved will manage unconsciously to make himself so disagreeable, demanding, and unlovable as to fulfill this fear. The therapeutic situation is partly defined as a different reaction, in that the therapist will not gratify totally this attempt on the patient's part and not supply the answer he is expecting. If the therapist does, however, play into the patient's pathology by becoming critical, rejecting, and "unloving" based on the patient's characterological difficulties and/or alcoholism per se, therapy has indeed become a replica of other situations in the patient's life.

A frequent transference/countertransference phenomenon in treatment of alcoholics is the patient's view of the therapist as his own superego, particularly the harsh and punitive aspects of that superego. The countertransference recognition of the possibility of manifesting critical, angry, and judgmental responses, especially regarding drinking behavior, is essential, as these responses would perpetuate a vicious cycle of drinking, anxiety due to guilt, and further punitive retribution for this behavior.

The therapist's withdrawal at the time of a patient's unheaval and an exacerbation of drinking behavior is an example of how the unconscious of the patient and the unconscious of the therapist might respond to one another. The alcoholic's self-hatred, guilt, depression and isolation are especially poignant at times of drinking[26] and may be transferred to the treating person. It is especially important to recognize these feelings and behaviors emanating from the patient and not withdraw from or criticize the patient at these times.

The capacity of the alcoholic patient to provoke a number of basically hostile countertransference reactions is well-known. One manifestation may be the referral of the patient to another therapist, or a referral for a group therapy under the guise of the patient needing "confrontation". Such a referral may mask a hostile wish toward a narcissistic patient that the group members would verbally retaliate in ways which the therapist would feel inhibited from doing, with the obvious motive of ridding himself of the troublesome patient.[27]

One of the most important factors deterring confrontation in an intervention with alcoholic patients is that the therapist's efforts will initially be met by anger and denial.[26] Non-intervention (thus, technically a countertransference avoidance) is justified by the therapist with the reasoning that confrontation about alcoholism or even broaching the subject of drinking will result in a patient's insultation, anger, and avoidance of further contact with the therapist.

Threatened Omnipotence

The rejection or nonrecognition of countertransference issues by the therapist may represent the rejection of the therapist's own unresolved struggle with anxiety and guilt with a residual amount of infantile omnipotence which dictates that the patient would absolutely comply with the orders of the therapist. This residue of omnipotent fantasy, when shown to be fallable, culminates in an unconscious rage at the patient who defies the therapist's knowledge and request.

Therapists who would never consider confronting a psychotic, neurotic, or character disorder patient with symptoms as *his fault* and controllable if he would only so *will,* glibly hurl these accusations at alcoholic patients. This may reflect a countertransference to a controlling and omnipotent fantasy in the patient of being able to drink despite the best efforts of people in their life, including the therapist. One patient angrily stated that neither her husband, lover, nor psychiatrist could keep her from drinking if she so decided. A countertransferential anger toward the patient can result when therapeutic omnipotence is assaulted verbally and directly or indirectly by refusal to comply with treatment. The alcoholic patient's resistance to treatment, epitomized by his return to the use of alcohol, represents a frustration for the therapist whose omnipotence is confronted and who may feel that his medical or therapeutic skill is insufficient.

The slow and repetitive nature of the work with alcoholics often provokes discouragement in the therapist. Regressive swings may exasperate the therapist, creating feelings of inadequacy experienced as anger toward the patient. This may be experienced as a defeat of the therapeutic intent or experienced as an assault against his own narcissism.

The recognition of alcoholism as a *treatable disease* should be balanced by setting *realistic expectations* in treating a chronic and perhaps relapsing disease. The often successful treatment of alcoholism is balanced by its chronicity and exacerbation in some patients, sometimes leading to the most marked countertransference reactions by the therapist. The failure of empathy, a transient partial identification with aspects of the patient, may manifest itself as countertransference when working with the chronic and relapsing alcoholic patient. An empathic appreciation of the amount of change implied for an alcoholic not to drink is required; this change represents an extreme life crisis which threatens one of the patient's ways of existing.

Counteridentification

Former alcoholics are heavily represented on staffs working with alcoholic patients. Thus, identification with the patient, reaction-formation on the part of the therapist toward manifestation of both defense and behavior in the patient, and projective identifications of both patient and therapist all compound the technical problems and threaten to erode the neutrality of the therapeutic situation. This issue may be exemplified by an incident in which a staff member, formerly an alcoholic, angrily stormed into an administrative staff meeting after having had an encounter with a "recidivist" alcoholic patient, suggesting that all "dependent alcoholics" be banned to an island exclusively for patients with problems of dependency and alcoholism. Alcoholic patients often too closely afront the denial and reaction formation of therapists who may be struggling with similar issues themselves, and to isolate those issues inside themselves, to an "island" in their psyche.

There is a tendency to displace treatment failure responsibility onto the patient by describing him as unmotivated if he is not willing to immediately give up his symptoms. The patient may be made to feel ashamed or guilty if he does not relinquish his symptoms as a requisite to treatment.

CONCLUSION

Countertransference may be a tool for understanding mental processes of the patient including the content, mechanism, and intensity of the patient's transference reactions. The recognition of the transference-countertransference constellation gives an added dimension to the understanding of the patient and additional information on which to base the type, manner, and timing of the interventions.

The danger and compromise occurs when the therapist does not pay sufficient attention to his own countertransference thoughts, feelings, and fantasies. These responses may then be unavailable for deepening understanding or for use in interpretation *per se* or supportive treatment. The therapist may also respond to countertransference by its nonrecognition and by acting out as a response.

The question of how much faith and reliance to put on countertransference reactions as therapists must be broached. Awareness of countertransference adds another dimension to the data derived from a patient and the process of his communication. However, there may be "blind spots" in the therapist as well as personal idiosyncrasies which may temper the transference-countertransference counterpart equation. One of the most glaring examples is the predetermined attitude of the physician toward the alcoholic patient.

We must also critically examine the deductions made from countertransference perceptions. For example, anger toward the patient may represent an original anger in a patient with a projective identification driven by guilt with an unconscious wish for retaliation. The therapist's task is first to become aware of a countertransference as a particular response toward a patient at a given time then to scrutinize the patient's part in bringing it about at this time and the purpose it serves for the patient, and lastly to contain any action on the part of the therapist which might emanate from this countertransference. By this process these reactions can be utilized for a deepening understanding of the patient. If the countertransference reaction has already transpired at the time of recognition, it is important to assess the effect of this reaction on the patient as additional information.

It is important to note the useful role of discussion, or even consultation in supervision with a colleague, of particular reactions toward an individual patient or toward particular groups of patients which persist despite introspection.

REFERENCES

1. Pursch, J. Physician's attitudinal changes in alcoholism. *Alcoholism: Clin. Exper. Res.* 2:358-361, 1978.
2. Schoolar, J., White, E., and Cohen, C. Drug abusers and their clinic-patient counterparts: a comparison of personality dimensions. *J. Consult. Clin. Psychol.* 39:9-15, 1972.
3. Haimann, P. On countertransference. *Int. J. Psycho-Anal.* 31, 1950.
4. Tower, L. Countertransference. *J. Amer. Psycho. Assoc.* 4:224-255, 1956.
5. Kernberg, O. Notes on countertransference. *J. Amer. Psychoan. Assoc.* 13, 1965.
6. Greenson, R., Loving, hating, and indifference toward the patient. *Int. Rev. Psa.* 1:259-266, 1974.
7. Moeller, M. Self and object in countertransference. *Int. J. Psycho.-Anal.* 58:365-374, 1977.
8. Reich, A. Further remarks on countertransference. *Int. J. Psycho-Anal.* 41: 1960.
9. Spitz, R. Countertransference: comments on its varying role in the analytic situation. *J. Amer. Psychoan. Assoc.* 4:256-265, 1956.
10. Reich, A. On countertransference. *Int. J. Psycho-Anal.* 32:3-7, 1951.
11. Racker, H. A contribution to the problem of countertransference. *Int. J. Psycho-Anal.* 34:313-324, 1953.
12. Glover, E. *The Technique of Psychoanalysis.* New York: International Universities Press, 1955.
13. Devito, R., Flaherty, L., and Mozdzierz, G. Toward a psychodynamic theory of alcoholism. *Dis. Nerv. Syst.* 31:43-49, 1970.
14. Yorke, C. A critical review of some psychoanalytic literature on drug addiction. *Brit. J. Med. Psychol.* 43:141-159, 1970.
15. Knox, W. Attitudes of psychiatrists and psychologists toward alcoholism. *Am. J. Psychiat.* 127:1675-1679, 1971.
16. Fann, W., Decker, N., Sands, P., and Miller, D. Alcoholism in a general hospital population. *Alcoholism.* 2:196, 1978.
17. Chafetz, M. Alcoholism and health professionals. *Psychiatric Annals.* 6:47-55, 1976.

18. Wolfe, I., Chaftez, M., Blane, H., and Hill, M. Social factors in the diagnosis of alcoholism and social and non-social situations. II Attitudes of physicians. *Q. J. Stud. Alcohol.* 26:72, 1965.

19. Chafetz, M. Alcoholism and alcoholic psychoses, in Freedman, A., Kaplan, H., and Sadock, B. (eds.), *Comprehensive Textbook of Psychiatry.* Baltimore: Williams and Wilkins, 1975, pp. 1336–1337.

20. Chafetz, M. Practical and theoretical considerations in the psychotherapy of alcoholism. *Q. J. Stud. Alcohol.* 281–291, 1959.

21. Silber, A. Rationale for the technique of psychotherapy with alcoholics. *Int. J. Psychoanal. Psychother.* 3:28–47, 1974.

22. Gustafson, J. The mirror transference in psychoanalytic psychotherapy of alcoholism: a case report. *Int. J. Psychoanal. Psychother.* 5:65–85, 1976.

23. Kohut, H. *The Analysis of the Self.* New York: International Universities Press, 1971.

24. Knight, R. Psychodynamics of chronic alcoholism. *J. Nerv. Ment. Dis.* 86:538, 1937.

25. Menninger, K. *Man Against Himself.* New York: Harcourt Brace, 1938.

26. DiCicco, L., Unterberger, H., and Mac, J. Confronting denial: an alcoholism intervention strategy. *Psychiat. Annal.* 8:54–64, 1978.

27. Doroff, D. Developing and maintaining the therapeutic alliance with the narcissistic personality. *J. Amer. Acad. Psychoanal.* 4:137–160, 1976.

CHAPTER 16

The Effects of Disulfiram on Peripheral and Central Norepinephrine Metabolism and Blood Pressure

C. RAYMOND LAKE
MICHAEL G. ZIEGLER
F. LESLIE MAJOR
G. LaVONNE BROWN
MICHAEL H. EBERT

INTRODUCTION

In 1948 two Danish physicians became ill at a cocktail party after ingesting disulfiram and subsequently reported on "a drug sensitizing the organism to ethyl alcohol.[1] Disulfiram was soon introduced for the treatment of alcoholism. ETOH is oxidized to acetaldehyde by alcohol dehydrogenase and further metabolized by acetaldehyde dehydrogenase. The drug produces an adverse reaction to ethanol by the inhibition of acetaldehyde dehydrogenase, which causes high blood levels of acetaldehyde shortly after alcohol ingestion.[2,3,4] The resulting acetaldehyde syndrome is characterized by vasodilation, orthostatic hypotension and a pulsating headache, apparently mediated by high blood

229

levels of acetaldehyde, an effective catecholamine releaser.[2,5,6] Disulfiram
by itself can have side effects of fatigue, tremor, reduced sexual potency,
headache, dizziness, and, in occasional patients, psychotic and confusional
states.[2,3,4,7,8] These effects may involve sympathetic nervous system
activation.

Disulfiram is a potent inhibitor of aldehyde dehydrogenase (KI $= 10^{-7}$)[5]
but also inhibits the enzyme dopamine-B-hydroxylase (DBH) somewhat
less effectively (KI $= 10^{-6}$) by chelating the copper ion essential to DBH
activity.[9] DBH converts dopamine to norepinephrine (NE) and is present in
nerve endings of the sympathetic nervous system where it is released
along with NE.[10,11] A 10^{-5}M concentration of disulfiram can completely
inhibit DBH activity[12] and high doses of disulfiram given to experimental
animals can acutely lower the NE content of heart and brain.[13,14] The
applicability of these *in vitro* and animal studies to the long-term use of
disulfiram in man is open to question because the usual human dose of
disulfiram is only 250 to 500 mg daily. DBH is present in great excess in the
body[15] and increased synthesis of DBH can be induced as sympathetic
nerve activity increases.[16,17]

Two studies have investigated the effect of disulfiram on plasma NE in
man, but these studies have serious defects. One used an insufficiently
sensitive fluorometric method to measure plasma NE[18] and reports basal
values of NE five times as high as we[19] or other investigators[20-23] have
found. The other study[24] reports plasma NE levels 250 times as large.
Neither of these studies employed a drug-free group as controls although
alcohol alters the metabolism of NE[25] and abstinence from alcohol after a
long period of drinking may affect NE metabolism.

Disulfiram can potentially inhibit sympathetic nervous function by
blocking the synthesis of NE or increase sympathetic function by
increasing blood aldehyde levels. We have previously investigated the
effect of the two doses of disulfiram most commonly used on pulse, blood
pressure, plasma DBH and NE levels in a group of alcoholic men as
compared with a drug-free control group of alcoholic men and found
significant activation of the peripheral sympathetic nervous system.[26] We
have since analyzed the effects of the drug on cerebrospinal fluid (CSF)
levels of NE in ten of these patients and report these findings here.

METHODS

Ten alcoholic men from the larger group previously reported[26] who
were otherwise in good health were admitted to the Alcohol Rehabilitation
Unit of the National Naval Medical Center and, after giving their written

informed consent, entered into this study. They were not allowed to consume alcohol and lived in the hospital for the duration of the study. None had severe symptoms of alcohol withdrawal and all were drug-free for at least four days before entering into the study. Their mean ($\pm$ SEM) age was 31 $\pm$ 3 years (range 18–47). Disulfiram was given in compressed tablets (Ayerst, Antabuse®) in a dose of 500 mg daily. All patients were studied before beginning drug therapy and after three weeks of treatment. The following evaluations were completed: The patients were asked to lie supine and relax in a quiet room. The needle of a "heparin lock" was inserted into an antecubital vein and the pulse rate was measured by palpation every five minutes and blood pressure was measured by auscultation. After at least 20 minutes, and not before the pulse rate was stable and the subject relaxed, the first blood sample was drawn with the subject recumbent. The subject then stood and after five minutes a second blood sample was taken and pulse rate and blood pressure were measured. We have previously shown that this blood drawing technique gives basal levels of plasma NE which do not further decrease after three hours of rest and which are reproducible in the same individual after several weeks.[19] Eighteen ml of blood was collected into acid citrate dextrose (ACD) anticoagulant, placed on ice and centrifuged in the cold within 30 minutes and the plasma separated and stored at −70°C until assayed for DBH and NE. A spinal tap was performed at about 9:00 AM, since there is a diurnal rhythm in CSF levels of NE.[27] The patients were on a low monoamine diet and were maintained at bed rest from midnight until the time of the lumbar puncture, which was done with the patient in the left lateral decubitus position. Since there is a gradient in NE levels in the lumbar space,[28] the 12th to the 16th ml of CSF out of the lumbar puncture needle was taken for analysis of NE. CSF was collected in a tube containing 10 mg of ascorbic acid and immediately frozen on dry ice and stored at −70°C until assayed, as previously described.[29] A control group for CSF levels of NE consisted of 30 normal controls and neurological patients with myopathy or no organic findings who underwent lumbar puncture at the NIH, as described for the alcoholic patients.

DBH activity was assayed by the method of Molinoff et al.,[30] using phenylethylamine as substrate in the presence of 3.5×10^{-6} M CuSO$_4$ at pH 5.5 with 4 ul of plasma in an incubation volume of 300 ul. In a preliminary experiment the addition of CuSO$_4$ gave a 100% increase in DBH activity in the plasma of patients, whether taking disulfiram or placebo. As CuSO$_4$ did not mask any inhibitory effect of disulfiram on DBH activity, CuSo$_4$ was added to all plasma samples prior to assay for DBH. The ACD anticoagulant did not interfere with the assay. DBH activity is expressed as one unit equal to one nanomole of phenyl-

TABLE 1.—Sympathetic Nervous System Function in Alcoholic Versus Control Subjects

Subjects (N)	Age[1] (yrs)	NE (pg/ml)			BP (torr)		Pulse (beats/min)		DBH[2] (units)
		Supine	Stand	CSF	Supine	Stand	Supine	Stand	
Controls (14)	30 ± 2	268 ± 44	477 ± 69	219 ± 29*	$\frac{113 \pm 3}{76 \pm 2}$	$\frac{107 \pm 4}{74 \pm 6}$	61.4 ± 2.2	73.9 ± 4.6	722 ± 42†
Alcoholics (10)	31 ± 3	214 ± 31	489 ± 49	235 ± 27	$\frac{119 \pm 3}{77 \pm 3}$	$\frac{118 \pm 4}{87 \pm 4}$	73.0 ± 3.0	93.2 ± 3.4	519 ± 42**
P (Student t Test)	NS	NS	NS	NS	NS	<0.05	<0.01	<0.01	<0.001

[1]Mean ± SEM

[2]One unit equals one nanomole of phenylethylamine converted to phenylethanolamine per ml of plasma per hour of incubation time.

*From a separate group of 30 normal controls and neurological patients with myopathy who underwent lumbar puncture at NIH (mean age=29 ± 2 years)

†From a large control group of 124 healthy volunteers

**From the entire group of 79 alcoholic patients originally studied[26] ethanolamine generated from phenylethylamine per ml of plasma per hour.

Plasma NE levels were measured by the radioenzymatic method of Lake et al.[19] which converts the endogenous NE to ^{3}H-epinephrine. The assay had a sensitivity (twice blank) of about 20 pg/ml of plasma.

Zung depression and anxiety self-rating scales were completed by each patient before and after three weeks of disulfiram.

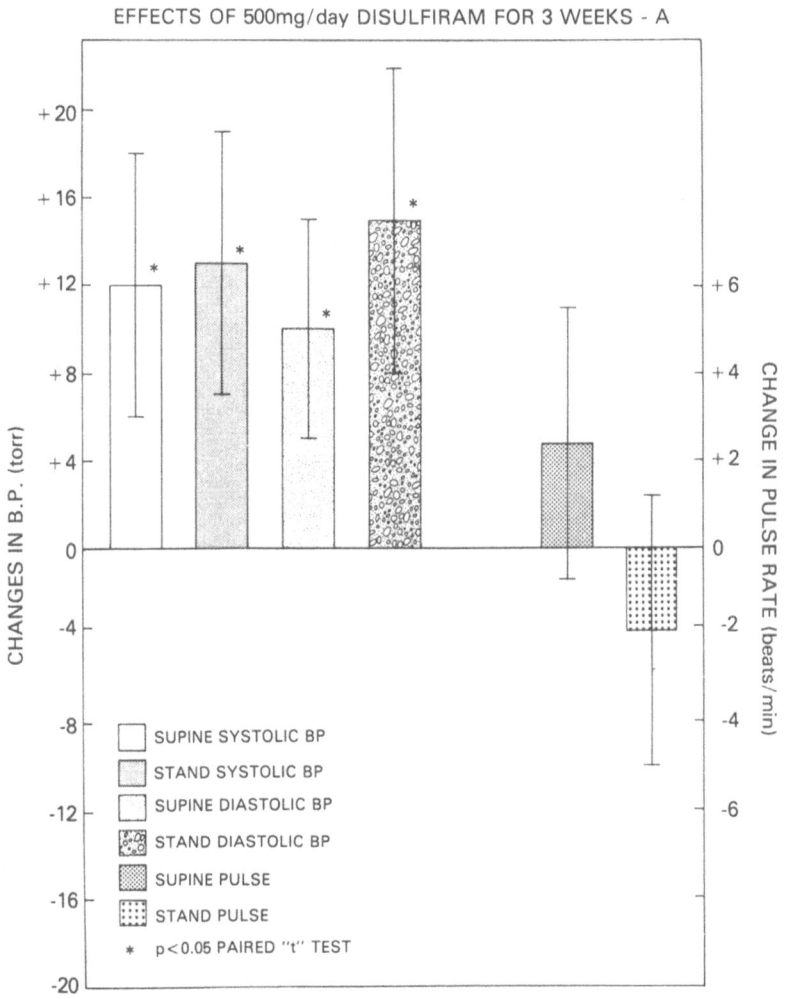

Figure 1. Mean ± SEM in blood pressure and pulse rate in ten alcoholic patients after treatment with 500 mg per day of disulfiram for three weeks.

RESULTS

The plasma and CSF NE values from the ten alcoholic patients did not differ significantly from a group of 14 normal controls of the same mean age (Table 1). The alcoholic patients had elevated pulse rates and standing blood pressures while plasma DBH activity was depressed. The patients showed significant depression (52 ±5) and anxiety (51 ±5) on the respective Zung scales. The changes after three weeks of disulfiram, 500 mg per day

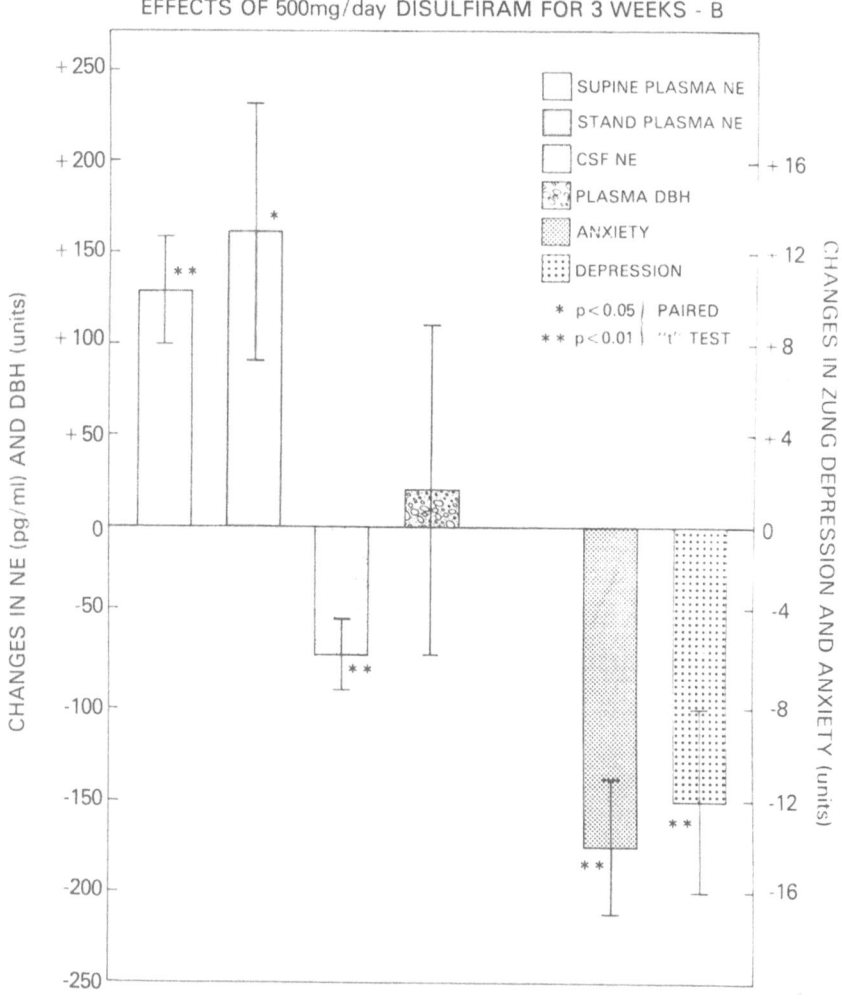

Figure 2. Mean ± SEM changes in NE, DBH, and Zung depression and anxiety scales in ten alcoholic patients after treatment with 500 mg per day of disulfiram for three weeks.

are given in Figures 1 and 2. Blood pressure but not pulse rate was significantly increased when compared by paired "t" test. Plasma levels of NE were also increased, but CSF NE was decreased in these same patients. The normal percent increments in plasma NE induced by standing was not altered by the disulfiram treatment. Before disulfiram the mean (± SEM) increase upon standing was 275 ± 42 pg/ml and after treatment, was 279 ± 56. One patient fainted after treatment.

The change in supine plasma NE from pre- to three weeks on disulfiram correlated significantly with the changes in supine systolic (L.R. = 0.71); p<0.01) and supine diastolic (L.R. = 0.71; p<0.01) blood pressures. Changes in standing plasma NE correlated with changes in standing systolic (L.R. = 0.51; p<0.05) and standing diastolic (L.R. = 0.54; p<0.05) blood pressures.

DISCUSSION

The function of the sympathetic nervous system in these alcoholic patients was intact as evaluated by measuring plasma levels of NE while the patients were supine and after standing. Plasma activity of DBH was low in the large group of 79 alcoholic patients in whom DBH was measured before treatment when compared to the activity in 124 healthy controls. These patients were also depressed but DBH is not abnormal in depressed populations.[31,32] Ewing et al.[33] reported that subjects with high DBH activity felt less drunk and sick after drinking than subjects with low DBH levels but concluded that DBH activity alone does not predict susceptibility to alcohol.[34] In newborn rats whose mothers were fed ethanol, Lau et al.[35] demonstrated low DBH which was not secondary to a direct inhibition of the enzyme. Also in rats, NE turnover was accelerated both during chronic ethanol administration and during withdrawal in the periphery and in brain, especially brain stem.[36,37] Rats given 6-hydroxydopamine centrally to destroy the dorsal NE bundle increased their consumption of ethanol.[38] After seven days of ethanol, DBH activity was decreased by about 40% in rats.[39] Another group found no difference in DBH activity between normals and alcoholic patients abstinent from alcohol for 3, 6, and 12 months after an admission for acute alcoholism (but DBH activity was lower, although not significantly, in the alcoholics at all three time points.)[40] However, the enzyme activity may return to normal after abstinence for three months. We have previously reported no change in DBH activity after only three weeks of abstinence.[26] These data do not explain the mechanism of significance of low DBH in our alcoholic population.

Alcoholism is related to several dietary deficiencies and DBH production may diminish as a result. Monoamine oxidase is another enzyme involved in catecholamine metabolism which has been noted to be reduced in alcoholic patients.[40] The effect may be nonspecific. Confirmation of low DBH in acute alcoholic patients awaits further studies, and if substantiated, further elucidation of the mechanism and the significance.

The concept that DBH is in excess and is not the rate limiting step,[10] is substantiated by these data since both resting levels of NE and the increment upon standing are normal concomitant with low DBH activity. DBH activity may have been inhibited by disulfiram, but not to the extent where NE production was significantly diminished. Nor could we detect any inhibition in the assay for the enzyme, but because of the substantial dilution of the plasma to be assayed, the assay may not detect some inhibitory effect by disulfiram. The absence of orthostatic hypotension previously reported[41] is consistent with a grossly intact sympathetic nervous system, although this group found absent or reduced sweating in their alcoholic patients. Our patients had elevated standing blood pressure as reported previously by others[41] and increased heart rate. Although the patients were judged not to have shown any signs of withdrawal after at least four days of hospitalization, this heightened cardiovascular activity may have been related to the withdrawal of alcohol.

As with the larger group of alcoholic patients treated for three weeks with 500 mg per day of disulfiram,[26] in the present group of ten patients blood pressure and plasma levels of NE increased significantly; concomitantly, CSF levels of NE decreased in these same ten patients treated with disulfiram. This inverse relationship of CSF and plasma NE levels may imply a central site of action of disulfiram. Central postsynaptic α-agonism (i.e., clonidine) causes a fall in peripheral levels of NE[42] and a fall in blood pressure by stimulating the inhibitory medullary α-adrenergic receptors.[43,44] Disulfiram may lower central NE turnover which is reflected by diminished NE measured in CSF without direct postsynaptic α-postsynaptic alpha-agonism. As a result, there may be less inhibitory impulses to the medullary cardiovascular regulatory center and greater outflow to the peripheral sympathetic nervous system, reflected by elevated plasma NE levels and blood pressure. Other mechanisms have been discussed[26] which may explain the peripheral increase: Disulfiram inhibits aldehyde dehydrogenase and even when subjects have no alcoholic intake, enough endogenous aldehyde may form to cause a detectable release of NE. The drug inhibits the magnesium-ATP dependent uptake of monoamines by chromaffin granules and this may result in an increase in circulating levels of NE. Neither hypothesis attends to the decrease in CSF NE. It is possible that brain DBH is more susceptible to disulfiram inhibition or is not causing an acceleration in peripheral sympathetic output.

The changes in plasma NE and blood pressure with disulfiram treatment correlated positively, suggesting a relationship between the increase in peripheral sympathetic nervous system activity and the elevation of blood pressure under these circumstances. In hypertensive patients we have not found such a relationship.[45] In the present study, the change in CSF NE with the drug did not relate significantly to changes in blood pressure, to changes in depression or anxiety, or to changes in plasma NE levels.

The relationship, if any, of the improvements in depression and anxiety to changes in NE levels can only be speculated and do not support the theory of diminished central NE turnover in depression.[46] If the decrease in CSF NE implies a diminished turnover of central NE metabolism concomitant with an improvement in depressive status, then the present data would seem to be incompatible with the NE part of the "permissive theory" of depression.[43] However, the correlations between change in either plasma or CSF NE with treatment and change in the rating scales were not significant. Since the present study did not include a group of unmedicated alcoholic patients who completed the rating scales and lumbar punctures, we cannot attribute the improvement to the drug. These effects are more likely secondary to the psychotherapeutic ward regimen.

In summary, alcoholic patients had elevated pulse rates and standing blood pressure, normal levels of NE in plasma and CSF, but low activity of DBH. The administration of 500 mg per day of disulfiram caused a decrease in CSF NE and an increase in plasma NE and blood pressure. As previously noted, alcoholic patients with hypertension should be carefully monitored if disulfiram is recommended, and patients taking 500 mg per day should also have their blood pressure followed and their dose reduced when possible.

ACKNOWLEDGMENTS

The authors would like to thank John Affronti, Anthony Sloane, Dorothy Parrish, and Audrey Reid for their technical assistance.

REFERENCES

1. Hald, J., and Jacobsen, E. A drug sensitizing the organism to ethyl alcohol. *Lancet.* 2:1001–1004, 1948.
2. Lundwall, L., and Baekeland, F. Disulfiram treatment of alcoholism. *J. Nerv. Ment. Dis.* 153:381–394, 1971.
3. Talbott, G.D., and Gander, O. Antabuse, 1973. *Md. State Med. J.* 22:60–63, 1973.
4. Acke, J. Evaluation du traitement au disulfirame de l'alcoolisme chronique. *Acta. Psychiatr.* Belg., 75:306–19, 1975.
5. Kitson, T.M. The disulfiram-ethanol reaction. *J. Stud. on Alcohol.* 38:96–113, 1977.
6. Walsh, M.J. Role of acetaldehyde in the interactions of ethanol with neuroamines, in Roach, M., and Micsaac, W. (eds.), *Biological Aspects of Alcohol,* University of Texas Press, 1971, pp. 233–266.
7. Knee, S.T., and Razini, J.: Acute organic brain syndrome: a complication of disulfiram therapy. *Am. J. Psychiat.* 131:1281–1282, 1974.
8. Liddon, S., and Satran, R. Disulfiram (Antabuse) psychosis. *Am. J. Psychiat.* 123:1284–1289, 1967.
9. Green, A. The inhibition of dopamine-B-oxidase by chelating agents. *Biochem. Biophys. Acta.* 81:394, 1964.
10. Viveros, O.H., Argueros, L., and Kirshner, N. Release of catecholamines and dopamine-B-oxidase from the adrenal medulla. *Life Sci.* 7:609–618, 1968.
11. Weinshilboum, R.M., Thoa, N.B., Johnson, D.G., and Kopin, I.J. Proportional release norepinephrine and dopamine-B-hydroxylase from sympathetic nerves. *Science* 174:1349–1351, 1971.
12. Goldstein, M., Anagnoste, B., Lauber, E., and McKereghan, M.B. Inhibition of dopamine-B-hydroxylase by disulfiram. *Life. Sci.* 3:763–767, 1964.
13. Musacchio, J.M., Goldstein, M., Anagnoste, B., Poch, G., and Kopin, I.J. Inhibition of dopamine-B-hydroxylase by disulfiram in vivo. *J. Pharmacol. Exp. Ther.,* 152:56–61, 1966.
14. Musacchio, J., Kopin, I.J., and Snyder, S. Effects of disulfiram on tissue norepinephrine content and subcellular distribution of dopamine tyramine and their B-hydroxylated metabolites. *Life. Sci.* 3:769–775, 1964.
15. Levin, E.Y., and Kaufman, S. Studies on the enzyme catalyzing the conversion of 3,4-dihydroxyphenylethylamine to norepinephrine. *J. Bio. Chem,.* 236:2043–2049, 1961.
16. Kvetnansky, R., Gerwitz, G.P., Weise, V.K., and Kopin, I.J. Enhanced synthesis of adrenal dopamine-B-hydroxylase induced by repeated immobilization in rats. *Mol. Pharmacol.* 7:81–86, 1971.
17. Weinshilboum, R.M., Kvetnansky, R., Axelrod, J., and Kopin, I.J. Elevation of serum dopamine-B-hydroxylase activity with forced immobilization. *Nature* 230:287–288, 1971.
18. Kaldor, A., Demeczky, L., and Juvancz, P. The effects of disulfiram on blood catecholamine level in man. *International Zeitschrift fur Klinische Pharmakologie Therapie und Toxicologie* 5:284–286, 1971.
19. Lake, C.R., Ziegler, M.G., and Kopin, I.J. Use of plasma norepinephrine for evaluation of sympathetic neuronal function in man. *Life. Sci.* 18:1315–1326, 1978.
20. Franco-Morselli, R. Elghozi, J.L., Joly, E., Di Giuilio, S., and Meyer, P. Increased plasma adrenaline concentrations in benign essential hypertension. *Brit. Med. J.* 2:1251–1254, 1977.
21. DeChamplain, J., Farley, L., Cousineau, D., and Van Aueringen, M-R. Circulating catecholamine levels in human and experimental hypertension. *Circ. Res.* 38:109–114, 1976.

22. DeQuattro, V., Miura, Y., Lurvey, A., Cosgrove, M., and Mendez, R. Increased plasma catecholamine concentrations and vas deferens norepinephrine biosynthesis in men with elevated blood pressure. *Circ. Res.* 36:118–126, 1975.

23. Pederson, E.B., and Christensen, N.J. Catecholamines in plasma and urine in patients with essential hypertension determined by double isotope derivative techniques. *Acta. Med. Scand.* 198:373–377, 1975.

24. Serebo, B. The suppression of noradrenaline and 3-hydroxytyramine (dopamine) excretion by disulfiram in alcohol dependent patients. *Brit. J. Addict.* 69:305–309, 1974.

25. Smith, A., and Gitlow, S. Effect of disulfiram and ethanol on catabolism of norepinephrine in man, in Maickel, R.P. (ed.), *Biochemical Factors in Alcoholism*. New York: Pergamon Press, 1962, pp. 53–60.

26. Lake, C.R., Major, L.F., Ziegler, M.G., and Kopin, I.J. Increased sympathetic nervous system activity in alcoholic patients treated with disulfiram. *Am. J. Psychiat.* 134:1411–1414, 1977.

27. Ziegler, M.G., Lake, C.R., Wood, J.H., and Ebert, M.H. Circadian rhythm in cerebrospinal fluid noradrenaline of man and monkey. *Nature* 264:656–658, 1976.

28. Ziegler, M.G., Wood, J.H., Lake, C.R., and Kopin, I.J. Norepinephrine and 3-methoxy-4-hydroxyphenyl glycol gradients in human cerebrospinal fluid. *Am. J. Psychiat.* 134:565–568, 1977.

29. Ziegler, M.G., Lake, C.R., Foppen, F.H., Shoulson, I., and Kopin, I.J. Norepinephrine in cerebrospinal fluid. *Brain Res.* 108:436–440, 1976.

30. Molinoff, P.B., Weinshilboum, R., and Axelrod, J. A sensitive enzymatic assay for dopamine-*B*-hydroxylase. *J. Pharmacol. Exp. Ther.* 178:425–431, 1971.

31. Shopsin, B., Freedman, L.S., Goldstein, M., and Gershon, S. Serum dopamine-*B*-hydroxylase (D*B*H) activity and affective states. *Psychopharmacologia* 27:11–16, 1972.

32. Lamprecht, F., Ebert, M.H., Turek, I., and Kopin, I.J. Serum dopamine-beta-hydroxylase in depressed patients and the effect of electroconvulsive shock treatment. *Psychopharmacologia* 40:241–248, 1974.

33. Ewing, J.A., Rouse, B.A., and Mueller, R.A. Alcohol susceptibility and plasma dopamine *B*-hydroxylase activity. *Research Commun. Chem. Path. and Pharmacol.* 8:551–554, 1974.

34. Ewing, J.A., Rouse, B.A., and Mills, K.C. Dopamine-*B*-hydroxylase activity as a predictor of response to alcohol. *Japan. J. Stud. Alc.* 10:61–64, 1975.

35. Lau, C., Thadane, P.V., Schanberg, S.M., and Slotkin, T.A. Effects of maternal ethanol ingestion on development of adrenal catecholamines and dopamine-*B*-hydroxylase in the offspring. *Neuropharm.* 15:505–507, 1976.

36. Pohorecky, L.A. Effects of ethanol on central and peripheral noradrenergic neurons. *J. Pharmacol. Exp. Ther.* 189:380–391, 1974.

37. Carlsson, A., and Lindovist, M. Effect of ethanol on the hydroxylation of tyrosine and tryptophan in rat brain *in vivo*. *J. Pharm. Pharmac.* 25:437–440, 1973.

38. Kiianmaa, K., Fuxe, K., Jonsson, G., and Ahtee, L. Evidence for involvement of central NA neurons in alcohol intake increased alcohol consumption after degeneration of the NA pathway to the cortex cerebri. *Neuroscience Letters*, 1:41–45, 1975.

39. Ng, L.K.Y., Lamprecht, F.V., Williams, R.B., and Kopin, I.J. Δ^9-Tetrahydrocannabinol and ethanol: differential effects on sympathetic activity in differing environmental setting. *Science* 180:1368–1369, 1973.

40. Sullivan, J.L., Stanfield, C.N., Schanberg, S., and Cavenar, J. Platelet monoamine and serum dopamine-*B*-hydroxylase activity in chronic alcoholics. *Arch. Gen. Psychiat.* 35:1209–1212, 1978.

41. Low, P.A., Walsh, J.C., Huang, C.Y., and McLeod, J.G. The sympathetic nervous system in alcoholic neuropathy: a clinical and pathological study. *Brain*, 98:357–364, 1975.

42. Lake, C.R., Ziegler, M.G., Coleman, M.D., and Kopin, I.J. The effects of clonidine on the sympathetic nervous system (SNS) function in hypertensive patients. *The Pharmacologist.* 20:228, 1978.

43. Kobinger, W. Central cardiovascular actions of clonidine, in Davies, D.V.S., and Reid, J.L. (eds.), *Central Action of Drugs in Blood Pressure Regulation.* Baltimore: University Park Press, 1978, pp. 181–193.

44. Reid, J.L. Clonidine and central noradrenal in turnover, in Davies, D.S., and Reid, J.L. (eds.), *Central Action of Drugs in Blood Pressure Regulation.* Baltimore: University Park Press, 1978, pp. 194–203.

45. Lake, C.R., Ziegler, M.G., Coleman, M.D., and Kopin, I.J. Age-adjusted plasma norepinephrine levels are similar in normotensive and hypertensive subjects. *N. Eng. J. Med.* 296:208–209, 1977.

46. Prange, A.J., Jr., Sisk, J.L., Wilson, I.C., Morris, C.E., Hall, C.D., and Carman, J.S. Balance, permission, and discrimination among amines: a theoretical consideration of the actions of L-tryptophan in disorders of movements and affect, in *Serotonin and Behavior* New York: Academic Press, 1973, pp. 539–548.

CHAPTER 17

The Use of Subhuman Primates in Alcoholism Research

H.L. ALTSHULER

INTRODUCTION

Recent progress in alcoholism research has been rapid, and there are indications that the scientific community is on the verge of a major expansion of knowledge about the mechanisms underlying the actions of ethanol which will lead to more rational approaches to the treatment of this complex and widespread disorder. Such progress depends upon the wisdom, insight, and vision of clinical investigators working together with creative and systematic laboratory scientists.

Clinical research has provided a great deal of information about all aspects of alcoholism and will continue to contribute much of the immediately applicable new facts about improved prevention and treatment of alcoholism. The limitations of clinical research are obvious ones, largely based upon the ethical questions concerning the use of human subjects for invasive experimental procedures. Indeed, recent years have witnessed rapid increases in the restrictions concerning the use of patients or volunteers for biomedical research. The use of experimental animals as research subjects provides the major means of expanding our fundamental knowledge by allowing systematic, multidisciplinary studies of the biochemical, physiological, and pharmacological aspects of the disorder. This chapter will provide an overview of the use of experimental animals, especially subhuman primates, in alcoholism research and provide selected examples of how these animals may be used most appropriately. In addition, the unique problems and advantages associated with the use of subhuman primates will be discussed, including the criteria for the rational selection of species and appropriate projects to insure the responsible use of these animals.

The Use of Experimental Animals in Alcoholism Research

Practically every species of animal that can be maintained in a laboratory has been used in alcoholism research, although laboratory rodents such as rats and mice are used most often.[1-12] There are many advantages to using rodents, especially the assurance that their early care and genetic background are well documented. Rodents are inexpensive and have short generation times that permit rapid establishment of inbred strains that have been selected for various response parameters. Although an exhaustive review of such applications is not possible here, it is important to emphasize that a wealth of information is developing concerning the establishment of rodent strains that exhibit specific responses to ethanol. Such studies provide potentially important means to increase our understanding of the genetic basis of alcoholism. Research in this area is moving quite rapidly, and new strains are being established with regularity.[13]

Other small laboratory mammals such as hamsters and gerbils have been used for alcoholism research.[14,15] Of particular interest are the studies conducted with a species of hamster that exhibits a high degree of ethanol preference and apparent biochemical resistance to the behavioral depressant effects of the compound.[16] This species should be extremely important in future research, especially in areas of research examining the neurochemical and neurophysiological basis of ethanol preference.

Invertebrate species have also been used to a limited degree in alcoholism research. Invertebrates such as Aplysia[17] are a frequent choice. Various fish also have been used.[18] Although such subjects are easy to work with and understand, relatively few laboratories use them for alcoholism research.

Other laboratory animals such as dogs,[19] swine[20] and other species have been used for a variety of alcoholism studies. Although there are many advantages to the use of such readily available animal models, there are disadvantages associated with ethical and methodological questions resulting from the extreme variability of such animals, especially regarding health, biological, and psychological background.

It has been suggested that subhuman primates are ideal animals for studies of the effects of ethanol on behavioral and central nervous system function.[21] Although that viewpoint has merit, the limitations that are associated with subhuman primate research are of major consequence. Although there is little question that the neuroanatomical, neurophysiological, and behavioral similarities between subhuman primates and humans recommend their extensive use, there are some crucial disadvantages. As in all aspects of research, these relative advantages and disadvantages must be weighed before selections are made.

Subhuman Primates as Subjects for Alcoholism Research

Subhuman primates have been proposed[21] to be the best animal species for alcoholism research because of the many similarities between the human and monkey nervous system and behavioral repertoire. Indeed, those considerations have merit, although the indiscriminate use of monkeys and apes for biomedical research has caused current problems that will hamper research for many years. There are certain types of experiments for which monkeys and apes are well suited and, in fact, provide the most effective and, occasionally, the only suitable experimental animal. On the other hand, there are many types of projects that have used monkeys when they were not appropriate. Frequently, those projects would have been improved by larger numbers of less complex and less expensive subjects. As a result of such indiscriminate use, a critical shortage of subhuman primates exists. The most severely affected species, the rhesus monkey, is the one that has been studied most thoroughly and about which most is known, especially concerning normative biomedical parameters. As a result of the current shortage, it has become absolutely mandatory for all investigators to reevaluate their subhuman primate models and critically reconsider their choice of species.

There are three general categories of subhuman primates that have been used in laboratory research: the rarely used prosimians, the simians, and the Great Apes. The simians have been used extensively as research subjects. The Great Apes consist of the larger, elaborately developed subhuman primate species, such as the gorilla, the chimpanzee, the orangutan, and the gibbon. There are remarkable similarities between human and Great Ape behavior. Unfortunately, Great Apes are extremely scarce, most endangered for their survival as a species, and prohibitively expensive.

The prosimians are a comparatively primitive group of subhuman primates and have not been used very often for alcoholism research, although there are certain types of protocols for which they are uniquely

TABLE 1.–Subhuman Primate Species Used for Alcoholism Research

NEW WORLD MONKEYS

Saimiri sciureus (squirrel monkey)— used occasionally for behavioral and metabolic studies; relatively small size.

Cebus capucinus (capuchin)— used infrequently in behavioral studies. Normative values for behavior and biomedical parameters are not well established.

OLD WORLD MONKEYS

Genus Macaca

M. mulatta (rhesus)— most widely used; availability critically scarce.

M. radiata (bonnet)— a reasonable substitute for the rhesus, but also scarce. Has been used for self-administration and electrophsiological studies.

M. nemestrina (pigtail)— useful for neurophysiological studies and might prove to be a reasonable substitute for the rhesus; also in short supply.

M. fascicularis (crab-eating)— being used with greater frequency to substitute for the rhesus; performs quite differently in most behavioral tasks but similar to rhesus in most physiological and biochemical parameters; availability at present quite good.

M. arctoides (stump-tailed)— larger but more gentle than the rhesus; also in quite short supply; has been used in cardiovascular research.

Papio Species (Baboons)

P. anubis and *P. cynocephalus*— have been used for studies of the metabolic and toxicological consequences of alcoholism.

P. papio— genetically epileptic; has been used rarely in alcoholism research, but might prove to be an interesting subject.

Cercopithecus

C. aethiops (vervet monkey)— appropriate size and adequate normative data; has been used very rarely; associated with Marburg virus.

Great Apes

Pan pan (chimpanzee)— has been used for alcohol-related behavioral and metabolic studies; extremely expensive and require special facilities.

biologically suited.[22] Other biomedical research areas such as oncology and reproductive physiology have capitalized on some of these unique features to great advantage. Although the prosimians may be of potential value for certain types of alcoholism research, their limited and primitive behavioral repertoire, their primitively organized central nervous system, and their small size are major hindrances to routine use. Further, they are unusually sensitive to some widespread viral diseases, adding additional reasons for the lack of enthusiasm for more frequent use of them for research.

The simians are usually subdivided into the Old World and New World monkeys. These species account for over 90% of the subhuman primate species used for biomedical research. Included in the Old World monkey group are macaques, baboons, and related African and Asian species. The New World monkeys, although usually smaller than the Old World species, are also used frequently, especially the squirrel monkey *(Saimiri sciureus)*, the capuchin *(Cebus* sp.), and the owl monkey *(Aotus aotus)*. The simians have been experimental subjects for almost all biomedical research disciplines, from pathbreaking research on infectious diseases (tuberculosis and malaria) and virology (poliomyelitis) to sociobiological studies.[23] Such a broad range of uses of these species was a partial cause of the current critical shortage and the subsequent interruption of many research programs. This problem will be discussed in greater detail.

The Great Apes are a fascinating and complex primate group. Their use in studies involving invasive and/or terminal procedures is strongly contraindicated. These animals, especially the chimpanzee, are appropriately used as subjects in a variety of sociobiological and behavioral studies, including a limited number pertaining to alcoholism.[24] They certainly could not be considered a preferred species for any type of research due to their scarcity, large size, and prohibitive cost.

Table 1[22,25,26] summarizes the species of subhuman primates that have been used most often in alcoholism research. The Old and the New World simians, principally the macaques, squirrel monkeys, and capuchins, are the most frequently used primate species in alcoholism research. The normative biomedical parameters for most species from these groups are reasonably well established,[22,26-28] and their behavioral repertoires are sufficiently similar to man's to allow meaningful generalizations from experimental data obtained in studies with them.

Choice of Subhuman Primates for Alcoholism Research: Criteria for Selection

Subhuman primates can serve as subjects for almost all types of biomedical research projects. Prior to recognition of the population depleting effects of the indiscriminate use of these animals, they were subjects in many projects that required euthanasia of very large numbers of animals. An extreme example of this may be found in the early history of the commercial production of polio vaccine. Early studies demonstrated that poliovirus grew quite successfully in tissue cultures derived from rhesus monkey kidneys. Subsequently, very large numbers of monkeys were imported for the sole purpose of immediate euthanasia and removal of their kidneys. Although many current vaccine production programs still require live rhesus monkey kidney cells, the increased sophistication of tissue culture techniques substantially reduced such wastefulness.

Many other examples of biomedical projects that resulted in the destruction of large numbers of monkeys could be given. Fortunately, most investigators have come to realize the seemingly obvious, that indiscriminate destruction of any wild animal species will reduce its future availability.

In summary, subhuman primates represent the best and occasionally the only suitable subjects for certain types of biomedical research. Unfortunately, they were not always used only for appropriate studies, and the result is a critical shortage of some monkey species, even for conservative and appropriate research applications. Ironically, the current shortage, while having very serious consequences in some research programs, is stimulating a reevaluation of the use of monkeys for medical research. That exercise will probably result in newer, more thoughtful, and more appropriate selection of animal species for use as laboratory subjects.

Animal Models of Alcoholism

Interest in and the need for an animal model of alcoholism has stimulated extensive research efforts, resulting in the equivalent of a specialty area of alcoholism research focused on animal models. The field is highly charged with controversy, stimulating extensive discussion of an appropriate definition of an animal model of alcoholism, the criteria for such a model, and suggestions that the model is not possible. Those controversies are beyond the scope of this chapter. In recent years, a general consensus has developed, agreeing that it would be illogical to seek a single animal model that could be a suitable subject for all types of alcoholism research.[29-31] Human alcoholism is so complex and variable that it is impossible to conceive of, or even define, an animal model that could incorporate all components. This discussion will illustrate how certain primate models are useful for studying experimental questions about specific aspects of alcoholism.

The Chronic Effects of Ethanol: Metabolic and Toxicological Studies

Among the most productive uses of primates in alcoholism research are the important studies conducted by Lieber and associates using baboons.[32,33] This group has done exhaustive studies of the metabolic and toxicological consequences of chronic ethanol ingestion by baboons. Ethanol was administered as a constituent of a liquid diet that had been formulated specifically to insure adequate nutrition for alcohol-consuming animals. That extremely important research has made an enormous impact on our understanding of the consequences of chronic ethanol ingestion, especially regarding the production of hepatic pathology. In addition, these experiments illustrate the use of subhuman primates in alcoholism research based on rational selection of the species, and for studies that do not destroy large numbers of animals. Furthermore, these studies pioneered the development of effective methods of administering ethanol to animals chronically.

Behavioral Studies

Several laboratories use subhuman primates as experimental subjects for psychopharmacological and behavioral studies of the addictive properties of ethanol and its actions as a reinforcer of behavior. Many use the self-administration model, which is a model that was developed to study other drugs of abuse and is based on the premise that drugs can serve as reinforcers of operant behavior.[34,35] Deneau[36] was the first to report that rhesus monkeys would self-administer ethanol intravenously and display patterns of ethanol intake that were similar to those exhibited by human alcoholics. The intravenous self-administration technique has been used by other investigators, including Winger and Woods,[31,37-40] Denoble and Begleiter,[41,42] and Altshuler et al.[43]

In the late 60s Yanagita and his group reported preliminary data about an intragastric self-administration procedure, reporting limited success and a number of technical difficulties.[44] Altshuler and his group[45-47] modified the early techniques extensively and reported its successful applications in studies of many drugs of abuse. Applications in ethanol-related studies were also demonstrated. It was reasoned that intragastric self-administration was more appropriate for alcohol studies than the intravenous self-administration method, since humans consume ethanol orally, and evaluations of its reinforcing properties should simulate that route as closely as possible.

That premise has been extended by Meisch and his group.[48-52] They reported that they have established ethanol as a reinforcer by the oral route in a limited group of rhesus monkeys, that the animals consume high doses of ethanol, and exhibit behavior quite similar to animals in intravenous or intragastric self-administration experiments.

Pieper reported[24] the use of chimpanzees for alcohol studies, including assessments of the acute and chronic behavioral effects of ethanol as well as preliminary studies of the metabolic disposition of ethanol.[24,53-55]

Some laboratories[56] use monkeys as subjects in electrophysiological experiments that are designed to describe and quantify the effects of ethanol on the electrical activity of surface and deep structures of the brain. Experiments such as these are extremely difficult to conduct, and their contribution to our full understanding of the effects of ethanol cannot be assessed for several years.

Several groups are attempting to develop subhuman primate models of the fetal alcohol syndrome,[57,58] a recently reported syndrome afflicting the offspring of alcoholic human mothers. Studies with other laboratory animals have supported the validity of the clinical observations, and demonstrated that ethanol can be a teratogen in other species. Attempts to produce subhuman primate models of FAS are just beginning, and information concerning their success or failure is not yet available.

In summary, subhuman primates have been used as subjects and animal models[59-63] in a wide range of alcoholism studies, including: (1) studies of the toxicological consequences of chronic ethanol consumption; (2) evaluations of the degree, nature and underlying contingencies of the behaviorally reinforcing properties of ethanol; (3) assessments of alcohol's effects on complex neurophysiological events; (4) evaluations of the mechanisms underlying tolerance and dependence; and (5) most recently, preliminary studies of its teratological effects. It is evident that the contribution of subhuman primates to the growth of our understanding of alcoholism has, and will continue to be, significant. The experiments summarized below are presented to illustrate, in a general way, the manner in which a specific research problem may be addressed by using subhuman primates as the most appropriate experimental subjects.

The Development of a Simian Intragastric Self-Administration Model of Alcoholism

The methodology for self-administration studies with monkeys was developed at the University of Michigan in the early 1960s[36,64] for studies of the intravenous self-administration of opiates and other drugs of abuse. The technical procedures were based on the procedures described by Weeks for work with rats. The technical details have been described many times, and will not be reiterated here. The procedures may be summarized by stating that an animal is fitted with an apparatus that allows it to obtain intravenous infusions of solutions through an indwelling intravenous cannula.

There have been only a handful of reports of experiments that used intravenous self-administration of alcohol with subhuman primates.[37-43] All report that alcohol serves as a reinforcer, albeit a less potent one than many other abused drugs. Questions have been raised about the wisdom of experimental designs based on intravenous self-administration,[46,51,52,65-67] and the problems of considering that approach to be a model of human drinking behavior.

Variations of the basic intravenous self-administration procedure have been attempted that sought to develop an animal model that self-administered drugs into its gastrointestinal tract, to simulate more closely human drinking.[44,68] Our laboratory[45-47] developed an intragastric self-administration procedure for use in monkeys. It has been applied successfully in studies of alcohol self-administration. Those results are summarized below, as well as some results from intravenous self-administration experiments.

METHODS

Over 65 rhesus monkeys ranging in weight from 3.5 to 6.5 Kg have served as subjects in alcohol self-administration studies during a 6 year period. Thirty-eight have been used in intragastric self-administration protocols, and approximately 25 have been used in intravenous self-administration protocols. All subhuman primates in our research facility were obtained from USDA approved vendors, and cared for according to the standards outlined by USDA, National Institutes of Health, and the American Association for Accreditation of Laboratory Animal Care. All animals received optimum medical care to insure that they were in the best of health when used as experimental subjects. The animals were maintained on a 12 hour light/dark cycle, consisting of a light phase extending from 7 am–7 pm and a dark phase from 7 pm–7 am. They were fed Purina® 25 monkey chow and had water available *ad lib*. The animals received frequent medical examinations, including clinical laboratory procedures, to monitor their health. They were TB tested monthly, and screened twice yearly for exposure to Herpes B virus. As will be described below, most animals that completed their usefulness as experimental subjects in these programs were subsequently used in other studies, and were eventually retired into our laboratory's breeding colony for an indefinite period of time.

Surgical Procedures. The surgical procedures for the implantation of both intravenous and intragastric cannulae are quite similar and have been described extensively in other places.[36,45-47] The main differences between the intragastric and intravenous surgical procedures were that the indwelling intravenous cannula was implanted directly into a vein (right or left internal jugular or right or left femoral), while the intragastric cannula was implanted into the animal's stomach by means of a Teflon® patch that served as a nontraumatic interface between the cannula and the serosal surface of the stomach.

Apparatus. The apparatus used in both intravenous and intragastric self-administration techniques were identical. The animals were housed in primate cages (Harford SM 2024) that had been modified to serve as self-administration chambers. Each chamber contained fittings for a flexible steel hose tether, two response levers, and two signal lights. The animals wore stainless steel harnesses[36] or cloth jackets (Medical Arts, Inc.) that served the dual purpose of restraining the animal and protecting the cannula.

The behavioral control unit was constructed of solid state components and provided automatic control over schedules of reinforcement and automated logging of responses on both digital counters and cumulative recorders. Infusions were delivered by Cole Parmer #7545 peristalic infusion pumps, coupled with Masterflex rate controllers such that the drug doses were a function of the rate and duration of the infusion. The system was calibrated daily.

Behavioral Procedures and Establishment of Control Data. The behavioral procedures for shaping the animals to respond in the intravenous self-administration mode and the intragastric self-administration mode were identical. Similarly, the necessary baseline control data were also obtained in exactly the same manner for both procedures. Approximately five days after surgery for the intravenous model, and 10 days for the intragastric model, saline was made available for self-administration according to a 24 hr/day period of availability on a fixed ratio 1 (CRF) schedule of reinforcement. The signal light above one of the two response levers was illuminated to indicate the active lever. Depressions of the active lever resulted in saline infusions (1 ml). Responses on the inactive lever, that is the lever located under the cue light that was not illuminated, were without consequence. The monkeys were allowed to respond randomly for saline infusions for an indefinite period of time until that random responding for saline had extinguished. During this phase of the studies and during all subsequent phases, the position of the active lever was changed regularly such that the left lever was active for several days, and the right lever on other days. The location of the active lever was indicated by the illuminated signal light.

After random responding for saline had extinguished, ethanol was made available in place of saline and the infusion pumps calibrated to provide each animal with ethanol doses of 100 mg/Kg/infusion following response on the active lever, according to a CRF schedule of reinforcement, 24 hr/day. The criteria for acquisition of self-administration varied somewhat according to each particular experiment. In general, the criteria for acquisition of ethanol self-administration with either method required that the animal was responding almost exclusively on the appropriate lever at rates sufficient to produce ethanol intake levels of at least 1 gm/Kg/day. Some studies required far more rigorous criteria for acquisition but, in general, the stated criteria dependably identified animals that were emitting drug seeking behavior for ethanol reinforcement.

Our early studies with the intragastric self-administration model were intended to assess the usefulness and applicability of the model. In those studies, the criteria for acquisition of ethanol intragastric self-administration were that the animal voluntarily began ethanol self-administration within 30 days of when the drug was first made available; that they responded at sufficient rates to result in daily ethanol doses of at least 1 gm/Kg/day; and, finally, that they maintained that response level (daily dose) for at least 30 consecutive days. Animals meeting those criteria were considered to have voluntarily initiated intragastric self-administration of ethanol. The criteria for spontaneous initiation of intravenous self-administration of ethanol were identical to those for intragastric self-administration.

Data Handling. The data obtained during these studies were analyzed in a number of ways, depending on the details of each study. The basic method of data analysis consisted of logging the number of responses emitted by each animal for ethanol reinforcement in a 24 hr period and converting the total number of responses to dosage information expressed as gm/Kg/24 hrs. Although in many of our studies we have added a variety of more sophisticated methods of data analysis, the results presented here were those that recorded daily ethanol intake data by individual animals, and computation of the mean and standard error of data obtained from a group of animals that had received similar experimental manipulations.

RESULTS

Intragastric Self-Administration Studies. Evaluation of the simian intragastric self-administration technique for its potential application to alcoholism research demonstrated that the technique effectively produces animals that self-administer ethanol into their gastrointestinal tract, and that it compares favorably with intravenous self-administration in most ways. Thirty-eight animals were tested for their proclivity to initiate intragastric self-administration of ethanol. Approximately two-thirds, 22, spontaneously initiated self-administration of alcohol when no additional experimental manipulations were required to establish responding. All but four of the group that did not spontaneously initiate self-administration eventually began alcohol intragastric self-administration after various experimental manipulations intended to assist acquisition had been performed. Table 2 summarizes those findings.

The simian intragastric self-administration model was used in several projects designed to evaluate the acute and chronic effects of ethanol. We have shown that the model is extremely durable and that animal subjects can be maintained for as long as two years. In addition, we have shown that the expected toxicological sequellae of chronic ethanol consumption develop during extended periods of alcohol intragastric self-administration, including gastritis, hepatitis, and the early manifestations of cirrhosis. The patterns of ethanol consumption by this model are remarkably similar to human alcohol intake patterns, especially those observed during the early stages of human alcoholism. We have reported that the patterns of ethanol intragastric self-administration resemble human binge-drinking patterns. Thus, monkeys will self-administer extremely high ethanol doses for several days, and then consume very little during the next 1–2 days. That pattern was repeated regularly, and the total alcohol dose consumed on the "binge" days increased over time.

TABLE 2.–Intragastric Self-Administration of Ethanol in Rhesus Monkeys, 1972-1978

38 MONKEYS IMPLANTED FOR ETHANOL STUDIES		
25 spontaneously initiated self-administration		
duration (months)	number of animals	
1–3	8	
3–6	7	
6–12	2	
12–18	4	these animals exhibited
18–24	3	abstinence syndrome on
>24	1	withdrawal from drug
13 did not spontaneously initiate self-administration		
9 animals did so after training with other drugs and/or forced addiction		
4 animals would not self-administer ethanol even after training and/or forced addiction		

Intravenous Self-Administration Studies. Our experiments with intravenous self-administration of ethanol in monkeys confirmed the reports of others[36-40,42] that monkeys will self-administer alcohol by that route. Intravenous self-administration studies are more difficult to conduct than intragastric studies, because the intravenous model is much less durable than the intragastric model, and is effected by many experimental variables that are controlled more easily in the intragastric model. However, the intravenous model is well suited for experiments designed to assess the effects of various experimental manipulations on the reinforcing effects of ethanol, since the short interval between responding and reinforcement increases the sensitivity of the procedure to detect alterations in reinforcement. Our recent report[43] on the effects of opiate antagonists on alcohol self-administration illustrates the usefulness of intravenous self-administration in such studies.

DISCUSSION

The summary of our self-administration studies is intended to illustrate one use of subhuman primates as animal models and experimental subjects for basic research projects dealing with alcoholism. It was not intended to be an exhaustive exposition of a particular hypothesis, nor a support of a particular model. It is, however, intended to illustrate the use of subhuman primates as subjects in experiments that they are uniquely suited for, as a means of increasing our understanding of alcoholism.

The results obtained during the early development of the intragastric self-administration model demonstrated that it is a valid and durable model for the study of voluntary ethanol consumption. The data pertaining to the durability of the model illustrate that it can be used in long-term experiments designed to study the influence of certain variables on long-term, voluntary ethanol consumption. Compelling questions pertaining to the interactions of alcohol-related pathology and continued voluntary alcohol intake remain unanswered. The intragastric self-administration model should be extremely useful in experiments attempting to obtain those answers.

Both the intravenous and the intragastric self-administration models are useful in other types of experimental designs. Our recent demonstration[43] that the opiate antagonist, naltrexone, causes suppression of intravenous alcohol self-administration raises many exciting possibilities about the neurochemical basis of ethanol reinforcement.

Intragastric and, to a lesser extent, intravenous self-administration procedures produce animal models that exhibit alcohol consumption patterns strikingly similar to the consumption patterns of some humans. When drug was availalbe 24 hr/day on a CRF schedule, binge-like intake patterns were observed. That pattern continued for many months, and provided a unique subject for lengthy studies of voluntary ethanol consumption. The choice of self-administration models should be determined by the goals of the proposed study, since each has unique advantages. That essential consideration does not apply only to choosing between self-administration models, but applies to the selection of animal subjects for all research projects.

The selection of specific animal models for research projects often presents a perplexing problem. Many factors must be considered, including cost, difficulty of housing, availability, and biological suitability. In addition, the range of potential subjects is changing and expanding rapidly. For example, several inbred strains of rodents exhibit certain unique responses to alcohol. They can provide a range of special models that are particularly suitable for certain experimental questions. Although the choices of subhuman primates do not include that degree of sophistication, there are important selection criteria that must be considered.

The selection of primate species for research projects is usually based on availability, cost, difficulty in handling and housing, and availability of normative physiological and biochemical baseline data. The rhesus monkey *(M. mulatta)* is the best documented subhuman primate species. Unfortunately, they have become extremely scarce due to the export embargo imposed by the Indian government in 1977. Only the baboon has been studied as thoroughly as the rhesus, and baboons are too large and difficult to handle for use in most research laboratories. Thus, the relative unavailability of the most suitable subhuman primate species introduces a major cautionary note regarding proposed research with such animals.

What, then, are appropriate reasons for selecting subhuman primates for subjects in biomedical research, especially as it pertains to alcoholism? It is my opinion that there are very few new investigations that can justify the use of subhuman primates. For the same reasons, it is not wise for new investigators to plan to establish research programs that depend on subhuman primates rather than one of the more available and less complex species. I suggest that, at least for the present time, the only types of studies that should plan to use subhuman primates as subjects are either those on-going research projects that have accumulated a substantial amount of data with these species, or the very rare studies for which no other animal would be suitable. In those cases, the use of other species could be extremely costly and disruptive of an investigator's research and might delay work that was on the verge of providing important new information about alcoholism. Even in such cases, it behooves the investigator to be extremely conservative about planning terminal studies and to make every attempt to use each animal in several studies and/or as breeding stock. All investigators using primates in their research must reconsider the need for them as subjects in their studies. If the need is valid and supportable, the investigator would be wise to select a subhuman primate species that is in good supply, reported to be thriving in their habitats, and where the habitat is within a stable and rational political jurisdiction.

I urge all investigators who use substantial numbers of subhuman primates in their research programs to establish small breeding programs as a way of providing partial replenishment of their use. Our experience with this venture has been that, although it is costly and time-consuming, it does insure a limited supply of replacement animals and can be conducted in most research animal facilities.

SUMMARY

In summary, subhuman primates have been and are presently being used as experimental subjects in a variety of research projects related to alcoholism. This chapter has attempted to survey those studies, presenting both the successes of such research efforts and the special problems associated with the use of subhuman primates as research subjects. The development of self-administration procedures was summarized, and the technique discussed as a potential animal model of alcoholism. Current problems pertaining to the availability of monkeys for research were discussed, and consideration of the selection of alternate species of experimental animals discussed. The problem of alcoholism is too immense and important to allow the current shortage of subhuman primate research subjects to produce a major slow-down of alcoholism research. Alcoholism has such devastating effects on its victims, their relatives, and society at large that present research efforts must be continued and intensified, regardless of the animal subjects used.

REFERENCES

1. Anderson, W.W., and Thompson, T. *Pharmacol. Biochem. Beh.* 2:447–454, 1974.
2. Cannon, D.S. et al. *Pharmacol. Biochem. Beh.* 2:831–837, 1974.
3. Cicero, T.J., Snider, S.R., Perez, V.J., and Swanson, L.W. *Physiol. Beh.* 6:191–198, 1970.
4. Cutler, M.G. *Neuropharm.* 15:495–501, 1976.
5. Geiger, J.F., Barker, L.M. *Q. J. Stud. Alcohol.* 37:950–958, 1976.
6. Goldstein, D.B. *J. Pharmacol. Exp. Ther.* 190:377–383, 1974.
7. Goldstein, D.B. *Fed. Proc.* 34:1953–1961, 1975.
8. Goldstein, D.B. *Life Sci.* 18:553–559, 1976.
9. Goldstein, D.B., Pal, N. *Science.* 172:288–293, 1971.
10. Lester, D. *Q. J. Stud. Alcohol.* 22:223–231, 1961.
11. Majchrowicz, E. *Psychopharmacology* 43:245–254, 1975.

12. Myers, R.D., in George, R., Okun, R., and Cho, A.K. (eds.), *Annual Review of Pharmacology and Toxicology.* Palo Alto, Calif.: Annual Reviews, 1978, pp. 125-144.
13. Eriksson, K. *Drug & Alc. Depend.* (In press).
14. Jarbe, T.U.C. *Arch. Internat. Pharmacodyn. Ther.* 227:118-123, 1977.
15. Ross, D., Hartman, R.J., and Geller, I. *Proc. West Pharmacol. Soc.* 19:326-330, 1976.
16. Thurman, R.G. *The Pharmacologist.* 20:160, 1978.
17. Barondes, S. *Drug & Alc. Depend.* (In press).
18. Faber, D. (personal communication).
19. Ellis, F.W., and Pick, J.R. *J. Pharmacol. Exp. Ther.* 175:88-93, 1970.
20. Brown, R.V., and Hutcheson, D.P. *Q. J. Stud. Alcohol.* 34:758-763, 1973.
21. West. L.J. *Ann. N.Y. Acad. Sci.* 197:13-15, 1972.
22. Terry, M.W., in Schrier, A.M. (ed.), *Behavioral Primatology—Advances in Research and Theory,* Vol. 1. New York: Wiley, 1977, pp. 1-32.
23. Goldfoot, D., in Schrier, A.M. (ed.), *Behavioral Primatology—Advances in Research Theory,* Vol. 1. New York: Wiley, 1977, pp. 139-184.
24. Pieper, W.A., Skeen, M.J., McClure H.M., and Bourne, P.G. *Science* 176:71-73, 1972.
25. Hershkovitz, P. *Living New World Monkeys (Platyrrhini),* Vol. 1. Chicago: University of Chicago Press, 1977, p. 1117.
26. Napier, J.R., and Napier, P.H. *A Handbook of Living Primates.* New York: Academic Press, 1967, pp. 456.
27. Altshuler, H.L., Stowell, R.E., and Lowe, R.T. *Lab. Ani. Sci.* 21:916-926, 1971.
28. Altshuler, H.L., and Stowell, R.E. *Lab. Ani. Sci.* 22:692-704, 1972.
29. Lester, D., and Freed, E.X. *Pharmacol. Biochem. Beh.* 1:103-107, 1973.
30. Mello, N.K. *Pharmacol. Biochem. Beh.* 1:89-101, 1973.
31. Woods, J.H., and Winger, G.D., in Mello, N.K. and Mendelson, J.H. (eds.), *Recent Advances in Studies of Alcoholism.* Washington: U.S. Government Printing Office, Publ. No. (HSM) 71-9045, pp. 413-436.
32. Lieber, C.S., and DeCarli, L.M., *Adv. Exp. Med. Biol.* 59:379-393, 1975.
33. Lieber, C.S., and DeCarli, L.M. *J. Med. Primatol.* 3:153-163, 1974.
34. Committee on the Problems of Drug Dependence, in Thompson, T., and Unna, K.R. (eds.), *Predicting Dependence Liability of Stimulant and Depressant Drugs.* Baltimore: University Park Press, 1977, pp. 303-318.
35. Thompson, T. in Thompson, T., and Unna, K.R. (eds.), *Predicting Dependence Liability of Stimulant and Depressant Drugs.* Baltimore: University Park Press, 1977, pp. 1-8.
36. Deneau, G., Yanagita, T., and Seevers, M.H., *Psychopharmacol.* 16:30-48, 1969.
37. Karoly, A.J., Winger, G.D., Ikomi, F., and Woods, J.H. *Psychopharmacol.* 58:19-25, 1978.
38. Winger, G.D., and Woods, J.H. *Ann. N.Y. Acad. Sci.* 215:162-175, 1973.
39. Woods, J.H., Ikomi, F., and Winger, G., in Roach, M.K., McIsaac, W.M., and Creaven, P.J. (eds.), *Biological Aspects of Alcoholism.* Austin: University of Texas Press, 1971, pp. 371-388.
40. Woods, J.H., and Winger, G.D. *Prev. Med.* 3:49-60, 1974.
41. Begleiter, H., Branchey, M.H., and Kissin, B. *Beh. Biol.* 7:137-142, 1972.
42. Denoble, V.J., and Begleiter, H. *Pharmacol. Biochem. Beh.* 8:391-397, 1977.
43. Altshuler, H.L., Feinhandler, D.A., and Phillips, P.E. *Life Sci.* (Submitted).
44. Yanagita, T. *Bull. Comm. on Problems of Drug Depend.* 5631-5640, 1968.
45. Altshuler, H.L., Weaver, S., and Phillips, P. *Life Sci.* 17:883-890, 1975.
46. Altshuler, H.L., and Talley, L., in Seixas, F.A. (ed.), *Currents in Alcoholism,* Vol. 1. New York: Grune and Stratton, 1977, pp. 243-253.
47. Altshuler, H.L., and Phillips, P.E., in Ho, B.T., Richards, D.W., III, and Chute, D.L. (eds.), *Drug Discrimination and State Dependent Learning.* New York: Academic Press, 1978, pp. 263-280.

48. Henningfield, J.E., and Meisch, R.A. *Pharmacol. Biochem. Beh.* 4:473–475, 1976.
49. Henningfield, J.E., and Meisch, R.A., in *Problems of Drug Dependence 1975.* Washington: National Academy of Science, 1976, pp. 924–929.
50. Meisch, R.A., and Henningfield, J.E. *Adv. Exp. Med. Biol.* B85:443–463, 1977.
51. Meisch, R.A., and Thompson, T., in Singh, J.M., and Lai, H. *Drug Addiction, Neurobiology and Influences on Behavior,* Vol. 3. Mount Kisco, N.Y.: Futura Publishers, 1974, 117 ff.
52. Meisch, R.A., Henningfield, J.E., and Thompson, T., in Gross, M.M. (ed.), *Alcohol Intoxication and Withdrawal.* New York: Plenum Press, 1975, pp. 323–342.
53. Pieper, W.A., in Majchrowicz, E. (ed.), *Biochemical Pharmacology of Ethanol.* New York: Plenum Press, 1975, 327 ff.
54. Pieper, W.A., and Skeen, M.J. *Adv. Exp. Med. Biol.* B85:43–55, 1977.
55. Pieper, W.A., and Skeen, M.J. *Pharmacol. Biochem. Beh.* 3:909–913, 1975.
56. Perrin, R.G., Kalant, H., and Livingston, K.E. *Electroenceph. Clin. Neurophysiol.* 39:157–171, 1957.
57. Elton, R.H., Greaves, D.A., Bunger, D.R., and Pyle, T.W. *Q. J. Stud. Alcohol.* 37:1548–1555, 1975.
58. Jacobson, S. (personal communication).
59. Cressman, R.J., and Cadell, T.E. *Q. J. Stud. Alcohol.* 32:764–774, 1971.
60. Elton, R.H., Malaby, J.E., Dau, D.L., and Arnold, R.V. *Q. J. Stud. Alcohol.* 36:1124–1130, 1975.
61. Glowa, J.R., and Barrett, J.E. *Pharmacol. Biochem. Beh.* 4:169–173, 1976.
62. Katz, J.L., and Barrett, J.E. *Pharmacol. Biochem. Beh.* 2:35–39, 1977.
63. Mello, N.K. *Physiol. Beh.* 7:77–101, 1971.
64. Schuster, C.R., and Thompson, T. *Ann. Rev. Pharmacol.* 9:483–502, 1968.
65. Smith, S.G., and Davis, W.M. *Pharmacol. Res. Commun.* 6:397–402, 1974.
66. Smith, S.G., Werner, T.E., and Davis, W.M. *Physiol. Psychol.* 4:91–93, 1976.
67. Smith, S.G., Werner, T.E., and Davis, W.M. *Psychopharmacol.* 53:223–226, 1977.
68. Yanagita, T., Ando, K., Takahashi, S., and Ishida, K. *Proc. Comm. on Problems of Drug Depend.* 6039–6051, 1969.

CHAPTER 18

Sexual Dysfunction in Male Alcoholics and its Objective Evaluation

ISMET KARACAN
SCOTT SNYDER
PATRICIA J. SALIS
ROBERT L. WILLIAMS
SABRI DERMAN

It is now generally recognized that alcohol abuse can lead to impotence. A large number of papers have dealt mainly with the role of alcohol consumption as a social lubricant, its influence on sexual potency, and its possible role in triggering erectile "failures" after heavy drinking, which can lead to more severe impotency problems. One of Shakespeare's most often quoted passages is "(Drink) provokes the desire, but it takes away the performance." Regrettably, this passage from *Macbeth* in large part represents our knowledge of the effects of alcohol on sexual behavior. The vast majority of research has been characterized by impressionistic, anecdotal, and subjective investigations and has notably lacked rigorous methodology.

Impotence is one of the rare health problems for which, until recently, the patient made his own diagnosis, estimated the effect of treatment, and decided whether the medical care had succeeded or failed. Although a physician can attempt to diagnose impotence by taking a careful history, performing laboratory tests for diseases that cause impotence, and giving psychological tests, his major source of information is still the patient himself, which limits the physician to highly subjective data. We have advanced the suggestion[1] that clinical use of the phenomenon of nocturnal penile tumescence (NPT) as a diagnostic tool can provide reliable objective data of male potency or impotence; therefore, the erectile disturbances of alcoholics can be evaluated with NPT recordings, and can indicate the presence and degree of the problem during alcohol abuse, sobriety, and treatment. In this chapter we will discuss the literature on the effects of alcohol on sexual performance and then present some preliminary data on the NPT characteristics of impotent alcoholics.

ALCOHOLISM AND SEXUAL PERFORMANCE

Moderate amounts of alcohol have long been noted to enhance sexual desire by lessening or removing inhibitions.[2] Ewing[3] suggested that this increased sexual freedom is due to the chemical depression of the rostral cerebrum by alcohol. That area of the brain was seen as the center for the self-critical and self-controlling faculties of people. Thus, alcohol has been seen as a social lubricant enabling greater sexual experimentation and performance because of its attenuation of the guilt and anxiety which are concomitants of sexual activity for many people.[4]

Another explanation for this "enhancement" may be that the threshold for male sexual performance is raised by alcohol, allowing the male partner a longer time to engage in foreplay and perhaps enhancing the couple's sexual performance by increasing the probability of the female experiencing orgasm.[5] Premature ejaculation in 23 of 200 men previously reporting difficulty improved with alcohol, probably by decreasing anxiety and guilt associated with sexual behavior.[3] These men reported that they had to control the amount of alcohol consumed carefully since excessive amounts resulted in either delayed ejaculation or even impotence.

The ingestion of excessive amounts of alcohol results almost invariably in impaired sexual performance, reducing heterosexual desire and activity.[6] Decreased libido as well as the absence of orgasm (particularly prevalent among women) may also result.[7] The scope of the problem is indicated by the fact that Masters and Johnson believe that alcohol is the second most frequent cause of secondary impotence.[8] Lemere[9] states that sexual impotence was noted in 8% of 17,000 alcoholics treated consecutively in a hospital setting. In one-half of these patients, the sexual impairment has continued after years of sobriety. Interestingly, libido was not affected and few females complained of sexual difficulties.

A variety of psychological and physiologic mechanisms have been invoked to explain why alcohol affects human sexual performance. The main psychological explanations for the effect of alcohol on sexual activity have come from social psychiatry. A person may use alcohol to avoid his or her partner, thus providing an excuse for the alcoholic's lack of affection and sexual desire. Alternatively, the nonalcoholic partner can become very self-righteous and condescending when the other's intoxication is discovered, and can reject the alcoholic and justify his or her own frigidity and aloofness.[3]

Since Abraham's report in 1926,[10] psychoanalysts have proposed associations between alcohol and a variety of sexual "perversions," most notably homosexuality. These are not usually considered to be causal relationships. Parker,[11] for instance, used psychometrics to compare alcoholics with moderate drinkers and observed that the former had significantly lower degrees of masculinity than the latter, but found no cause and effect relationship between alcohol use and homosexuality.

The prevailing physiological explanations for the effect of alcohol on sexual ability come from the often overlapping fields of endocrinology and neurology. Since Silvestrini's observation in 1926[12] of testicular atrophy and gynecomastia in male alcoholics with liver disease, alcohol-induced endocrinologic changes have been offered as an important, if not causal, factor in these effects.[2] These end-organ effects are probably due to a derangement in androgen metabolism, most notably testosterone.[13] Recent studies suggest that the fall in testosterone levels during alcohol consumption is accompanied by a rise in plasma LH levels; however, it is not known whether these endocrinologic changes actually cause the sexual dysfunction noted with alcohol use. It is conceivable that alcohol-induced alterations in hypothalamic-pituitary relationships may affect hormonal factors which are even more directly responsible for sexual behavior. A recent comprehensive review of the effects of alcohol on pituitary-gonadal hormones and sexual function in males is available.[14]

Other studies indicate that neurologic deficits are primarily responsible for the effects of alcohol. Damage to a nervous system arc consisting of the cerebral cortex (origin of sexual thoughts), anterior portion of the temporal lobe (regulates libido intensity), hypothalamus, spinal cord reflex centers (responsible for erection), and peripheral nerves (transmitters of sensory and vasomotor impulses to and from the genital organs) has been postulated to impair erectile capacity.[10]

Some physiological studies of the effects of alcohol on heterosexual desire and activity have been completed. Rubin and Henson[5] have shown that penile tumescence is significantly reduced by alcohol ingestion and the decrease corresponds to the amount of alcohol consumed. In this study, the first drink of young-adult male alcoholics reduced their mean erection from 50% to 45% of maximum as measured by a penile transducer. The third drink reduced the mean erection from 49% to 23% of maximum. The third drink was also the point at which mean latency to full erection was increased from 1.5 to 3 minutes. The main effect of low (0.5–0.6 ml/kg) amounts of alcohol was on the maintenance of erection and not on the rate of development of arousal or maximum degree of erection attained, although high blood alcohol levels did correspond to greater impairment of sexual arousal. Arousal was not totally eliminated, however, even with blood alcohol levels as high as 106–156 mg/100 ml. Some subjects reported enhanced sexual arousal, indicating how subjective reporting can be at variance with objective physiological data.

Farkas and Rosen[15] studied the effects of acute administration of alcohol on the penile tumescence of healthy adult male university students. A slight increase in penile tumescence was noted with blood alcohol concentrations less than 0.025%, and with a concomitant maximal penile diameter increase; however, there was a much greater decrement in both tumescence rate and penile diameter as blood alcohol levels surpassed the 0.025% level.

In women, vaginal pulse pressure has been measured and found to be decreased by alcohol ingestion. Wilson and Lawson[16] studied university women between the ages of 18 and 22. Vaginal pulse pressure was measured by means of a photoplethysmograph and was found to diminish with increasing blood alcohol level. Sexual arousal, as measured by the Thematic Apperception Test and the subjects' self-reports, indicated no correlation between blood alcohol levels and sexual excitement.

All three of these studies[5,15,16] utilized erotic materials in the form of films, pornographic literature, and the like to sexually arouse their subjects after alcohol ingestion. The studies did not account for character variables such as guilt, morality, or religious persuasion, which can profoundly influence sexual response to pornographic material. Measurement of NPT instead of daytime sexual arousal decreases the significance of some of these variables.

AN OBJECTIVE ASSESSMENT OF ERECTILE FUNCTION IN IMPOTENT ALCOHOLICS

In a preliminary study of the NPT characteristics of impotent alcoholics we examined six men who presented with a chief complaint of inability to attain and/or maintain an erection. They underwent evaluation of NPT in our Sleep Disorders Center as part of the diagnostic work-up. In the course of the evaluation it was concluded clinically that the patients had histories of significant alcohol misuse or abuse. The group represented all such patients evaluated to date. The patients were 45 to 55 years of age. All but one patient was separated or divorced; the exception has been married to his second wife for 22 years. Occupations ranged from unemployed because of disability to businessman. At the time of the evaluation two patients continued to drink; the other four claimed to have been abstinent for variable periods of time (maximum four years). All patients denied taking any drugs during the evaluation period.

The patients were evaluated according to our standard procedure,[1] which included monitoring of sleep and NPT (base and tip) patterns on three consecutive nights and administration of selected psychological tests. For this report we analyzed NPT data from the penis tip for the second evaluation night. The NPT data were scored as described elsewhere.[17]

Each patient was matched by age ($\pm$ one year) with a healthy control subject who had undergone three consecutive nights of NPT monitoring under similar conditions. (These subjects were among those described in previous reports.[18,19]) For each control subject, data from the second and third nights were averaged to form a single observation. Data from the two groups of six men were compared with two-tailed t-tests for independent samples ($df = 10$). A probability of 0.05 was the limit for statistical significance.

Table 1 shows the results of comparisons between the two groups of men for the major NPT characteristics. On the average the two groups

TABLE 1.–NPT Characteristics of Six Impotent Alcoholic Patients and Six Age-Matched Healthy Control Subjects

Characteristic	Patients		Controls		
	Mean	S.D.	Mean	S.D.	p
Age (years)	50.8	4.9	50.8	4.4	—
Minutes of sleep	372.5	64.5	371.8	36.2	NS
Minutes of NPT	94.5	30.4	103.8	34.6	NS
Minutes of full NPT	32.3	35.5	84.2	36.5	<.05
Number of full NPT episodes	0.8	1.0	2.7	0.8	<.01
Minutes of partial NPT	62.2	54.5	19.5	15.7	NS*
Number of partial NPT episodes	2.8	1.2	1.0	0.6	<.01
Maximum change in penile tip circumference (millimetres)	15.8	7.2	23.1	3.7	NS*

*$p < .10$

obtained equivalent amounts of sleep. Although the impotent patients as a group displayed slightly fewer minutes of NPT, the difference was not significant. On the other hand, the group of impotent patients displayed significantly less full NPT (minutes and number) and more partial NPT (significant for number, trend for minutes) than the controls. As expected from these results, the maximum circumference change tended to be reduced in the group of patients.

Closer inspection of data for individual patients (Table 2) revealed, however, two distinct subgroups of patients—those whose NPT was clearly abnormal in the complete absence of full NPT, and those who exhibited at least some full NPT. Three patients fell into each subgroup. The patients who had no full NPT displayed variable and, in two cases, somewhat extreme total amounts of NPT. The number of partial NPT episodes (3.3) in the patients approximated the total number of episodes (3.7) in the control subjects, but the amount of partial NPT in the patients was clearly very high. The maximum circumference change in the patients never reached half of the control-group average.

For the patients who exhibited full NPT, the total amount of NPT was, on the average, 20 minutes less than for the control subjects. All three patients obtained less full NPT (average of 20 minutes and one episode) than the average for the controls. Amounts and numbers of partial NPT episodes were more variable, but the average amount was equivalent to that of controls while the average number was greater. The maximum circumference change was close to the control value for all three patients.

Although speculation and discussion of relationships among alcohol consumption, enhanced sexual desire, and impaired sexual performance have a long history, systematic research on these relationships has only recently begun. To date, little of this research has employed an objective means of assessing erectile function. The research that has done so has involved presentation of erotic material, a procedure fraught with potential contaminants, to university students. The study we described here thus represents the first known attempt to examine a population of critical interest—impotent alcoholics—in a way that removes the contaminants associated with previous procedures.

The study constituted a preliminary examination of whether alcohol misuse or abuse is associated with significant disturbances in NPT that could indicate an organic basis for the frequent complaint of impotence in alcoholics. The study was preliminary for several reasons. Among other things, the sample size was quite small, periods of alcohol misuse or abuse were variable, and periods of alcohol abstinence were variable. In addition, although alcohol abuse may reasonably be expected to produce organic deficits that lead to impotence, the alcoholic is as susceptible, if not more

TABLE 2.–NPT Characteristics of Impotent Alcoholic Patients Without and With Full NPT

Patient	Age (yr)	Min. Sleep	Min. NPT	Min. Full	No. Full	Min. Partial	No. Partial	Max. Circ.
				Characteristic				
Without								
1	55	446	60	0	0	60	3	11
2	51	352	107	0	0	107	3	11
3	42	448	147	0	0	147	4	8
Mean	49	415	105	0	0	105	3	10
S.D.	7	55	43	—	—	43	0.6	2
With								
4	55	292	90	70	2	20	2	20
5	53	377	72	62	2	10	1	19
6	49	320	90	61	1	29	4	27
Mean	52	330	84	64	2	20	2	22
S.D.	3	43	10	5	0.6	9	1.5	4

so, to psychogenic impotence as any other man. Despite these complicating factors, the study provided suggestive evidence that deserves examination in more controlled investigations.

The major suggestive finding was the relatively high incidence of disturbed NPT in the impotent alcoholics. Our extensive examinations of normal men[18,19] revealed that it is extremely unlikely for NPT to be disturbed in men who do not complain of impotence. In contrast, 50% of our small sample of impotent alcoholics displayed clearly abnormal NPT. It will, of course, be of great interest to us to determine whether this rate is confirmed in a more extensive series of patients. If it is, we will have additional evidence for our hypothesis that, because NPT is significantly disturbed in impotent patients who have a high probability of organic deficits, NPT can be considered a valid index of erectile capacity and therefore of use in the differential diagnosis of organogenic and psychogenic impotence.

The degree of NPT disturbance in one subgroup of patients was striking — a total absence of full erection during sleep and exaggerated amounts of partial erection. The data suggest that the mechanisms that initiate and maintain regular NPT episodes were intact in the patients, but that the mechanisms that allow maximal engorgement of the penis were defective. We do not at present have sufficient data to indicate whether the defect may be neural,[1] vascular,[1,20] hormonal, or other.

For the three patients whose NPT was generally normal, our clinical decision was to conclude that impotence was not organically determined. On the other hand, there are some indications in the data of NPT deterioration and possible slight organic involvement. Total amount of NPT was in the low-normal range, as were the amount of full NPT and the number of such episodes. Amount and number of partial NPT were variable, but Patient 6 had an unusually high number of partial episodes. Perhaps these slight abnormalities indicate the initial phase of organic involvement. It will be interesting to follow these patients to determine whether full-scale NPT disturbance eventually develops and is associated with exacerbation of impotence.

Although the number of patients with disturbed NPT was impressive for the alcoholic patients, it was considerably smaller than the number (80%) in our recent study of 35 impotent diabetics.[17] Deterioration of erectile mechanisms may, therefore, be rather more likely with diabetes than with alcohol abuse. If further studies confirm the rate for alcoholics, diagnostic and research strategies may be aided. In the clinical setting, it will be helpful to know that an impotent diabetic probably has organic involvement, whereas an impotent alcoholic may or may not have organic involvement. In the research setting, it may be more profitable to focus research into the physiological mechanisms of erectile dysfunction on diabetics and research into psychological and mixed etiologies of impotence on alcoholics.

For both the impotent alcoholics and the impotent diabetics, it is important to realize that aspects of self-selection probably biased our patient samples. Most of our patients are evaluated in anticipation of receiving a radical form of treatment—implantation of a penile prosthesis.[21] The sample may therefore be loaded with patients who are resistant to more conservative forms of treatment and/or who have greater degrees of organic involvement.

In summary, our preliminary study of six impotent patients with histories of alcohol abuse suggests that such abuse may damage physiological erectile mechanisms, and this damage may account for impotence in at least half of alcoholics who complain of impotence. Further controlled investigations are needed to confirm and extend this finding.

REFERENCES

1. Karacan, I., Salis, P.J., and Williams, R.L. The role of the sleep laboratory in the diagnosis and treatment of impotence. In Williams, R.L., and Karacan, I. (eds.), *Sleep Disorders: Diagnosis and Treatment.* New York: Wiley, 1978, pp. 353–382.
2. Carver, A.E. The interrelationship of sex and alcohol. *Int. J. Sex.* 2:78–81, 1948.
3. Ewing, J.A. Alcohol, sex, and marriage. *Med. Aspects Hum. Sex.* 2:43–50, 1968.
4. Fox, R. A psychiatrist discusses drinking and sex. *Sex. Beh.* 1:67–69, 87, 1971.
5. Rubin, H.R., and Henson, D.E. Effects of alcohol on male sexual responding. *Psychopharmacology* 47:123–134. 1976.
6. Levine, J. The sexual adjustment of alcoholics. A clinical study of a selected sample. *Q. J. Stud. Alcohol* 16:675–680, 1955.
7. Viamontes, J.A. Alcohol abuse and sexual dysfunction. *Med. Aspects Hum. Sex.* 8:185–186, 1974.
8. Masters, W.H., and Johnson, V.E. *Human Sexual Inadequacy.* Boston: Little, Brown, 1970.
9. Lemere, F., and Smith, J.W. Alcohol-induced sexual impotence. *Am. J. Psychiat.* 130:212–213, 1973.
10. Abraham, K. The psychological relations between sexuality and alcoholism. *Int. J. Psycho-Anal.* 7:2–10, 1926.
11. Parker, F.B. A comparison of the sex temperament of alcoholics and moderate drinkers. *Am. Sociol. Rev.* 24:366–374, 1959.
12. Silvestrini, R. Gynecomastia in men with cirrhosis of the liver. *Ref. Med.* 42:701–704, 1926.
13. Galvao-Seles, A., Anderson, O.C., Burke, C.W., Marchall, J.C., Corker, C.S., Brown, R.L., and Clark, M.L. Biological activity of androgens. *Lancet* 1:173–177, 1973.
14. Mendelson, J.H., Mello, N.K., and Ellingboe, J. Effects of alcohol on pituitary-gonadal hormones, sexual function, and aggression in human males. In Lipton, M.A., DiMascio, A., and Killam, K.F. (eds.), *Psychopharmacology: A Generation of Progress.* New York: Raven Press, 1978, pp. 1677–1692.

15. Farkas, G.M., and Rosen, R.C. Effect of alcohol on elicited male sexual response. *J. Stud. on Alcohol* 37:265–272, 1976.
16. Wilson, G.T., and Lawson, D.M. Effects of alcohol on sexual arousal in women. *J. Abnorm. Psych.* 85:489–497, 1976.
17. Karacan, I., Salis, P.J., Ware, J.C., Dervent, B., Williams, R.L., Scott, F.B., Attia, S.L., and Beutler, L.E. Nocturnal penile tumescence and diagnosis in diabetic impotence. *Am. J. Psychiat.* 135:191–197, 1978.
18. Karacan, I., Williams, R.L., Thornby, J.I., and Salis, P.J. Sleep-related penile tumescence as a function of age. *Am. J. Psychiat.* 132:932–937, 1975.
19. Karacan, I., Salis, P.J., Thornby, J.I., and Williams, R.L. The ontogeny of nocturnal penile tumescence. *Waking Sleeping* 1:27–44, 1976.
20. Karacan, I., Ware, J.C., Dervent, B., Altinel, A., Thornby, J.I., Williams, R.L., Kaya, N., and Scott, F.B. Impotence and blood pressure in the flaccid penis: Relationship to nocturnal penile tumescence. *Sleep* 1:125–132, 1978.
21. Scott, F.B. The surgical treatment of erectile impotence. In Williams, R.L., and Karacan, I. (eds.), *Sleep Disorders: Diagnosis and Treatment.* New York: Wiley, 1978, pp. 401–409.

CHAPTER 19

The Search for Psychopathic States in Alcoholics and Other Drug Abusers

DAVID C. KAY

DEFINING THE PATHOLOGY OF DRUG ABUSE

Several viewpoints exist as to the definition and pathology of alcoholism and other drug abuse problems. Within the scope of this discussion, the term *drug abuse* will include all problems with any psychoactive drug, including alcohol: biological problems, psychological problems, and/or social problems. The competition in ideas as to the essential pathology of drug abuse has become sufficiently intense that many theorists support a multi-factorial approach. However, no therapy based on any viewpoint (including the multi-factorial) has yet consistently yielded a permanent improvement in large numbers of those individuals caught in the web of compulsive drug use. In fact, increasing numbers of people are now becoming involved in one or another pattern of psychoactive drug abuse. This review will attempt to emphasize a biological viewpoint of drug abuse which recently has gained more experimental support, and which has potential use in a rational therapy of drug abuse.

The pathology issue might become more clear if we consider the question, "When is an alcoholic not an alcoholic?" Answers to this question range from "Never—once an alcoholic, always an alcoholic", to

"Until the next episode—a person is only alcoholic when drinking and in trouble." It is obvious that *drug-taking* is a phasic (episodic) phenomenon, and that intoxication (which usually requires several drug-taking occurrences) is also phasic in most people. Such phasic intoxication is seen even with free access during experimental alcohol studies.[1] Possibly the question above might be rephrased, "Is an individual equally liable at every moment to return to a prior pattern of drug abuse?" This latter question can be answered in the negative for sedative-hypnotics such as alcohol, both in humans and in animals; the course of such chronic drug intake and intoxication is episodic, for no certain reason. Repetitive drug-seeking behaviors, such as "hustling" (seeking money for drugs) or "copping" (seeking sources for drugs) might well be measurable, but also are episodic (usually at a higher amount or rate than that of drug-taking or of intoxication).

If some tonic phenomenon could be discovered by which to estimate the tendency to take drugs (craving) even when not using them, the assessment of pathology in drug abusers could become more scientific. Especially desirable as such a measure of craving would be some biological phenomenon with a tonic component, comparable to blood sugar level (as a measure of status of a diabetic).

Alcoholism and other types of drug abuse have been defined by several theorists as a *disease*. Webster's unabridged dictionary defines disease as "an alteration of state of the human body ..., interrupting or disturbing the performance of the vital functions." It would appear critical to the concept of disease that a *change in state* occurs, and it is clear from the discussion above that although *drug-taking* and *drug-seeking* may be reliable markers (signs or symptoms) of the disease of drug abuse, neither can be used as the essential definition of the pathologic state. However, one form of treatment for alcoholism and other drug abuse diseases still consists of a protracted period of voluntary or involuntary abstinence from the drug, as if such an experience of life without drug-taking would confer further ability to avoid drug-taking.

Other theorists have identified the essential pathology in the drug itself, labeling alcohol or opiates as "hard" (pathological), while other drugs are "soft" (nonpathological). Drug dependence problems have been identified by drug type by the World Health Organization[2] and the American Psychiatric Association,[3] which implies that the drug defines the disease. Although such classifications can be heuristic descriptive tools, the history of drug abuse has been replete with evidence that abuse of one psychoactive drug has been significantly associated with the abuse of other drugs. This must be recognized as evidence of an essential pathology which transcends any specific drug. Identification of the drug as the essential pathologic component has been used as justification for both prohibitionistic and permissive attitudes toward various psychoactive drugs. The essential pathology of drug abuse has been identified by some theorists as existing in the drug-abusing subculture, or in the social relationships of the drug abuser. However, such a subpopulation is not always viewed as pathologic; some see drug "use" as an expression of an alternate life style. Apart from drug availability (provision or denial of drug), the association of an individual's social relationships to his drug-taking behavior has not yet been competent to predict his craving for drugs (unless he is taking them). Also, alcoholism is a good example of a drug abuse problem which transcends population subcultures and specific social relationships.

Finally, the essential pathology of drug abuse has been located by some in the personality of the individual abuser. The search for the "alcoholic personality" or "addict personality" has not revealed a personality pattern specific for any of these drug abuse problems, although some commonality in alcoholics, opiate addicts and criminals has been found, as will be discussed below.

It is recognized that chronic drug abuse may result in diseases (damage) in an individual's *body, social relationships* and *personality.* The critical question is what disease is present *before* such secondary diseases emerge? It might well be that drug abuse represents a spontaneous but unsuccessful *treatment* for such a primary disease. This chapter reviews some progress in a search for a disease underlying drug abuse.

THE CONCEPT OF PSYCHOPATHIC PERSONALITY

The type of antisocial behavior now labeled as psychopathic has been recognized for centuries. It was considered a type of mental disorder by the time of Pinel,[4] who used the label of *manie sans delire* to describe aimless antisocial behavior.[5,6] J. C. Pritchard[7] coined the term *moral insanity* for such antisocial behavior, and Esquirol[8] included this behavior among his *monomanias.*

Morel,[9] Magnan,[10] and Lombroso[11] espoused the idea of *moral degeneracy;* that certain individuals have a hereditary predisposition to moral pathology. Koch[12] developed the term *psychopathic inferiority* and Kraepelin[13] the terms *psychopathic state* and *psychopathic personality.* However, such German authorities[14] have applied those terms to many personality disorders besides that expressed in antisocial behavior. English and American authorities have generally used the term of *psychopathic personality* in the sense of Pritchard (a disorder associated with antisocial behavior) and we shall use that term in such a fashion throughout this discussion. *Sociopathic personality disturbance: antisocial reaction* was introduced as a modern equivalent in the 1952 edition of the A.P.A. Diagnostic and Statistical Manual,[15] and *antisocial personality* in the DSM II.[3]

Cleckley[16] has provided the most extensive clinical profile of the psychopath. He considers sixteen features (Table 1) to be characteristic. As can be seen by studying this list, Cleckley's definition rests on several clinical judgments, rather than just observable phenomena. However, it appears to be internally consistent and clinically reproducible. He views the psychopath (sociopath) as having a disorder equivalent to psychosis, but with a "mask of sanity".

Robins[18] uses the behavioral description of psychopathy developed at Washington University. They exclude the criteria of schizophrenia, chronic brain syndrome, or mental retardation. Behavioral criteria for psychopaths include: (1) chronic failure to confirm with social norms; (2) failure to maintain close personal relationships; (3) a poor work record; (4) engaging in illegal activities; (5) problems maintaining support; (6) sudden changes in plans; and (7) a low frustration tolerance. Except for the last two, these criteria primarily are historical, and should reflect the most persistent patterns of psychopathic behavior.

The Washington University criteria have also been dominant in the current A.P.A. definition (Table 2) of *antisocial personality disorder*.[19] Such objective criteria should at least ensure definition of a consistent group of individuals for research and clinical studies. A major difficulty, however, which would stem from this dominant historical approach is the resultant inability to discover significant therapeutic shifts because the history cannot be changed.

There has been a recent revival in interest in the psychopath, as evidenced in four books.[20-23] Discussion of the psychopath has even penetrated into the general press.[24] Yochelson and Samenow[25,26] also have examined this problem from a distinctively different viewpoint. This discussion will emphasize the interaction of concepts of psychopathy with concepts of drug abuse, and will accentuate contributions to this area by investigations at the Addiction Research Center.

MEASUREMENT OF PSYCHOPATHIC PERSONALITY

The most prevalent measure of psychopathy in the United States is the Psychopathic Deviate (*Pd*) scale of the Minnesota Multiphasic Personality

Inventory (MMPI). This scale consists of 50 items (Table 3) which were initially derived[27] from a largely juvenile population undergoing psychiatric evaluation for delinquent behavior (non-capital offenses). Major features of this population include "repeated and flagrant disregard for social customs and mores, an inability to profit from punishing experiences as shown in repeated difficulties of the same kind, and an emotional shallowness in relation to others, particularly in sexual and affectional display."[28]

Probably as a reflection of the original derivation of its items, the *Pd* scale tends to be more sensitive to low levels of psychopathy (a short history of antisocial behavior), and not so sensitive to changes such as drug effects in individuals with a high level of psychopathy (a long history of antisocial behavior). It includes many expressions of angry rebellion, especially directed toward the family (items 16, 21, 24, 35, 42, 91, 96, 110, 127, 134, 141, 216, 224, 235, 237, 244, 245). It also includes expressions of depressed ideation and mood (items 61, 67, 84, 94, 102, 106, 107, 248) despite a public bravado (items 82, 171, 180, 201, 267, 284). Especially, a discomfort with sexual feelings (items 20, 37, 231, 239) is seen in this scale, which is appropriate in rebellious and confused juveniles, but would be surprising in older antisocial adults.

The Mania (*Ma*) of the MMPI (Table 4) has also been used as a measure of psychopathy, usually in association with the *Pd* scale. This scale consists of 46 items which were developed[27] to estimate the "overactivity, emotional excitement and flight of ideas" of hypomania.[28] Several items (21, 59, 97, 109, 111, 127, 143, 157, 167, 171, 180, 181, 212, 222, 250, 267, 268, 271, 277, 289, 298) are used in other measures of psychopathy, or are comparable.

Two newer MMPI scales have been developed which are better candidates for measuring degree of psychopathy in older delinquents. The Antisocial (*Ant*) scale (Table 5) was developed by Haertzen and associates[29] from the Social Maladaption factorial scale (MMPI items 38, 118, 289, 294) in the factor analyses of the *Pd* scale by Astin[30] and Monroe.[31]This Antisocial scale (Table 5) consists of 25 items with a major emphasis on historical items.[11] It has been validated in several ways; it differentiates degree of criminality and level of addiction.[29] In both its trait and state format, this state differentiates addicts and alcoholics from non-drug-using controls, when the *Pd* scale does not.[32]

When seeking an MMPI scale which would differentiate prisoner populations on the basis of Cleckley-like clinical dimensions, Spielberger and associates[33] developed a Sociopathy (*Spy*) scale (Table 6). The major characteristic of this 20-item scale is toughness. Individuals rating high on this scale deny any physical weakness (items 332, 412, 533), deny shyness (items 91, 99, 138, 171, 172, 201, 391, 509) and glorify aggressiveness (items 28, 96, 181, 250).

A psychopathic (*Pyp*) scale (Table 7) has also been developed for the Addiction Research Center Inventory (ARCI). This 71-item scale[34] was revised from the one developed by Haertzen and Panton[35] in 785 subjects in order to distinguish psychopathic (criminal, addict, alcoholic) groups from non-psychopathic (normal, mentally ill) groups. In its modified form,[34] it has a high KR-20 (.754) and is useful as a measure of individual difference. Criminals and addicts are the most deviant, and best differentiated from normals and mentally ill in this scale, with alcoholics intermediate. Such a scale differentiated these groups better than did reported scales on the MMPI, CPI, GZTS and 16 P.F.[35]

The ARCI itself is a 550-item questionnaire which contains many items that are presumptive indicators of psychopathic deviation. It has been developed to demonstrate specific patterns of drug effects, as well as characteristics of personality and clinical diagnoses.[34]

The California Psychological Inventory[36] also has scales which tend to reflect psychopathic tendencies. The Socialization (*So*) scale (Table 8) was originally developed as a delinquency scale, although it is now scored in the opposite direction. The 54 items of the Socialization scale are scored opposite in Table 8 to their usual direction, so that items in that table are comparable in direction to the other psychopathy scales. Ten of these items are comparable to MMPI items in the *Pd* scale and 5 items to those of the *Ma* scale. Excitement, impulsivity and supiciousness are more evident in this scale than in some others.

The Responsibility (*Re*) scale of the CPI (Table 9) also can be used as a measure of psychopathy. The 42 items of the Responsibility scale are scored opposite in Table 9 to their usual direction, so that such items are also comparable to the other psychopathy scales. Only 3 *Re* items are related to the *Pd* scale and 3 to the *Ma* scale. Most of this scale's items are quite different from those in the other psychopathy scales.

Such psychological measures of psychopathy as described in the seven scales above have overlap in the specific items included, as well as equivalent statements or logical opposite statements. The *Ant* scale has 16 items (64%) with equivalents in the other scales, followed by the *Pd* scale (30 items; 60%), *Spy* scale (12 items; 60%), *So* scale (25 items; 46%), *Ma* scale (20 items; 44%), *Pyp* scale (27 items; 38%) and the *Re* scale (15 items; 36%).

The *Pd* scale has the most equivalent items in other scales, especially in the *So* and *Pyp* scales. The *Ant* and *Spy* scales both have 6 equivalent items in the *Pd* scale, but only have one equivalent item in common. The *Pyp* scale has the lowest ratio of total equivalent items per length, while the *Ant* scale has the highest ratio. Such equivalent items could be expected to contribute to higher correlations between these psychological measures of psychopathy.

The seven psychological scales described above (*Pd, Ma, Ant, Spy, Pyp, So, Re*) vary in their sampling of a history of antisocial problems, and also vary in their sampling of other historical phenomena. A historical bias could thus be introduced in those items once an individual had experienced such historical events. The MMPI *Ant* scale contrasts markedly with the MMPI *Spy* scale in this dimension: the *Ant* scale is highest and the *Spy* scale lowest (32% vs 0%) in antisocial historical bias; the *Ant* scale also is greater in general historical bias (56% vs 20%). It is evident, therefore, that these two scales measure quite different aspects of the psychopathic personality. Of the two standard MMPI scales the *Pd* is higher than the *Ma* scale in antisocial (12% vs 2%), but equivalent in general (38% vs 39%) historical bias. This contrast in the *Ma* scale reflects the inclusion of items needed to capture episodic hypomanic behavior.

In the non-MMPI scales, the CPI *So* scale is higher than the *Re* scale in antisocial (17% vs 10%) and general (41% vs 29%) historical bias. The stress in the ARCI *Pyp* scale on current state is reflected in its low antisocial (4%) and general (17%) historical bias. It can be seen that these psychological measures vary considerably in historical bias, and thus in their use of such data in their definition of psychopathy.

SOCIOPATHIC HISTORY IN THE DEFINITION OF PSYCHOPATHY

One of the most consistent and reproducible dimensions in defining a psychopath is a long and repetitive history of social problems (sociopathy, in the sense of *social pathology*). This phenomenon has led to the Washington University and American Psychiatric Association criteria for diagnosis of antisocial personality disorder, enumerated above and discussed below. A history of antisocial problems is included to varying degrees in psychological tests of psychopathy, as discussed above.

The clearest evidence for the existence of sociopathic personality as a psychiatric disorder is presented by Robins,[18] who argues that a common set of symptoms appearing in persons with a similar age of onset, a similar family history of the disorder, and a similar course of the disorder, constitutes a psychiatric disease. Sociopathic personality (Table 10)

occurs in children whose fathers have a high incidence of the disease and whose siblings and offspring also appear to have an elevated incidence. The symptoms follow a predictable course, beginning early in childhood with illegal behavior and school discipline problems and continuing into adulthood as illegal behavior, marital instability, social isolation, poor work history, and excessive drinking.[18]

These investigators studied the outcome 30 years later of 524 child guidance clinic patients and 100 controls. Of the patients, 406 had been referred for antisocial behavior and 118 for other reasons. Using criteria developed at the Washington University Department of Psychiatry (Table 10), they considered (but did not mandate) the diagnosis of sociopathic personality in these adults only if the individual demonstrated violations of societal goals in at least 5 of the 19 life areas described. All but one of these criteria (truancy) referred to behavior after age 18. It is important to note that they did not include in their criteria the 1952 DSM idea that these persons "profit neither from experience nor punishment, and maintain no real loyalties to any person, group or code."[15]

The investigators[18] located 90% of the 624 subjects (and records on 98%); 94 of these adult subjects were diagnosed as having a sociopathic personality. A majority of these 94 individuals had histories of poor work functioning (85%), financial dependency (79%), repeated arrests (75%), poor marital stability (74%; 81% of those married), heavy drinking (72%), school problems and truancy (71%), impulsive behavior (67%), sexual promiscuity or perversion (64%), recklessness as an adolescent (62%), vagrancy (60%), physical aggression (58%) and social isolation (56%). Poor marital history, impulsiveness, vagrancy, and the use of aliases distinguished the adult subjects with sociopathic personality from those with anxiety neurosis, hysteria, schizophrenia or alcoholism. The group diagnosed as alcoholics (29 men) were very similar to the sociopaths: 70% of the alcoholics had adult antisocial symptoms in at least five life areas, although these problems were not as severe as those of the sociopathic group. It must be recognized that these two diagnoses were exclusive: if an individual had enough evidence to be diagnosed sociopathic, his alcohol problems would be described as part of his sociopathy (Table 10) rather than being the basis of an additional diagnosis of alcoholism.

Antisocial behavior as a child was significantly associated with sociopathic personality as an adult. However, 406 children had antisocial behavior referrals and only 94 adults were diagnosed as sociopathic. This is a reflection of the stricter criteria for the adult diagnosis, as well as a reflection of differing outcomes of those with antisocial childhood problems. Antisocial symptoms in children were powerful predictors of sociopathy, hysteria, and alcoholism. They also predicted the level of antisocial behavior in adults who were psychotic, or who had less antisocial behavior than that necessary to be diagnosed as sociopathic. Sociopathic personality could be predicted about equally by three childhood measures: (1) the variety (number of areas) of antisocial behavior, (2) the number of episodes of antisocial behavior, or (3) the seriousness of the antisocial behavior (court involvement). Many measures of poverty or deprivation were not predictors of sociopathic disease independent of the child's antisocial behavior.[18]

Hewett and Martin[37] have also found evidence for a long history of problems in alcoholics and opiate addicts, in contrast to control subjects with little drug use. They developed a Personal History Questionnaire (PHQ) with scales to assess alcohol and drug abuse, adult sociopathy, adult non-sociopathic difficulties, and developmental (childhood and adolescent) difficulties. They found that both groups of drug abusers scored greater than controls in PHQ measures of developmental and adult *non-sociopathic* difficulties: drug abusers had more adult depression, sleep disorder, daytime restlessness, and perceptual dysfunction. They also had more childhood and adolescent learning problems, sleep disorders, and daytime restlessness.

Childhood antisocial behavior was greater than controls in drug abusers. As adults, they had more antisocial behavior, criminal behavior, work instability, legal difficulties (both misdeameanors and felonies), and problems with alcohol and other drugs. Incidentally, these drug abusers had significantly higher scores on several standard MMPI scales (*Pd, Sc, Ma, Pt* and D), while the *Ant* scale differentiated them best (addict >alcoholic >control).[37]

Thus, there is strong evidence for a psychopathic (sociopathic) trait or disease in an substantial number of individuals on the basis of a persistent history of difficulties. However, evidence is less clear as to variations (especially improvement) in such individuals. The larger population of other children and adults with antisocial behavior,[48] including drug abuse problems, would appear a better group in which to look for potential measures of spontaneous or induced (treatment) improvement.

RELATION OF DRUG ABUSE TO PSYCHOPATHY

The relationship of alcoholism, opiate abuse and psychopathy was early recognized in scientific studies of addiction. Kolb[38] found that 39% of the 230 opiate addicts whom he examined had either a history of spree drinking (20.5%) or of continuous excessive drinking (18.7%). Besides the spree drinkers (inebriate personality), he[39] also described thrill-seekers (psychopathic diathesis) and habitual criminals (psychopathic personality) as types of addicts. Felix[40] later included all these groups within a psychopathic personality class.

It has been a common finding to note an elevated Pd (MMPI) scale in alcoholics and opiate addicts, even though many different personality patterns are clinically apparent. Astin[30] described five nonorthogonal factors in the Pd scale in opiate addicts: Self-esteem, Hypersensitivity, Social Maladaptation, Emotional Deprivation and Impulse Control. Monroe et al.[31] modified and expanded such an analysis, and derived six major orthogonal factors: Intrapunitiveness, Denial of Shyness, Hypersensitivity, Impulse Control, Emotional Deprivation and Social Maladaptation. These factors have proved useful in distinguishing between psychopaths, but they have an uncertain relationship to psychopathy because the direction of item response in their derivation was ignored.

Hill et al.[41] analyzed the MMPI patterns of 571 alcoholics, opiate addicts and criminals. Their composite profiles were markedly similar (Figure 1). Only the differences in the D (2) scale appear practically significant: alcoholics and addicts were higher than criminals in this scale.

Principle axis and rectangular factor analyses extracted five factors, with the first three well-defined. The first factor defined an "undifferentiated

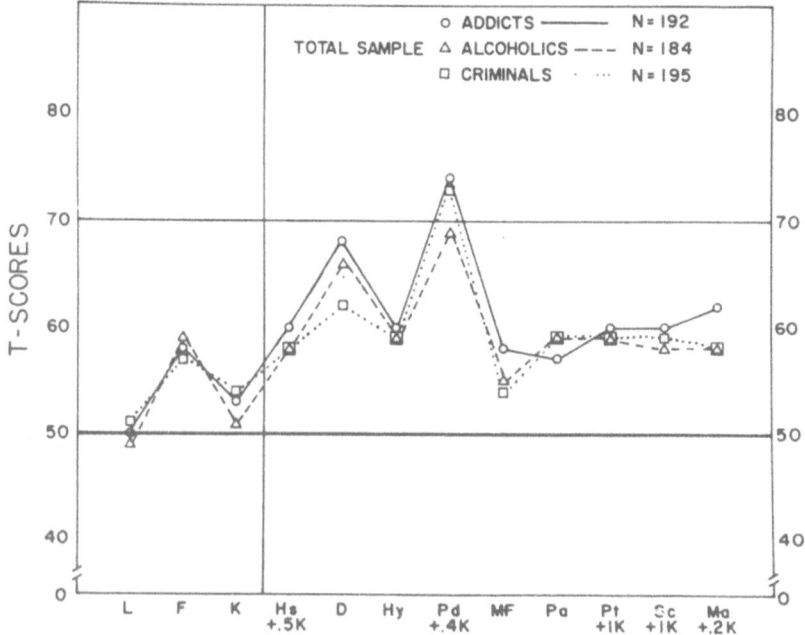

Figure 1.   Composite MMPI profiles of alcoholics, opiate addicts and criminals (total n = 571). Published from Hill et al. (41) by permission.

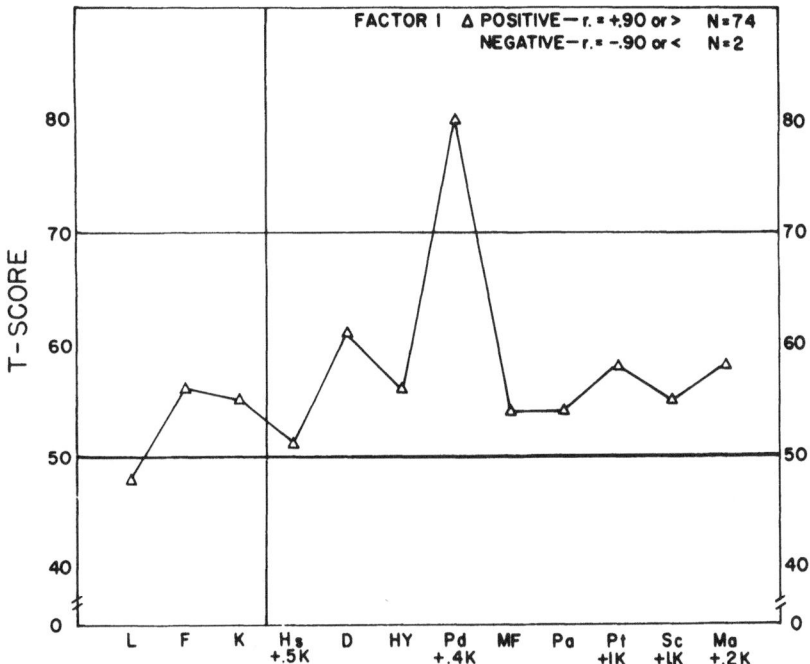

Figure 2. Composite profile of Factor 1 (The undifferentiated psychopath). Published from Hill et al. (41) by permission.

psychopath" (Figure 2), with a single elevation of the *Pd* scale. Alcoholics were lower in loading on this factor.

The second factor defined two patterns: a "primary psychopath" (Figure 3), with elevations of *Pd* (4) and *Ma* (9), and a "depressed neurotic psychopath", (Figure 3) with a marked elevation of *D* (2) and with *Hy* (3) and *Pt* (7) comparable to *Pd* (4). Alcoholics tend toward higher loadings for the depressed psychopath pattern, while criminals had higher loadings for the primary psychopath pattern (opiate addicts were intermediate). The third factor differentiated neurotic from schizoid patterns.[41] Thus, three basic patterns of behavior (aggressive, depressed, withdrawn) can be seen to interact with a more general psychopathic factor.

Components of the MMPI profile seen above in alcoholics, opiate addicts and criminals[41] have also been seen by other authors.[42-45] Haertzen[46] found that opiate addicts have an elevated *Pd* scale regardless of demographic status (age, sex, ethnicity) or institutional status (prisoner, probationer, civil commitment, volunteer). Abusers of stimulants, sedative-hypnotics or hallucinogens also have similar MMPI scale elevations.[47-50] Hill[51] postulates drug abuse to result from the interaction of an *available drug* and a *social deviant*[52] individual (drug abuse of all types is

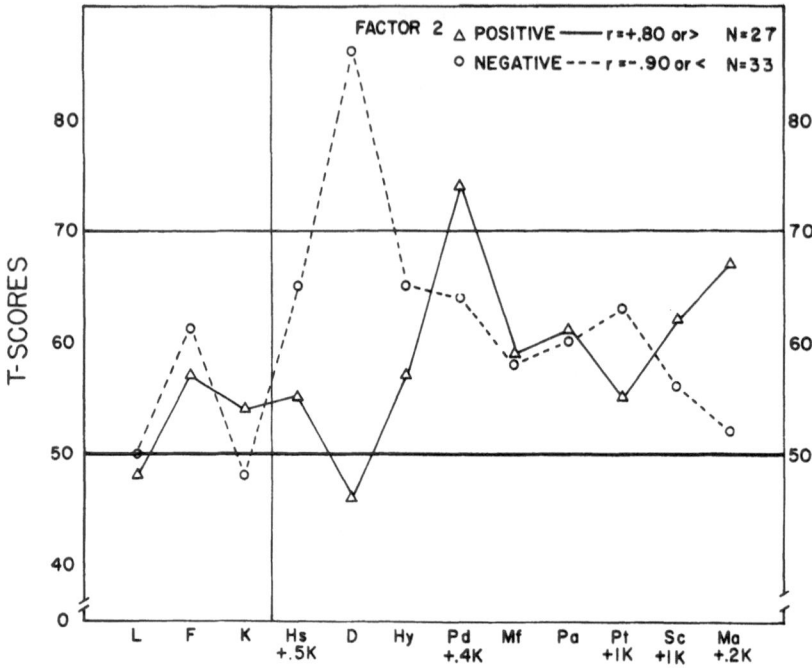

Figure 3.   Composite profiles of Factor 2 (Positive pole: primary psychopath; negative pole: depressed neurotic psychopath). Published from Hill et al. (41) by permission.

associated with a common personality defect); This concept of generalized social deviance is like that of Robins.[18]

DRUG EFFECTS ON PSYCHOPATHS

It is clear that various psychoactive drugs differ in their effects on psychopathic individuals. The Addiction Research Center Inventory (ARCI) has been constructed on the basis of this differentiation.[34,53] Opiates were early described[54,55] as a means of decreasing the aggressiveness of psychopaths, in contrast to the increase in belligerence during alcohol intoxication.

The *MBG* scale in the ARCI[34] measures euphoria: feeling popular, pleasant, talkative, happy. It characterizes the initial reaction to both morphine and amphetamine in psychopaths. The *PCAG* scale measures fatigue, weakness, slowness, sluggishness, and low motivation. It characterizes the initial reaction to pentobarbital, chlorpromazine and alcohol in psychopaths. The *LSD* scale measures anxiety, tension, depersonalization and difficulty in concentration. It characterizes the initial reaction to LSD and other hallucinogenic drugs in psychopaths.[34] Of course, some of these same drug effects have also been seen in nonpsychopathic individuals, but the scales have been developed on the basis of their differentiation in chronic opiate addicts.

Opiate drugs differ in effects on motivation from sedative-hypnotics. Hill et al.[56] found that pentobarbital increased working for reward under a high incentive condition, and decreased such work under a low incentive condition. However, morphine produced work more like that under control for both incentive conditions (morphine made these opiate addicts less subject to external motivation).

In contrast to their differing initial effects, chronic effects of psychoactive drugs appear more similar in psychopaths. Chronic methadone[57] did not persistently elevate the *MBG* scale, but did elevate the *PCAG* scale, tiredness, and social withdrawal, while decreasing measures of popularity and efficiency. The hypochondriasis, hysteria and schizophrenia scales of the MMPI were increased during chronic administration of methadone, which reflected the subject's social withdrawal and somatic preoccupations. Increasing dysphoria is characteristic during chronic administration of morphine.[58]

Chronic administration of sedative-hypnotics is also characterized by decreasing[59] euphoria and increasing dysphoria. Chronic alcohol intake[59] is associated with increased tension, anxiety, craving for drug, depression (including suicidal ideation), suspiciousness, and social withdrawal. Isbell et al.,[1] in the first experimental demonstration of an alcohol abstinence syndrome, also noted increased psychopathology in their subjects during chronic intoxication, together with elevations of hysteria and schizophrenia scales on the MMPI. Chronic barbiturate administration is associated with similar phenomena: increased personal neglect, confusion, irritability (including fights), accidents, depression, hyperactivity or withdrawal, and suspiciousness.[60,61] Similar chronic experiments with stimulants and hallucinogens have not been done as yet, but anecdotal accounts would indicate comparable dysphoric states occur with those drugs, too. In an early study of marihuana and pyrahexyl, Williams et al.[62] reported general lassitude, increased personal neglect, decreased ability to concentrate, and decreased inhibitions during chronic drug use. No MMPI or other personality inventory was utilized in that study. Even more marked effects are seen in psychopaths during abstinence after chronic intake of psychoactive drugs; those data will be reviewed later in this discussion.

PROTRACTED ABSTINENCE – AN INDUCED BIOLOGICAL STATE

Characteristic abstinence patterns are seen upon withdrawal of opioids[57,63] or sedative-hypnotics.[1,60,61] Up to the first 6–9 weeks after withdrawal of morphine or other opioids, humans experience a relative hypertension, tachycardia, hyperthermia, mydriasis, hyperpnea, anorexia, restlessness and weight loss; nausea, emesis, diarrhea, muscle cramps, sweating, rhinorrhea and insomnia are also part of this acute abstinence pattern. The MMPI increases in *Hs, Sc,* and *Hy* scales.[57] The ARCI shows an increase in the *PCAG, weak, tired, social withdrawal* and *chronic opiate* (negative feeling state) scales, with a decrease in the *MBG, efficiency* and *competitive* (positive feeling state) scales and an increase in *alcohol withdrawal* and *opiate withdrawal* scales.[57]

About 8–9 weeks after withdrawal of an opioid, a different pattern begins to emerge. In humans this is characterized by relative hypotension,[63] bradycardia, hypothermia, miosis, tachypnea,[57,63] decreased respiratory center sensitivity to CO_2[64], increased delta sleep and REM sleep,[65] increased cold pressor response,[66] and increased norepinephrine secretion.[67] In the rat, there is seen increased metabolic rate and increased fluid intake,[68] with "wet-dog shakes" and increased sleep[69] and increased aggression.[70] In the dog, there is seen mydriasis, hypopnea and hyperalgesia.[71]

The existence of such a protracted abstinence was first established by Martin and associates in the rat,[68] and then in the human[57,63] and the dog.[71] In humans such a drug-induced disease is associated with a tendency toward increased *D, Hs, Pd, Pt* and *Sc* scales of the MMPI, and with increased negative feeling states and decreased positive feeling states on scales of the ARCI.[57] Protracted abstinence lasts more than four months in humans.[57]

A comparable search has not been accomplished for protracted abstinence after sedative-hypnotics such as alcohol, although several physiological measures are known to be persistently abnormal after drug withdrawal in alcoholics. Withdrawal of barbiturates[60,61] and of alcohol[1,34] is known to be initially associated with a characteristic abstinence pattern.

Upon initial withdrawal of alcohol, tremulousness, nausea, perspiration and insomnia are followed by marked tremor, weakness, vomiting, diarrhea, hyperreflexia, fever and hypertension. The most severe abstinence is associated with convulsions ("rum fits") and delirium,[1] as well as abnormalities (spikes and slow-wave bursts) in the EEG. Upon initial withdrawal of barbiturate,[60,61] weakness, tremor, great anxiety, anorexia, nausea and vomiting, rapid weight loss, tachycardia, tachypnea, fever, hypertension, postural hypotension, grand mal convulsions and psychosis developed. The psychosis was characterized by anxiety, agitation, insomnia, confusion, disorientation (time and place), delusions, and auditory and visual hallucinations. Anxiety temporarily decreased after each convulsion. No gross abnormalities could be detected 2-3 months after withdrawal of alcohol or barbiturates, although the existence of a (subtle) protracted abstinence syndrome was not postulated at that time.

THE CONCEPT OF PSYCHOPATHIC STATE

The phenomena of protracted abstinence, as detailed above, have been defined primarily in the biological sphere, with some indication that psychological status (feeling state) and behavior are involved. In evolving a hypothesis about the pharmacological factors in drug abuse, Martin[72,73] recognized that the state of protracted abstinence might well be a model for feeling states in individuals *before* as well as *after* chronic psychoactive drug intake.

Because such a psychological state appeared to be dominated by a particular type of unpleasant feeling state ("hypophoria") that was reversible by psychoactive drugs, Martin hypothesized that drug abusers (including both opiate addicts and alcoholics) were afflicted by an increased need-state;[72] cf. Robins.[18] This increased need-state would lead to the several behaviors labeled as "psychopathic" or "sociopathic". He designed five scales to include pertinent dimensions of this pathological state (Table 11): Impulsivity, Egocentricity, Need, Hypophoria and Sociopathy.

His Maturation scale (Mat) is actually scored positively for immaturity. The use of the maturation concept incorporates the idea that these behaviors and feelings are evidence of immaturity, which would diminish with age as such needs diminished.

Martin and associates[72] tested this instrument and others in three populations: 53 alcoholics, 24 opiate addicts and 54 controls (who used very little of any psychoactive drug). All *Mat* scales (except Egocentricity) and the total Maturation Scale clearly differentiated controls from drug abusers, and most scales differentiated addicts from alcoholics. In the MMPI, the *Pd, Ma* and *D* scales also differentiated controls from drug abusers, as did plasma levels of testosterone and LH.

As part of this endeavor to define the current feeling states of non-using alcoholics and addicts, Haertzen[32] developed the Social Experience Questionnaire (SOEX). This questionnaire was constructed by systematic revision of several MMPI, CPI and ARCI psychopathy scales (described in this chapter earlier) so that only comparable current feelings, thoughts, motives and actions were assessed. This instrument was then tested also in 53 alcoholics, 28 opiate addicts and 54 low-drug using controls. It was found to significantly differentiate controls from drug abusers in 58% of its 560 items. Thus, the current status of drug abusers' life, experience and condition, including mood (current contextless feelings) is different from non-abusers.

Haertzen conceived the SOEX as measuring the current *state* of *psychopathy,* and thus *psychopathic state.*[32,74] He further refined the concept by developing six rational psychopathic state scales (Table 12). These short scales were derived from comparable long scales which had been judged to measure the (1) search for highs, (2) impulsivity, (3) egocentricity, (4) increased needs, (5) hypophoria and (6) sociopathic attitudes. After long scales had been developed and then tested in the three populations, this short (90 item) version (the Psychopathic State Inventory; PSI) was developed with items which best correlated with the parent (long) scales as well as best differentiating drug abusers from controls.[74] It should be noted that the items in the PSI scales are not greatly equivalent to the items in rational scales developed with the same names by Martin.[72] The PSI scales have had the benefit of both rational development (of a large pool of SOEX items) and of pragmatic testing prior to definition.

THE CONCEPT OF HYPOPHORIA

A crucial element of this discussion of psychopathic states is Martin's concept of hypophoria. Martin defined this negative feeling state as comparable to depression, but without feelings of unworthiness, sleep disorders, anorexia, decreased libido or inability to experience joy.[72,73] The Hypophoria scale in the *Mat* "includes items relating to a general negative perception of life; a poor self-image; feelings of being disrespected, disapproved of and unappreciated; feelings of inefficiency or ineptness; and withdrawal from competition, worry and anger".[72] He conceptualized this feeling state as a reaction to social frustration of the increased need-state of sociopathic individuals.[73] Although he defines hypophoria as a feeling state, Martin includes elements of attitudes (poor self-image, unpopular, inefficient, withdrawal) that are quite complex.

Hewett[37] reviews the work of Winokur[75-80] in support of a "depressive spectrum disease" which appears more related to alcoholism than it is to primary depression. She finds evidence in the personal history of drug abusers for persistent low moods without severe depression; these started at an early age before the onset of drug abuse. She concludes that these data are evidence for the existence of an "affective-antisocial spectrum disorder characterized by early onset, low moods, and alcohol abuse, drug abuse and/or antisocial behaviors".[37]

Haertzen[74] utilized the concept of hypophoria to encompass "negative feeling states such as depression" and developed the Hypophoria scale in the PSI with items which were correlated with low mood items. These items (Table 12) do not include much about secondary "feelings", such as judgments about how others react.

In considering hypophoria, Cowan and Kay[81] distinguished four elements in this concept; lack of confidence, unpopularity, anergia, and joylessness. After they segregated SOEX items which appeared to express these four elements, factor analysis demonstrated only two components; Defeated (lack of confidence, unpopularity and anergia) and Joyless. The Defeated scale differentiated both drug abuser groups from controls, but not from each other; the Joyless scale differentiated control and alcoholic groups from addicts, but not from each other.

Reid[82] also conceptualizes the psychopath (aneothopath) as suffering a type of mood disorder ("sadness"), but considers it primary rather than reactive to social constrictions. He sees that the "nothing which ... lies at the center of the psychopath is a lack of energy, of living force", with defensive avoidance of such an endogenous depression.

POTENTIAL OF THE CONCEPT OF PSYCHOPATHIC STATE

Several benefits would result if the search for definable psychopathic states is successful. First, the use of such a "tonic" state measure could provide a much better estimate of significant shifts in psychopathic (sociopathic) disorders, rather than tabulating historical events or waiting for episodic ("phasic") phenomena such as drug intake.

Second, treatment programs for alcoholism, opiate addiction and other psychopathic disorders would benefit from the use of measures of psychopathic state to assess the degree and duration of improvement from various treatments. This could be accomplished without requiring drug intake (usually a measure of failure) to be the measure of success.

Third, such psychological measures of psychopathic state could provide validation for biological and behavioral markers of minor types of psychopathy, and thus lead to better understanding of the neuropathology of psychopathic states.

TABLE 1.–Characteristics of the Psychopath[17]

1. Superficial charm and good "intelligence".
2. Absence of delusions and other signs of irrational thinking.
3. Absence of "nervousness" or psychoneurotic manifestations.
4. Unreliability.
5. Untruthfulness and insincerity.
6. Lack of remorse or shame.
7. Inadequately motivated antisocial behaviour.
8. Poor judgment and failure to learn by experience.
9. Pathologic egocentricity and incapacity for love.
10. General poverty in major affective relations.
11. Specific loss of insight.
12. Unresponsiveness in general interpersonal relations.
13. Fantastic and uninviting behaviour with drink and sometimes without.
14. Threats of suicide, rarely carried out.
15. Sex life impersonal, trivial, and poorly integrated.
16. Failure to follow any life plan.

TABLE 2.–Antisocial Personality (A.P.A. DSM III)[19]

A. Current age at least 18 and a history of continuous and chronic antisocial behavior in which the rights of others are violated.

and

B. Onset before age 15, as indicated by a history of two or more of the following:
1. Truancy (positive if at least five days per year for at least two years, not including the last year of school).
2. Expulsion from school.
3. Delinquency (arrested or referred to juvenile court because of behavior).
4. Running away from home overnight at least twice while living in a parental or parental surrogate home.
5. Persistent lying.
6. Unusually early or aggressive sexual behavior.
7. Unusually early drinking to excess.
8. Thefts.
9. Vandalism.
10. Required to repeat school grades, or grades markedly below those expected on the basis of estimated or known "IQ."
11. Chronic violations of rules at home and/or at school (other than truancy).

and

C. At least three of the following since age 15:
1. Poor occupational performance over several years, as shown by either (a) frequent job changes (three or more jobs in five years not accounted for by nature of job or economic or seasonal fluctuation), (b) significant unemployment (six months or more in ten years when expected to work), or (c) serious absenteeism (average three or more days late or absent per month). N.B.: Poor academic performance for the last few years of school may substitute for this criterion in individuals who, by reason of their age or circumstance, have not had an opportunity to demonstrate occupational adjustment.

(Continued)

TABLE 2. (Continued)

2. Three or more non-traffic arrests, or one felony conviction.
3. Two or more divorces or separations (whether married or not).
4. Repeated physical fights or assaults (not required by job or to defend someone).
5. Repeated thefts, whether caught or not.
6. Illegal occupation (e.g., prostitution, pimping, drug sales).
7. Repeated defaulting on debts or other major financial responsibilities (e.g., child support).
8. Traveling from place to place without a prearranged job or clear goal, or without a clear idea of when the travel will terminate.

and

D. No period of five years or more during which the individual behaved in a conforming manner, with the exception of time spent bedridden, confined to a hospital or penal institution, or under treatment.

and

E. Does not meet established criteria for a diagnosis of Schizophrenia or severe Mental Retardation.

TABLE 3.–(50 Items) Psychopathic Deviate (Pd) Scale–MMPI[27]

8.F	My daily life is full of things that keep me interested.
16.T	I am sure I get a raw deal from life.
20.F	My sex life is satisfactory.
21.T	At times I have very much wanted to leave home.
24.T	No one seems to understand me.
32.T	I find it hard to keep my mind on a task or job.
33.T	I have had very peculiar and strange experiences.
35.T	If people had not had it in for me I would have been much more successful.
37.F	I have never been in trouble because of my sex behavior.
38.T	During one period when I was a youngster I engaged in petty thievery.
42.T	My family does not like the work I have chosen (or the work I intend to choose for my life work.)
61.T	I have not lived the right kind of life.
67.T	I wish I could be as happy as others seem to be.
82.F	I am easily downed in an argument.
84.T	These days I find it hard not to give up hope of amounting to something.
91.F	I do not mind being made fun of.
94.T	I do many things which I regret afterwards (I regret things more or more often than others seem to.)
96.F	I have very few quarrels with members of my family.
102.T	My hardest battles are with myself.
106.T	Much of the time I feel as if I have done something wrong or evil.
107.F	I am happy most of the time.
110.T	Someone has it in for me.
118.T	In school I was sometimes sent to the principal for cutting up.
127.T	I know who is responsible for most of my troubles.
134.F	At times my thoughts have raced ahead faster than I could speak them.
137.F	I believe that my home life is as pleasant as that of most people I know.

(Continued)

TABLE 3. (Continued)

141.F	My conduct is largely controlled by the customs of those about me.
155.F	I am neither gaining nor losing weight.
170.F	What others think of me does not bother me.
171.F	It makes me uncomfortable to put on a stunt at a party even when others are doing the same sort of things.
173.F	I liked school.
180.F	I find it hard to make talk when I meet new people.
183.F	I am against giving money to beggars.
201.F	I wish I were not so shy.
215.T	I have used alcohol excessively.
216.T	There is very little love and companionship in my family as compared to other homes.
224.T	My parents have often objected to the kind of people I went around with.
231.F	I like to talk about sex.
235.F	I have been quite independent and free from family rule.
237.F	My relatives are nearly all in sympathy with me.
239.T	I have been disappointed in love.
244.T	My way of doing things is apt to be misunderstood by others.
245.T	My parents and family find more fault with me than they should.
248.F	Sometimes without any reason or even when things are going wrong I feel excitedly happy, "on top of the world".
267.F	When in a group of people I have trouble thinking of the right things to talk about.
284.T	I am sure I am being talked about.
287.F	I have very few fears compared to my friends.
289.F	I am always disgusted with the law when a criminal is freed through the arguments of a smart lawyer.
294.F	I have never been in trouble with the law.
296.F	I have periods in which I feel unusually cheerful without any special reason.

TABLE 4.–(46 Items) Mania (Ma) Scale—MMPI[27]

11.T	A person should try to understand his dreams and be guided by or take warning from them.
13.T	I work under a great deal of tension.
21.T	At times I have very much wanted to leave home.
22.T	At times I have fits of laughing and crying that I cannot control.
59.T	I have often had to take orders from someone who did not know as much as I did.
64.T	I sometimes keep on at a thing until others lose their patience with me.
73.T	I am an important person.
97.T	At times I have a strong urge to do something harmful or shocking.
100.T	I have met problems so full of possibilities that I have been unable to make up my mind about them.
101.F	I believe women ought to have as much sexual freedom as men.
105.F	Sometimes when I am not feeling well I am cross.
109.T	Some people are so bossy that I feel like doing the opposite of what they request, even though I know they are right.
111.F	I have never done anything dangerous for the thrill of it.

(Continued)

TABLE 4. (Continued)

119.F	My speech is the same as always (not faster or slower, or slurring; no hoarseness).
120.F	My table manners are not quite as good at home as when I am out in company.
127.T	I know who is responsible for most of my troubles.
134.T	At times my thoughts have raced ahead faster than I could speak them.
143.T	When I was a child, I belonged to a crowd or gang that tried to stick together through thick and thin.
148.F	It makes me impatient to have people ask my advice or otherwise interrupt me when I am working on something important.
156.T	I have had periods in which I carried on activities without knowing later what I had been doing.
157.T	I feel that I have often been punished without cause.
166.F	I am afraid when I look down from a high place.
167.T	It wouldn't make me nervous if any members of my family got into trouble with the law.
171.F	It makes me uncomfortable to put on a stunt at a party even when others are doing the same sort of things.
180.F	I find it hard to make talk when I meet new people.
181.T	When I get bored I like to stir up some excitement.
194.T	I have had attacks in which I could not control my movements or speech but in which I knew what was going on around me.
212.T	My people treat me more like a child than a grown-up.
222.T	It is not hard for me to ask help from my friends even though I cannot return the favor.
226.T	Some of my family have habits that bother and annoy me very much.
228.T	At times I feel that I can make up my mind with unusually great ease.
232.T	I have been inspired to a program of life based on duty which I have since carefully followed.
233.T	I have at times stood in the way of people who were trying to do something, not because it amounted to much but because of the principle of the thing.
238.T	I have periods of such great restlessness that I cannot sit long in a chair.
240.T	I never worry about my looks.
250.T	I don't blame anyone for trying to grab everything he can get in this world.
251.T	I have had blank spells in which my activities were interrupted and I did not know what was going on around me.
263.T	I sweat very easily even on cool days.
266.T	Once a week or oftener I become very excited.
267.F	When in a group of people I have trouble thinking of the right things to talk about.
268.T	Something exciting will almost always pull me out of it when I am feeling low.
271.T	I do not blame a person for taking advantage of someone who lays himself open to it.
277.T	At times I have been so entertained by the cleverness of a crook that I have hoped he would get by with it.
279.T	I drink an unusually large amount of water every day.
289.F	I am always disgusted with the law when a criminal is freed through the arguments of a smart lawyer.
298.T	If several people find themselves in trouble, the best thing for them to do is to agree upon a story and stick to it.

TABLE 5.–(25 Items) Antisocial (Ant) Scale—MMPI[29]

*38.T	During one period when I was a youngster I engaged in petty thievery.
45.T	I do not always tell the truth.
56.T	As a youngster I was suspended from school one or more times for cutting up.
85.T	Sometimes I am strongly attracted by the personal articles of others such as shoes, gloves, etc., so that I want to handle or steal them though I have no use for them.
95.F	I go to church almost every week.
103.T	I have little or no trouble with my muscles twitching or jumping.
*118.T	In school I was sometimes sent to the principal for cutting up.
143.T	When I was a child, I belonged to a crowd or gang that tried to stick together through thick and thin.
156.F	I have had periods in which I carried on activities without knowing later what I had been doing.
167.T	It wouldn't make me nervous if any members of my family got in trouble with the law.
175.T	I seldom or never have dizzy spells.
195.T	I do not like everyone I know.
202.F	I believe I am a condemned person.
203.T	If I were a reporter I would very much like to report news of the theater.
243.T	I have few or no pains.
251.F	I have had blank spells in which my activities were interrupted and I did not know what was going on around me.
272.T	At times I am all full of energy.
277.T	At times I have been so entertained by the cleverness of a crook that I have hoped he would get by with it.
*289.F	I am always disgusted with the law when a criminal is freed through the arguments of a smart lawyer.
*294.F	I have never been in trouble with the law.
*296.T	I have periods in which I feel unusually cheerful without any special reason. (False on *Pd* scale)
311.T	During one period when I was a youngster I engaged in petty thievery.
412.T	I do not dread seeing a doctor about a sickness or injury.
419.T	I played hooky from school quite often as a youngster.
471.T	In school my marks in deportment were quite regularly bad.

*Items also on the *Pd* or *Ma* scales.

TABLE 6.–(20 Items) Sociopathy (Spy) Scale—MMPI[33]

*21.T	At times I have very much wanted to leave home.
28.T	When someone does me a wrong I feel I should pay him back if I can, just for the principle of the thing.
91.T	I do not mind being made fun of.
*96.F	I have very few quarrels with members of my family.
99.T	I like to go to parties and other affairs where there is lots of loud fun.
138.F	Criticism or scolding hurts me terribly.
148.F	It makes me impatient to have people ask my advice or otherwise interrupt me when I am working on something important.

(Continued)

TABLE 6. (Continued)

*171.F It makes me uncomfortable to put on a stunt at a party even when others are doing the same sort of things.
172.F I frequently have to fight against showing that I am bashful.
181.T When I get bored I like to stir up some excitement.
*183.F I am against giving money to beggars.
*201.F I wish I were not so shy.
250.T I don't blame anyone for trying to grab everything he can get in this world.
280.T Most people make friends because friends are likely to be useful to them.
332.F Sometimes my voice leaves me or changes even though I have no cold.
378.F I do not like to see women smoke.
391.T I love to go to dances.
412.T I do not dread seeing a doctor about a sickness or injury.
509.F I sometimes find it hard to stick up for my rights because I am so reserved.
533.T I am not bothered by a great deal of belching of gas from my stomach.

*Items also on the *Pd* or *Ma* scales.

TABLE 7.–(71 Items) Psychopathic (Pyp) Scale—ARCI[34]

17.T Occasionally when I am mad at someone I will give him the "silent treatment".
25.F I am embarrassed by dirty stories.
28.T I would be able to make a smart remark if anyone got overbearing with me.
36.T Sometimes strange places seem familiar to me.
41.T I can think of a lot of things to say when I want to impress someone.
44.F I believe a person should never tell a lie.
47.T It takes a lot of argument to convince most people of the truth.
52.T Telling lies does not bother most people.
53.T Most people are not sincere in being friendly.
61.T For some reason the idea of home depresses me.
65.F Time seems to be passing faster than usual.
78.T I am very particular about the way my hair is cut.
85.T It bothers me to have someone wake me up.
89.T A serious movie would appeal to me more than a comedy.
93.F I wish I were more feminine.
103.T My life story would make an interesting book.
108.T I would like to wear expensive clothes.
117.F I would rather have many acquaintances than a few good friends.
118.T I know who is responsible for most of my troubles.
134.T I like to read newspaper articles on crime.
135.T I would like to listen to music all day.
136.F I would like to be a private secretary.
142.T It does not bother me to hurt someone I do not know.
148.F I am easily downed in an argument.
149.T I am sometimes so preoccupied that I can look at a person and not see him.
154.T I sometimes wonder what hidden reason people may have for doing something nice for me.
159.T I am often said to be hot-headed.
163.T Most people are really dangerous.

(Continued)

TABLE 7. (Continued)

165.F	Thinking of the opposite sex does not appeal to me now.
174.T	If I weren't pretty sharp, a great many people would beat me out of things.
181.F	I am against giving money to beggars.
193.T	I try to avoid ignorant people.
197.F	I couldn't get mad at anyone right now.
198.F	Everything seems to taste good to me.
202.T	I wish I could retire and do nothing for the rest of my life.
205.T	Criminals are usually caught by accident.
215.T	I like to let people know what I think of them.
230.T	I have not lived the right kind of life.
238.T	Most people inwardly dislike others.
250.F	Most people are trying to do what is right.
258.T	I am a good sexual partner.
274.F	As I think back on it, my father had my best interests at heart.
292.T	It does not bother me particularly to see animals suffer.
299.F	Right now I feel as if all my needs are satisfied.
310.T	I have been in trouble with the law.
311.F	For some reason I am very appealing to members of my own sex.
333.T	I am very sensitive about my appearance.
335.T	Nothing gives me more pleasure than to beat a "sucker."
340.F	Right now I would enjoy conversation more than sex.
343.F	I have not been in trouble with the law.
347.T	I am smart enough to do just about anything I want, if I set my mind to it.
368.T	I do not blame a person for taking advantage of someone who lays himself open to it.
370.F	Most women are faithful to their husbands.
373.F	I am very strongly attracted by members of my own sex.
385.T	I feel there are many jobs that are beneath my level of dignity.
393.T	My family does not like the work I have chosen (or the work I intend to choose for my life work.)
414.F	I like to talk about everything that is the least bit interesting.
420.F	I am often afraid of the dark.
451.T	My parents have often objected to the kind of people I went around with.
455.F	Sexual things disgust me.
466.F	I seldom do dangerous things for the thrill of it.
468.F	I do not like to see women smoke.
486.T	I am in favor of giving money to beggars.
493.T	I like to think about how many people of the opposite sex find me attractive.
501.T	I am more concerned with my health than with my personal appearance.
508.T	I believe other people have more weaknesses than they are willing to admit.
516.T	There have been times when I have hurt my best friend because I did not care at the time.
517.F	I feel as if I had just had a good meal.
525.T	I am not easily downed in an argument.
533.T	Once in a while I laugh at a dirty joke.
535.F	I would rather watch someone else than have sexual intercourse myself.

TABLE 8.–(54 Items) Low Socialization Scale—CPI*[36]

12.T	I often feel that I made a wrong choice in my occupation.
36.T	When I was going to school I played hooky quite often.
62.F	I think Lincoln was greater than Washington.
93.T	I would do almost anything on a dare.
94.T	With things going as they are, it's pretty hard to keep up hope of amounting to something.
123.F	I think I am stricter about right and wrong than most people.
144.F	I am somewhat afraid of the dark.
156.T	I hardly ever get excited or thrilled.
164.T	My parents have often disapproved of my friends.
168.F	My home life was always happy.
170.T	I often act on the spur of the moment without stopping to think.
180.F	My parents have generally let me make my own decisions.
182.T	I would rather go without something than ask for a favor.
184.T	I have had more than my share of things to worry about.
192.F	When I meet a stranger I often think that he is better than I am.
198.F	Before I do something I try to consider how my friends will react to it.
212.F	I have never been in trouble with the law.
214.T	In school I was sometimes sent to the principal for cutting up.
223.F	I keep out of trouble at all costs.
245.F	Most of the time I feel happy.
257.T	I often feel as though I have done something wrong or wicked.
284.F	It is hard for me to act natural when I am with new people.
302.T	I have often gone against my parents' wishes.
317.F	I often think about how I look and what impression I am making upon others.
323.F	I have never done any heavy drinking.
327.T	I find it easy to "drop" or "break with" a friend.
334.F	I get nervous when I have to ask someone for a job.
336.T	Sometimes I used to feel that I would like to leave home.
338.T	I never worry about my looks.
339.T	I have been in trouble one or more times because of my sex behavior.
315.T	I go out of my way to meet trouble rather than try to escape it.
367.F	My home life was always very pleasant.
369.T	I seem to do things that I regret more often than other people do.
373.F	My table manners are not quite as good at home as when I am out in company.
385.T	It is pretty easy for people to win arguments with me.
386.T	I know who is responsible for most of my troubles.
389.F	I get pretty discouraged with the law when a smart lawyer gets a criminal free.
393.T	I have used alcohol excessively.
394.F	Even when I have gotten into trouble I was usually trying to do the right thing.
395.F	It is very important to me to have enough friends and social life.
396.T	I sometimes wanted to run away from home.
398.T	Life usually hands me a pretty raw deal.
405.T	People often talk about me behind my back.
409.F	I would never play cards (poker) with a stranger.
416.T	I don't think I'm quite as happy as others seem to be.
420.T	I used to steal sometimes when I was a youngster.

(Continued)

TABLE 8. (Continued)

428.T	My home as a child was less peaceful and quiet than those of most other people.
429.F	Even the idea of giving a talk in public makes me afraid.
431.T	As a youngster in school I used to give the teachers lots of trouble.
435.T	If the pay was right I would like to travel with a circus or carnival.
436.T	I never cared much for school.
439.F	The members of my family were always very close to each other.
444.T	My parents never really understood me.
457.T	A person is better off if he doesn't trust anyone.

*Scored opposite to Socialization (So) scale.

TABLE 9.–(42 Items) Low Responsibility Scale—CPI*[36]

16.T	There's no use in doing things for people; you only find that you get it in the neck in the long run.
18.F	A person who doesn't vote is not a good citizen.
20.T	I have had very peculiar and strange experiences.
22.F	When a person "pads" his income tax report so as to get out of some of his taxes, it is just as bad as stealing money from the government.
26.T	It's a good thing to know people in the right places so you can get traffic tags, and such things, taken care of.
36.T	When I was going to school I played hooky quite often.
43.T	It's no use worrying my head about public affairs; I can't do anything about them anyhow.
49.T	When someone does me a wrong I feel I should pay him back if I can, just for the principle of the thing.
51.F	Every family owes it to the city to keep their sidewalks cleared in the winter and their lawn mowed in the summer.
61.F	I liked school.
73.T	Maybe some minority groups do get rough treatment, but it's no business of mine.
75.T	We ought to worry about our own country and let the rest of the world take care of itself.
77.T	When I get bored I like to stir up some excitement.
90.T	As long as a person votes every four years, he has done his duty as a citizen.
105.T	I am fascinated by fire.
113.T	School teachers complain a lot about their pay, but it seems to me that they get as much as they deserve.
121.T	I was a slow learner in school.
126.F	I do not dread seeing a doctor about a sickness or injury.
129.T	I think I would like to drive a racing car.
138.F	I seldom or never have dizzy spells.
139.T	It is all right to get around the law if you don't actually break it.
162.F	Every citizen should take the time to find out about national affairs, even if it means giving up some personal pleasures.
164.T	My parents have often disapproved of my friends.
179.F	When I work on a committee I like to take charge of things.
189.T	In school my marks in deportment were quite regularly bad.
193.F	I would be ashamed not to use my privilege of voting.

(Continued)

TABLE 9. (Continued)

205.T	I enjoy a race or game better when I bet on it.
206.T	I have often found people jealous of my good ideas, just because they had not thought of them first.
210.T	I very much like hunting.
212.F	I have never been in trouble with the law.
213.F	It makes me angry when I hear of someone who has been wrongly prevented from voting.
221.F	People have a real duty to take care of their aged parents, even if it means making some pretty big sacrifices.
234.F	We ought to pay our elected officials better than we do.
235.F	I can honestly say that I do not really mind paying my taxes because I feel that's one of the things I can do for what I get from the community.
253.T	When prices are high you can't blame a person for getting all he can while the getting is good.
261.T	We ought to let Europe get out of its own mess: it made its bed, let it lie in it.
278.F	If I get too much change in a store, I always give it back.
283.F	I like to read about science.
286.F	I have never done anything dangerous for the thrill of it.
288.T	As a youngster I was suspended from school one or more times for cutting up.
294.T	I feel that I have often been punished without cause.
300.T	Police cars should be especially marked so that you can always see them coming.

*Scored opposite to Responsibility (Re) scale.

TABLE 10.–Criteria for The Diagnosis of Sociopathic Personality[18]

A. POOR WORK HISTORY—at least six of the following: 6 + jobs within ten years, successive jobs at less pay or less prestige, fired for incompetence or personality conflict, unemployment for more than a month at a time, quitting because of fights or arguments, much time out for illness, chronic absenteeism, job troubles from drinking, no job of as much as three years' duration in the last ten years.

B. POOR MARITAL HISTORY—two or more divorces, marriage to wife with severe behavior problems, repeated separations.

C. EXCESSIVE DRUGS—addiction to barbiturates, bromides, morphine, benzedrine, or dexedrine, or a period of experimentation with drugs for non-medical purposes.

D. HEAVY DRINKING—medical complications, arrests, firing, serious family complaints due to alcohol, or chronic intake of 3 + drinks at least three times a week or seven drinks per sitting.

E. REPEATED ARRESTS—three or more non-traffic arrests.

F. PHYSICAL AGGRESSION—arrest record for fighting, reports of wife or child beatings, self-report of many fights.

G. SEXUAL PROMISCUITY OR PERVERSION—arrests on charges pertaining to sex, interview claims of extreme promiscuity (50 different sexual partners), interview reports of homosexuality.

H. SUICIDE (ATTEMPTS)—death by suicide, police record, hospital, or interview reports of suicide attempts.

(Continued)

TABLE 10. (Continued)

I. IMPULSIVE BEHAVIOR—frequent moving from one city to another, more than one elopement, sudden army enlistments, unprovoked desertion of home.

J. SCHOOL PROBLEMS AND TRUANCY—four or more of the following plus repeated truancy; did not leave school at graduation point, two years older than average in the last year at school, attended four or more grammer schools, left school voluntarily before completing expected level, failed one full year or more, complaints re discipline from teachers, fights with students, expulsion or suspension.

K. PUBLIC FINANCIAL CARE—totally or partially supported by relatives, friends, social agencies, or public institutions.

L. POOR ARMED SERVICES RECORD—enlistment of less than one year's duration, demotions, repeated AWOL, court-martial, punishments, desertion, dishonorable discharge.

M. VAGRANCY—period of several months or more of travel around the country without prearranged employment.

N. MANY SOMATIC SYMPTOMS—at least ten somatic symptoms scored from interview on medical-psychiatric inventory or fewer if severe or disabling.

O. PATHOLOGICAL LYING—fantastic history given which does not apparently serve the function of omitting or white-washing reports of antisocial behavior.

P. LACK OF FRIENDS—does not participate in activities of any informal social group, sees friends less than once in two weeks, has no or only one close friend, sees less than ten people socially.

Q. USE OF ALIASES—interview report or police record showing use of an assumed name.

R. LACK OF GUILT ABOUT SEXUAL EXPLOITS AND CRIMES—interviewer's impression from the way in which patient reports his history.

S. RECKLESS YOUTH—age span of 18 to 20 years reported as characterized by seven or more of these: feeling carefree, leisure time spent almost entirely in social activity, little time spent at home, self-report as reckless or wild, drove fast, fought, drank excessively, changed jobs frequently, spent money extravagantly.

TABLE 11.–(67 Items) Maturation Scale—Mat[72]

Impulsivity Subscale

3.T   I have done something different today on the spur of the moment.
32.T   Right now I would enjoy gambling.
41.T   I feel that I could be hot-headed today.
58.T   The members of my family would not like my goals for work today.
59.T   I have the urge to do something shocking.
64.T   It is possible that I would do something on a dare today.

Egocentricity Subscale

7.T   People could say that I lack warmth in my personal relations.
23.T   I will try to get my fair share today.
31.T   It wouldn't bother me to hurt my best friend because I don't care today.
57.T   My capacity for love is decreased.
48.F   I have been thinking there is some love in my family.
49.F   I'd give some of my money to my parents if they wanted it.
50.F   My capacity for love is increased.

(Continued)

TABLE 11. (Continued)

Need Subscale

12.T	My current sexual behavior could get me in trouble.
29.T	Talk about sex would appeal to me now.
46.T	I am in the mood for some type of sexual activity with those of my own sex.
47.T	I have reason to feel more concerned with my health than personal appearance.
62.T	Someone could criticize me for eating too much today.
65.T	I have a condition or illness which requires medical diagnosis.
14.F	Right now I feel as if all my needs are satisfied.
28.F	I have few or no pains.
43.F	I am more in the mood to watch someone else than to have sexual intercourse myself.
56.F	Thoughts of the opposite sex have not been on my mind today.
67.F	I have been exposed to no temptation today.

Hypophoria Subscale

4.T	I envy the happiness I see in those around me.
5.T	I have had more than my share of worries today.
6.T	I would find it somewhat hard to talk to someone new.
9.T	I am sensitive about my personal appearance today.
11.T	It would make me feel uneasy now to talk to a group.
19.T	The friendliness that people have shown today does not seem sincere.
37.T	I wish I could retire and do nothing for the rest of my life.
38.T	If my family were with me now, they would treat me like a child.
39.T	The idea of home is depressing to me.
51.T	I feel that I have had a raw deal out of life today.
52.T	My parents would object to some of the people I have talked with today.
60.T	I don't seem to be as happy as those about me.
1.F	I have been excited at times today.
8.F	I am full of energy.
17.F	Something happened today to make me think I'll amount to something.
18.F	Things around me seem more pleasing than usual.
20.F	I couldn't get very mad at anyone now.
24.F	I notice that I have increased respect for myself.
22.F	Today I say things in the easiest possible way.
25.F	My experiences today have kept me interested.
26.F	I make up my mind with ease today.
27.F	Time seems to be passing faster than usual.
33.F	I would not be easily downed in an argument now.
35.F	I have been thinking how pleasant my home life was.
54.F	My relatives would sympathize with me today.
55.F	I have been feeling happy today.
61.F	I would be happy all the time if I felt as I do now.

Sociopathic Subscale

2.T	I see no reason for worrying about public affairs today.
15.T	People could say that some of my recent behavior has indicated poor judgment.
40.T	Some of my actions today would be against my parents' wishes.
42.T	The suffering of animals is no concern of mine.
44.T	I would get pleasure from beating a "sucker".

(Continued)

TABLE 11. (Continued)

45.T	I would be entertained by the cleverness of a crook.
53.T	It would not bother me to hurt a stranger.
66.T	Some of my recent behavior has indicated poor judgment.
10.F	I wouldn't do any heavy drinking today if I had the chance.
13.F	It is important for me today to keep up my friendships.
16.F	Every person should make his bed every day even if he dosen't feel very good.
21.F	This is one day that I'll keep out of trouble.
30.F	If I had to do it, I would put in extra time today to increase my rewards.
34.F	I feel shame when I don't do my job as well as I could.
36.F	I will live up to the promises I have made to others today.
63.F	I would vote today if a presidential election were held.

TABLE 12.–(90 Items) Psychopathic State Inventory—PSI*[74]

EGOCENTRIC SCALE (Ego)[a]

8.T	I have been getting some ideas about who is responsible for some of my troubles. (S 36)
14.T	I have been thinking of the ways that people may be impressed by me. (S 51)
21.T	I am wearing myself out by feeling sorry for myself. (S 93)
25.T	I seem to be in search of my real self now days. (S 115)
26.T	I felt impatient with someone for interrupting me today. (S 123)
31.T	The friendliness that people have shown today does not seem sincere. (S 176)
34.T	If I were sleeping, it would irritate me to be awakened. (S 189)
41.T	I am worried about myself. (S 251)
52.F	Someone has been nice to me today. (S 302)
54.T	Ignorant people should keep out of my way today. (S 335)
77.T	I did more things for myself than for others today. (S 493)
81.T	I have been thinking about past disappointments in love. (S 507)
85.T	I would like to let a few people know what I think of them. (S 535)
87.T	I cannot keep my mind on things that don't concern me. (S 551)
90.T	Some things that puzzle other people seem quite clear to me now. (S 557)

HIGH SCALE (Hi)[b]

10.F	I wouldn't do any heavy drinking today even if I had the chance. (S 44)
11.T	It would be better if I were high. (S 46)
15.T	I can stand sorrow best when I am high. (S 60)
30.T	Night reminds me of when I got high. (S 146)
32.T	It makes me feel like a failure when I can't get high. (S 160)
39.T	I feel as if I must relax completely. (S 246)
42.T	I am thinking more about the pleasures of the past than the things I might do in the future. (S 258)
51.T	Night reminds me of joy for a day gone by. (S 299)
56.T	I seem to be in search of a high all the time. (S 344)
57.T	A pleasant feeling reminds me of being loaded. (S 346)
69.T	A pleasant feeling reminds me of what I want. (S 420)
71.T	I daydream about how loaded I have been. (S 444)
74.T	I am never happier than when I am high. (S 446)

(Continued)

TABLE 12. (Continued)

85.T	I feel more like getting high today. (S 544)
88.T	If I were drunk now I would feel happy. (S 546)

HYPOPHORIA SCALE (Hyp)[c]

2.F	I am enjoying myself. (S 9)
12.T	I have a feeling of just dragging along rather than coasting. (S 47)
19.T	I have difficulty in sleeping because of the irritations where I live now. (S 89)
23.T	I am very lonely. (S 101)
27.F	My work today has kept me interested. (S 124)
33.T	I wish I were not so lonely. (S 177)
35.T	There is something wrong with my outlook and relationship to the rest of the world. (S 191)
37.T	I am moody. (S 214)
38.T	Other people think that I am unaware of things. (S 215)
59.F	My movements are free, relaxed, and pleasurable. (S 362)
61.F	My experiences today have kept me interested. (S 388)
64.T	I am against feeling the way I do. (S 399)
65.T	I don't seem to be as happy as those about me. (S 401)
82.F	I feel happy right now. (S 509)
84.F	I feel cheerful. (S 529)

IMPULSIVITY SCALE (Imp)[d]

1.F	I have not done anything today just for the thrill of it. (S 8)
3.T	My life seems dull to me now that I'm not where the action is. (S 10)
7.F	I become nervous when riding fast and reckless. (S 31)
16.T	I would enjoy more freedom to act. (S 70)
18.T	My life seems dull to me now because of lack of freedom. (S 71)
24.T	I feel as if I could be hot-headed today. (S 105)
44.T	I am greatly bothered by people who interfere with my efforts. (S 270)
48.T	I get most impatient when I can't get what I want. (S 292)
49.T	My thoughts have been getting ahead of my speech. (S 297)
62.T	It makes me feel like a failure when I can't do the things I want to do. (S 392)
63.T	If it were not for stimulation from others, I would feel bored. (S 394)
70.T	The best way for me to handle impatience is to leave. (S 423)
73.F	My conversations with others have kept me interested. (S 476)
75.T	My life seems at a standstill to me now. (S 486)
80.T	I would make a smart remark now to anyone who got over-bearing with me. (S 505)

NEED SCALE[e]

4.T	If it were not for my own activity, life would be boring. (S 16)
6.T	My daydreams today have been mostly about women. (S 28)
9.T	It makes me impatient to be broke. (S 37)
13.T	I have been thinking of the times when I wanted to go home. (S 50)
22.T	My mind seems to tell me what I shouldn't do, but my weakness seems to do it. (S 94)
43.T	I have been thinking of ways to relieve my bodily misery. (S 260)
45.T	I am more horny than usual. (S 280)
46.T	I have been complaining about the food. (S 287)
47.T	I wish I were alone. (S 289)
53.F	Most of my needs are met every day. (S 320)

(Continued)

TABLE 12. (Continued)

55.F	Right now I feel as if all my needs are satisfied. (S 339)
67.T	I have been thinking of how many people of the opposite sex find me attractive. (S 407)
68.T	I have reason to feel more concerned with my health than with my personal appearance. (S 413)
76.T	If I were sleeping, it would irritate me to be awakened. (S 489)
83.T	I have a peculiar craving for ice cream or something cold. (S 510)

SOCIOPATHY SCALE (Soc)[f]

5.T	I have been thinking of ways to get around the law. (S 25)
17.T	If I were less alert, some people would try to beat me out of something. (S 72)
20.T	I daydream about the street. (S 92)
28.T	I am troubled by some injustice that involves me. (S 136)
29.T	It would not bother me to hurt a stranger. (S 138)
36.T	I resent having someone threaten what little security I have. (S 205)
40.T	Some of my actions today would be against my parents' wishes. (S 250)
50.T	I know of someone who was so clever in breaking a rule that I hope he gets by with it. (S 298)
58.T	I think of times when I played hooky from school. (S 359)
60.T	It would not bother me to stop seeing the friends I have been seeing lately. (S 376)
66.T	If I got mad at someone today, I would give him the "silent treatment". (S 405)
72.T	I daydream about what I will do when I will get home. (S 448)
78.T	I would get pleasure from beating a "sucker". (S 496)
79.T	I think about the day when I will quit taking orders. (S 504)
89.T	I feel suspicious of some nice things someone has done for me. (S 555)

*Each scale's items are arranged chronologically by PSI number, with Social Experience Inventory (SOEX) item number indicated within parenthesis.
a. SOEX Scale 81.   d. SOEX Scale 79.
b. SOEX Scale 76.   e. SOEX Scale 83.
c. SOEX Scale 84.   f. SOEX Scale 87.

REFERENCES

1. Isbell, H., Fraser, H.F., Wikler, A., Belleville, R.E., and Eisenman, A.J. An experimental study of the etiology of "rum fits" and "delirium tremens." *Q. J. Stud. Alcohol.* 16:1–33, 1955.
2. World Health Organization, Expert Committee on Addiction Producing Drugs. *Report on the Thirteenth Session,* Tech. Rep. Ser. No. 273, WHO, Geneva, 1964.
3. American Psychiatric Association. *Diagnostic and statistical manual: Mental disorders (DSM II),* Washington, D.C., 1968.
4. Pinel, P. *Traite medico-philosophique sur l'alienation mentale,* Paris: *J. Ant. Brosson,* 1809.
5. Maughs, S. A concept of psychopathy and psychopathic personality: its evaluation and historical development. *J. Clin. Psychopath.* 2:465–499, 1941.
6. Pichot, P. Psychopathic behavior: a historical overview, in Hare, R.D., and Schalling, D. (eds.), *Psychopathic Behavior: Approaches to Research.* New York, Wiley, 1978, pp. 55–70.
7. Pritchard, J.C. *A Treatise on Insanity and Other Disorders Affecting the Mind.* London: Sherwood, Gilbert & Piper, 1835.

8. Esquirol, E. *Des Maladies Mentales Considerees sous les Rapports Medical, Hygienique et Medico-legal.* Paris: J.B. Bailliere, 1838.
9. Morel, B.A. *Traite des Degenerescences Physiques Intellectualles et Morales de l'Espece Humaine et des Causes qui Produisent ces Varietes Maladives.* Paris: J.B. Bailliere, 1857.
10. Magnan and Legrain. *Les Degeneres (Etat Mental et Syndromes Episodiques).* Paris: Rueff et Cie, 1895.
11. Lombroso, C. *Crime, Its Causes and Remedies.* Translated by Horton, H.P. Boston: Little Brown, 1911.
12. Koch, J.L.A. *Die Psychopathischen Minderwertigkeiten. Erste Abteilung. Einleitung—Die Angeborenen Andauernden Psychopathischen Minderwertigkeiten.* Ravensburg: Otto Maier, 1891.
13. Kraepelin, E. *Psychiatrie, Ein Lehrbuch fur Studierende und Aerzte. Siebente, vielfach umgearbeitete Auflage. II. Band. Klinische Psychiatrie,* Leipzig: J.A. Barth, 1915.
14. Schneider, K. *Die Psychopathische Personlichkeiten,* 9. Aufl. Wein: Franz Deuticke, 1950.
15. American Psychiatric Association. *Diagnostic and Statistical Manual: Mental Disorders (DSM I),* Washington, D.C., 1952.
16. Cleckley H. *The Mask of Sanity,* lst ed., St. Louis: Mosby, 1941.
17. Cleckley H. *The Mask of Sanity,* 5th ed., St. Louis: Mosby, 1976.
18. Robins, L.N. *Deviant children grown up: a sociological and psychiatric study of sociopathic personality.* Baltimore: Williams and Wilkins, 1966.
19. American Psychiatric Association: *Diagnostic and Statistical Manual: Mental Disorders (DSM III),* Washington, D.C. (1979).
20. Hare, R.D. *Psychopathy: Theory and Research.* New York: Wiley, 1970.
21. Reid, W.H. *The Psychopath: A Comprehensive Study of Antisocial Disorders and Behaviors.* New York: Brunner/Mazel, 1978.
22. Hare, R.D., and Schalling, D. *Psychopathic Behavior: Approaches to Research.* New York: Wiley, 1978.
23. Smith, R.J. *The Psychopath in Society.* New York: Academic Press, 1978.
24. Harrington, A. The coming of the psychopath. *Playboy* 18(12):203-335, 1971.
25. Yochelson, S., and Samenow, S.E. *The Criminal Personality. Volume I: A Profile for Change.* New York: J. Aronson, 1976.
26. Yochelson, S., and Samenow, S.E. *The Criminal Personality. Volume II: The Change Process.* New York: J. Aronson, 1977.
27. McKinley, J.C., and Hathaway, S.R. The MMPI: V. Hysteria, hypomania and psychopathic deviate. *J. Appl. Psychol.* 28:153-174, 1944.
28. Dahlstrom, W.G., and Welsh, G.S. *An MMPI Handbook: A Guide To Use in Clinical Practice and Research,* Minneapolis: University of Minnesota Press, 1960.
29. Haertzen, C.A., Hill, H.E., and Monroe, J.J. MMPI scales for differentiating and predicting relapse in alcoholics, opiate addicts, and criminals. *Int. J. Addict.* 3:91-106, 1968.
30. Astin, A. A factor study of the MMPI psychopathic deviate scale. *J. Consult. Psychol.* 23:550-554, 1959.
31. Monroe, J.J., Miller, J.S., and Lyle, W.H. Extension of psychopathic deviancy scales for the screening of addict patients. *Educ. & Psychol. Measurement* 24:47-56, 1964.
32. Haertzen, C.A., Martin, W.R., Hewett, B.B., and Sandquist, V. Measurement of psychopathy as a state, *J. Psychology* 100:201-214, 1978.
33. Spielberger, C.D., Kling, J.K., and O'Hagan, S.E.J. Dimensions of psychopathic personality: antisocial behavior and anxiety, in Hare, R.D., and Schalling, D. (eds.), *Psychopathic Behavior: Approaches to Research.* New York: Wiley, 1978.
34. Haertzen, C.A. *An Overview of Addiction Research Center Inventory Scales (ARCI): an*

appendix and manual of scales. Rockville, Md.: DHEW Publication No. (ADM) 74–92, 1974.

35. Haertzen, C.A., and Panton, J.H. Development of a "psychopathic" scale for the Addiction Research Center Inventory. *Int. J. Addict.* 2:115–127, 1967.

36. Gough, H.G. *California Psychological Inventory Manual.* Palo Alto: Consult. Psychol. Press, 1957.

37. Hewett, B.B., and Martin, W.R. Psychometric comparisons of sociopathic and psychopathological behaviors of alcoholics and drug abusers versus a low drug control population. *Int. J. Addictions* 15(1): 1980 (In Press).

38. Kolb, L. Types and characteristics of drug addicts. *Ment. Hyg.* 9:300–313, 1925.

39. Pescor, M.J. The Kolb classification of drug addicts. *Public Health Repts, Suppl.* 155:1–10, 1939.

40. Felix, R.H. An appraisal of the personality types of the addict. *Am. J. Psychiat.* 100:462–467, 1944.

41. Hill, H.E., Haertzen, C.A., and Davis, H. An MMPI factor analytic study of alcoholics, narcotic addicts and criminals. *Q. J. Stud. Alcohol.* 23:411–431, 1962.

42. Black. F.W., and Heald, A. MMPI characteristics of alcohol and illicit drug abusers enrolled in a rehabilitation program. *J. Clin. Psychol.* 31:572–5, 1975.

43. Frame, M.C., and Osmond, W.M.G. Alcoholism: psychopathic personality and psychopathic reaction type. *Med. Proc. Jhbg.,* 2:257–261, 1956.

44. Hewitt, C.C. A personality study of alcohol addiction. *Q. J. Stud. Alcohol.* 4:368–386, 1943.

45. Rosen, A.C. A comparative study of alcoholic and psychiatric patients with the MMPI. *Q. J. Stud. Alcohol.* 21:253–266, 1960.

46. Haertzen, C.A. Clinical psychological studies, in Martin, W.R., and Isbell, H. (eds.), *Drug Addiction and the U.S. Public Health Service,* Washington, D.C.: U.S. Government Printing Office, 1978, pp. 155–168.

47. Cox, C., and Smart, R.G. Social and psychological aspects of speed use: a study of types of speed users in Toronto. *Int. J. Addict.* 7:201–217, 1972.

48. Penk, W.E., and Robinowitz, R. Personality differences of volunteer and nonvolunteer heroin and nonheroin drug users. *J. Abnorm. Psych.* 85:91–100, 1976.

49. Schoolar, J.C., White, E.H., and Cohen, C.P. Drug abusers and their patient counterparts: a comparison of personality dimensions. *J. Consult. Clin. Psychol.* 39:9–14, 1972.

50. Smart, R.G., and Jones, D. Illicit LSD users: Their personality characteristics and psychopathology. *J. Abnorm. Psych.* 75:286–292, 1970.

51. Hill, H.E. The social deviant and initial addiction to narcotics and alcohol. *Q. J. Stud. Alcohol.* 23:562–582, 1962.

52. Cameron, N., and Margaret, A. *Behavioral Pathology.* Boston: Houghton Mifflin, 1951.

53. Hill, H.E., Haertzen, C.A., Wolbach, A.B., and Miner, E.J. The Addiction Research Center Inventory: Standardization of scales which evaluate subjective effects of morphine, amphetamine, pentobarbital, alcohol, LSD-25, pyrahexyl and chlorpromazine. *Psychopharmacologia,* 4:167–183, 1963.

54. Kolb, L. Drug addiction in its relation to crime. *Ment. Hyg.* 9:74–89, 1925.

55. Pescor, M.J. A statistical analysis of the clinical records of hospitalized drug addicts. *Publ. Health Repts. Suppl.* 143:1–30, 1943.

56. Hill, H.E., Belleville, R.E., and Wikler, A. Motivational determinants in modification of behavior by morphine and pentobarbital. *AMA Arch. Neurol. Psychiat.* 77:28–35, 1957.

57. Martin, W.R., Jasinski, D.R., Haertzen, C.A., Kay, D.C., Jones, B.E., Mansky, P.A., and Carpenter, R.W. Methadone—a reevaluation. *Arch. Gen. Psychiat.* 28:286–295, 1973.

58. Haertzen, C.A., and Hooks, N.T. Changes in personality and subjective experience

associated with the chronic administration and withdrawal of opiates. *J. Nerv. Ment. Dis.* 148:606–614, 1969.

59. Mendelson, J.H., La Dou, J., and Solomon, P. Psychiatric findings, in Mendelson, J.H. (ed.), *Experimentally Induced Chronic Intoxication and Withdrawal in Alcoholics. Quart. J. Stud. Alcohol.* Suppl. 2, 1964, pp. 40–52.

60. Isbell, H., Altschul, S. Kornetsky, C.H., Eisenman, A.J., Flanary, H.G., and Fraser, H.F. Chronic barbiturate intoxication: an experimental study. *Arch. Neurol. Psychiat.* 64:1–28, 1950.

61. Fraser, H.F., Isbell, H., Eisenman, A.J., Wikler, A., and Pescor, F.T. Chronic barbiturate intoxication: further studies. *AMA Arch. Int. Med.* 94:34–41, 1954.

62. Williams, E.G., Himmelsbach, C.K., Wikler, A., Ruble, D.C., and Lloyd, B.J. Studies on marihuana and pyrahexyl compound. *Publ. Health Rep.* 61:1059–1083, 1946.

63. Martin, W.R., and Jasinski, D.R. Physiological parameters of morphine dependence in man — tolerance, early abstinence, protracted abstinence. *J. Psychiat. Res.* 7:9–17, 1969.

64. Martin, W.R., Jasinski, D.R., Sapira, J.D., Flanary, H.G., Kelly, O.A., Thompson, A.K., and Logan, C.R. The respiratory effects of morphine during a cycle of dependence. *J. Pharmacol. Exp. Therap.* 162:182–189, 1968.

65. Kay, D.C. Human sleep and EEG through a cycle of methadone dependence. *Electroenceph. Clin. Neurophysiol.* 38:35–43, 1975.

66. Himmelsbach, C.K. Studies on the relation of drug addiction to the autonomic nervous system: results of cold pressor tests. *J. Pharmacol. Exp. Therap.* 73:91–98, 1941.

67. Eisenman, A.J., Sloan, J. W., Martin, W.R., Jasinski, D.R., and Brooks, J.W. Catecholamine and 17-hydroxycorticosteroid excretion during a cycle of morphine dependence in man. *J. Psychiat. Res.* 7:19–28, 1969.

68. Martin, W.R., Wikler, A., Eades, C.G., and Pescor, F.T. Tolerance to and physical dependence on morphine in rats. *Psychopharmcologia* 4:247–260, 1963.

69. Khazan, N., and Colasanti, B. Protracted rebound in rapid eye movement sleep time and EEG voltage output in morphine-dependent rats upon withdrawal. *J. Pharmacol. Exp. Therap.* 183:23–30, 1972.

70. Gianutsos, G., Hynes, M.D., Puri, S.K., Drawbaugh, R.B., and Lal, H. Effect of apomorphine and nigrostriatal lesions on aggression and striatal dopamine turnover during morphine withdrawal: evidence for dopaminergic supersensitivity in protracted abstinence. *Psychopharmacologia* 34:37–44, 1974.

71. Martin, W.R., Eades, C.G., Thompson, W.O., Thompson, J.A., and Flanary, H.G. Morphine physical dependence in the dog. *J. Pharmacol. Exp. Therap.* 189:759–771, 1974.

72. Martin, W.R., Hewett, B.B., Baker, A.J., and Haertzen, C.A. Aspects of the psychopathology and pathophysiology of addiction. *Drug. Alc. Depend.* 2:185–202, 1977.

73. Martin, W.R., Haertzen, C.A., and Hewett, B.B. Psychopathology and pathophysiology of narcotic addicts, alcoholics, and drug abusers, in Lipton, M.A., DiMascio, A., and Killam, K.F. (eds.), *Psychopharmacology: A Generation of Progress.* New York: Raven Press, 1978, pp. 1591–1602.

74. Haertzen, C.A., Martin, W.R., Ross, F.E., and Neidert, G.L. Psychopathic State Inventory (PSI): Development of a short test for measuring psychopathic states. *Int. J. Addict.* 14(8): 1979 (In Press).

75. Pitts, F.N., and Winokur, G. Affective disorder — VII: Alcoholism and affective disorder. *J. Psychiat. Res.* 4:37–50, 1966.

76. Winokur, G., Cadoret, R., Dorzak, J., and Baker, M. Depressive disease: a genetic study. *Arch. Gen. Psychiat.* 24:135–144, 1971.

77. Winokur, G., Cadoret, R., Baker, M., and Dorzak, J. Depression spectrum disease versus pure depressive disease: some further data. *Brit. J. Psychiat.* 127:75–77, 1975.

78. Winokur, G. The division of depressive illness into depression spectrum disease and pure depressive disease. *Int. Pharmacopsychiat.* 9:5–13, 1974.

79. Woodruff, R.A., Guze, S.B., Clayton, P.J., and Carr, D. Alcoholism and depression. *Arch. Gen. Psychiat.* 28:97–100, 1973.

80. Cadoret, R., and Winokur, G. Depression in alcoholism. *Ann. N.Y. Acad. Sci.* 233:34–39, 1974.

81. Cowan, J.D., Kay, D.C., Neidert, G.L., Ross, F.E., and Belmore, S. Defeated and joyless: potential measures of change in drug abuser characteristics (in preparation).

82. Reid, W.H. The sadness of the psychopath, in Reid, W.H. (ed.), *The Psychopath: A Comprehensive Study of Antisocial Disorders and Behaviors.* New York: Brunner/Mazel, 1978, pp. 7–21.

The views expressed by the author do not necessarily reflect the opinions, official policy or position of the Addiction Research Center, the National Institute on Drug Abuse, the Alcohol, Drug Abuse and Mental Health Administration, or the U.S. Department of Health, Education and Welfare.

CHAPTER 20

Nondrug Detoxification

CHARLES L. WHITFIELD

With nondrug detoxification we now have an extra therapeutic choice: the choice *not* to give CNS depressant chemicals to our alcoholic patients. I believe that in selected patients this choice may have several advantages, which I will discuss below.

Detoxification has come to mean being at hand during alcohol withdrawal to treat or prevent dangerous difficulties, such as hallucinations, seizures and delirium tremens.[1-7] This usually means that a registered nurse and/or physician must be present, which today is expensive.

Alcoholics know that depressant chemicals are effective in treating their withdrawal symptoms. We helpers know this also. Since we knew that alcohol was also a toxic drug, and for other reasons, we looked for and found less toxic substitute depressant drugs such as paraldehyde, barbiturates and for nearly 20 years, the benzodiazepines. These drugs fit in well with the general "better living thru chemistry" trend in medicine, and remained so until the early 1970s.

In 1970, I learned that Simpson in Des Moines had successfully treated the withdrawal in 100 actively-drinking chronic alcoholics without psychoactive drugs.[7,8] On visiting his facilities, I discovered that treatment consisted of:

1. The traditional treatment for delirium, plus
2. One or more "talk downs", using what I call the "3-R's": Reassurance, Reality orientation, and Respect.

I tried this on my own patients, and was pleasantly surprised that it worked.[1] Others and I have found that this therapy works for 95% of all alcoholics undergoing detoxification. These are ambulatory or semi-ambulatory and otherwise uncomplicated chronic alcoholics.

In this paper, I will first describe the recognition and the components of the alcohol withdrawal syndrome. Then I will describe how this nondrug, though medically and "people" oriented approach, can be used in a social setting and in a hospital.

RECOGNITION OF ALCOHOL WITHDRAWAL

The four major manifestations of alcohol withdrawal in alcohol dependent patients are tremor, hallucinosis, seizures ("rum fits") and delirium tremens. These may be found in other conditions, from meningitis to withdrawal from other sedative-hypnotic drugs. The history of a recent bout of heavy or alcoholic drinking lasting at least a week,[3] though nearly always longer, and the absence of other conditions, usually serve to make the diagnosis of alcohol withdrawal.

About half of ambulatory alcoholic patients who stop drinking have *none* of these four major manifestations.[1,2] Although it may be desirable for alcoholics to be observed under expert supervision during the first three days of their withdrawal from alcohol, it is by no means mandatory. Indeed, if an intelligent nonmedical helper (friend, relative, fellow AA member) will stay with the patient for the majority of those first three days, the patient may not need expert supervision. However, if the patient elects to be detoxified at home, it is highly desirable that the nonmedical helper keep in close contact with a physician with expertise in the management of alcohol withdrawal.

Alcoholic Tremulousness

Tremors have been observed to occur in about half of alcoholic patients withdrawing from the drug (Table 1). In their mildest form they appear in the morning, after a night's abstinence. But they may be severe, and usually reach maximum intensity about 24 hours after the last drink. By then the tremor is usually coarse and generalized, though it may fluctuate greatly in severity.[4] This tremulousness, as does the entire withdrawal syndrome, responds well to reassurance by an authority figure.[1]

In addition, anorexia, nausea and sometimes vomiting are present in varying degrees.[4] Generalized weakness may be prominent. Also possible are tinnitus, hyperacusis, itching, muscle cramps, mood disturbance and sleep disturbance.[9] The patient is alert, startles easily, and usually craves alcohol or other drugs to quiet his symptoms.[4]

These tremors are *not* delirium tremens or even "pre-DTs." In my review of the medical literature to date I have never seen a documented reference made to such a condition as "pre-DTs," although from time to time I hear the term used. Also, in observing our 1,024 ambulatory patients undergoing withdrawal, we have not observed such a phenomenon.[1]

Alcoholic Hallucinosis

In our series of 1,024 consecutive, otherwise uncomplicated, ambulatory patients undergoing withdrawal, 39% gave a history of having had hallucinations upon previous withdrawal.[1] With *nondrug* detoxification (described below) only 4% actually had hallucinations. In 266 hospitalized patients observed around 1950, hallucinations were observed in about 13%.[2]

The hallucination is almost never the mythical "pink elephant". Rather, it is usually one of insects, small animals, or voices. In a series of 50 consecutive patients with alcoholic hallucinosis, 58% were purely visual, 16% were purely auditory and 26% were a mixture of visual and auditory.[5]

Alcohol Withdrawal Seizures

Classically called "rum fits," these seizures occurred in 12% of hospitalized patients.[2] By contrast, only 1% of our 1,024 ambulatory patients had a seizure, although 17% of them had given a history of having had such. Three of the 12 patients we observed gave a history of idiopathic epilepsy.[1] When such a seizure occurs it is nearly always a major motor one with loss of consciousness (90%) and usually occurs in a patient with a *history* of alcohol *withdrawal seizures.*[3]

In a study of 241 patients with alcohol withdrawal seizures, nearly all began after age 25.[3] The shortest drinking sprees were 5 and 7 days, but most patients had been drinking much longer. Nearly half (42%) had only one seizure, but most patients had two or more seizures (24% had 2, 14% had 3, 9% had 4, and 3% had status). Nearly all (90%) occurred or began within 48 hours of the last drink.

Patients without classical "rum fits" may have seizures on stopping drinking after as few as 5 or 6 drinks. These patients usually have a history of either idiopathic or post-traumatic epilepsy and usually have abnormal EEGs. Those with classical "rum fits" generally have normal EEGs.

Although nurses and aides should watch the patient carefully after a withdrawal seizure, it is rare for a patient to die from withdrawal seizure alone. If the patient does not recover fairly rapidly after a seizure, he should be checked by a physician.

Delirium Tremens

Delirium tremens is an advanced state of alcohol withdrawal that should be diagnosed by only specific criteria. These two criteria are extreme hyperactivity of:

1. The psychomotor system, and
2. The autonomic nervous system.[2,6]

Hyperactivity of the *psychomotor* system is manifested by extreme agitation and restlessness, usually with hallucinosis and disorientation. Hyperactivity of the *autonomic* nervous system may be manifested by sweating, tachycardia, (greater than 120 to 130/minute), dilated pupils, and low grade fever.[2,6]

Simpson and others have theorized that DTs may in part be an iatrogenic disease.[7,8] Similar to the psychosis which commonly occurs after one type of complete sensory deprivation of normal healthy individuals,[10] alcohol dependent patients on withdrawal may become delirious when their sensory link with reality is severed by various means, such as high dose sedatives, intravenous fluids, restraints and a generally cold, unsympathetic environment.

While there is fragmentary data to show that alcohol withdrawal seizures may be associated with hypomagnesemia, there is no convincing evidence that delirium tremens is associated with hypomagnesemia.[3]

THE PROPERLY-MANAGED DETOXIFICATION CENTER

Contrary to traditional opinion and practice,[13] there is now strong evidence that detoxification is carried out better, cheaper and more rapidly in a properly managed detoxification center than in a general hospital.[1,7,8,14,15,20]

O'Briant,[14] Simpson et al.,[7,8] and Kendis[15] each had a series of over 5,000 admissions for detoxification. Kendis used chlordiazepoxide (Librium) 25 mg qid. and observed only 4 mild cases of DTs. O'Briant in California and Simpson in Des Moines used almost no psychoactive drugs and observed no ambulatory patient with DTs.[8,14] We have used no psychoactive drugs in 1,024 ambulatory patients and have observed only one patient to develop DTs.

This relative absence of DTs is at first puzzling because, as you may recall, the frequently quoted incidence for DTs in chronic alcoholics withdrawn from alcohol in various settings is from 5 to 10%. Also, the death rate from DTs varies from 1% to as high as 35%.[16,17] The death rate from DTs in Kendis, O'Briant, Simpson and our series totaling more than 15,000 patients[1,7,8,14,15] is zero, although the previous statistics suggested that between 15 and 5,000 deaths were expected.[16,17]

Reasons for Low Number of Withdrawal Symptoms

Probable reasons for our having such a low incidence (0.098%) of DTs and a zero death rate[1] are:

1. The patients were ambulatory and, except for their alcoholism and acute withdrawal, were otherwise uncomplicated.
2. Complicated or seriously ill patients, such as those with coma, severe acute abdominal pain, signs of pneumonia, significant trauma or drug overdose were referred to a hospital.
3. Each detoxification center had a specially trained staff to provide a lot of attention and supervision for their patients.[1]

During the observation of our 1,024 ambulatory patients, the detoxification center staff saw an additional 90 (8%) alcoholic patients who were complicated by a problem requiring immediate medical attention and so were not admitted to the detoxification center initially. These were triaged to the hospital emergency department. Their problems were most often overdose with other drugs, moderate to severe dyspnea, narcotic dependence, acute abdomen, alcohol-Antabuse reaction, and psychosis. The patients requiring emergency department referral after admission to the detoxification center had various problems: complicated seizures, severe hypertension, suicide gesture, and rarely, severe hallucinosis and paranoia.

There is no doubt that with one or more serious medical complications present in a hospitalized alcoholic undergoing withdrawal that the incidence of DTs will be higher (Table 1). One of the major reasons for this

TABLE 1.–Withdrawal Manifestations Observed in 1,024 Otherwise
Uncomplicated Ambulatory Patients (1976)[1] as Compared with 266
Hospitalized Patients (1950)[2]

| | Ambulatory | | Hospitalized |
	% by History	% with Non-drug Detox Management	Patients (%)
Tremors	—	37.0	47.0
Hallucinosis	39	4.0	13.0
Seizures	17	1.0	12.0
Delirium Tremens	27	0.1	5.3

higher incidence in such complicated patients may well be the *sensory
deprivation* to which we physicians and nurses often subject such
patients.[7,10]

Methods to Achieve Lower Number of Withdrawal Symptoms

But how does one achieve this low DT and death rate in ambulatory
patients? Basically, one can accomplish such and achieve quicker recovery
by:

1. Providing a non-threatening, positive environment.
2. Using reality orientation, i.e. doing all possible environmentally,
   verbally and physically to restore the patient's link with reality.
3. Avoiding the use of all psychoactive drugs, especially sedatives
   and "tranquilizers".
4. Keeping the patient ambulatory and eating a regular diet as far as
   possible.
5. Encouraging the patient to perform purposeful activity, such as
   small or even token duties, and most importantly to participate in
   lecture/discussion and group therapy discussions, which are held
   1 or 2 times daily.

In our series of 1,024 patients, the detoxification center staff had 2
patients admitted in florid, classical DTs from the jail. In both of these
patients, using these above techniques, the symptoms and signs of DTs
disappeared gradually over about 30 minutes.[1]

As a common example: a disoriented appearing and tremulous patient
walks up to the nursing station, the staff office, or to a staff member. He
may ask for help in a specific way, such as, "I want some Librium", or ask
in a nonspecific way, or may ask only nonverbally. You, the staff member,
observe that he is in distress, and begin to "tune in" to that distress by

observation and empathy. You might then tell the patient your interpretation of the distress. Take him off to the side, or sit right there with him and take his pulse (touching, sensory input, physical reassurance) or touch his shoulder. Ask his orientation to person, place, time, and personal condition (more sensory input). Then provide the "Three Rs" — reassurance, reality orientation and respect. If he is hallucinating, talk about it to him. Have him walk (all senses, including proprioception) with you into another room. If he is improving, have him "help you" with purposeful activity, such as emptying ashtrays or trashcans in the room. Tell him why he is there and that you know he is feeling bad, and that he is going to get better soon. With your positive and benign persistence, the person will nearly always improve, manifested by a lessening of his tremulousness, a slowing of his pulse and a clearing of his sensorium. Had you just given a depressant drug, you might have attributed his improvement to the drug.

Simpson and coworkers, O'Briant and I almost never give psychoactive drugs. Indeed, the only medications we give routinely are vitamins. For patients with a history of withdrawal seizures, phenytoin (diphenylhydantoin) has been recommended. Only one controlled study has been done using Dilantin in alcohol withdrawal. It showed that 100 mg by mouth three times daily decreased the seizures significantly ($p < .005$) in patients with a *history* of seizures.[18] Other controlled studies may be necessary to substantiate these results.

Also, we *avoid hospitalization unless there is a clear indication.* I believe from the results of these studies and from my own experience treating alcoholics that there are only three indications for hospitalization of alcoholics:

1. Any condition that would require hospitalization in any patient, such as uncontrolled bleeding or coma,
2. A severe Antabuse-alcohol reaction.
3. Alcoholism that is refractory to outpatient treatment.

In my opinion, uncomplicated alcohol withdrawal is not usually an indication for hospitalization. Rather, *these patients should be admitted to a properly-managed detoxification center,* such as described above, if available. The term "properly-managed" is of extreme importance: the detoxification center staff must be properly trained and supervised, and they must be sympathetic toward and sincerely interested in helping alcoholics.[1,14,18]

Further Efficacy of Avoiding Psychoactive Drugs

In addition to the results from the above 3 series of over 15,000 detoxified ambulatory patients, the possible efficacy of avoiding psychoactive drugs has also been shown in a study of 400 VA Hospital patients undergoing symptoms of alcohol withdrawal, although the authors did not write about this point of view.[19] Patients were treated in a double-blind fashion with chlordiazepoxide (Librium), chlorpromazine (Thorazine), hydroxyline (Vistaril), thiamine, or placebo. Overall, placebo or thiamine, or both, were equal or superior to the other treatments, especially in the areas of greater self-care capability and social competence. However, DT's or seizures occurred in only 2% of the chlordiazepoxide-treated patients, in contrast to 10% in the other groups.[19] Dilantin was not given in this study.

PROCEDURE FOR NONDRUG PATIENT DETOXIFICATION

Based on the above data,[1,7,8,9,12] I would formulate the following procedure or standing orders for the detoxification of the ambulatory, otherwise uncomplicated patient undergoing alcohol withdrawal (Table 2).

TABLE 2.–Suggested Procedure for Nondrug Detoxification

1. Diet and fluids as desired (regular diet)
2. No restraints
3. Vital signs (temperature, BP, pulse) every 4 hours
4. History and physical examination by a physician or designee within 24 hours of admission to the center
5. Thiamine 100 mg, folate (as Leucovorin) 1 mg IM by RN on admission, then same amount by mouth daily thereafter
6. Multiple vitamin by mouth daily
7. Tylenol, antacid as needed
8. No psychoactive drugs
9. Provide a nonthreatening, positive environment
10. Keep patient active, as tolerated
11. Reality orientation, reassurance and respect in abundance
12. Call physician or take patient to emergency department as indicated

Medications prescribed by personal physicians should not be continued during time in the center unless they are clearly indicated for a condition that is ongoing. Thus antibiotics, antituberculosis drugs, antidiabetic and heart medications should usually be continued. Antihypertensive drugs and any or all psychoactive drugs should be discontinued while in the center.[1,20] Individual counseling should be available for at least 2 hours a week from skilled counselors or social workers. AA, daily group therapy, and other treatment aids should be readily available.

In such a center, using physician and emergency department back-up, patient deaths appear to be unusual (Table 3), curable medical illness

TABLE 3.–Data on 2 Series of Alcoholic Patients Detoxified in a Properly-Managed Center[1,20]

	6,000 Patients[20]	1,024 Patients[1]
Deaths	1	0
Referrals to hospital	2–5%	8%
a) Retained by hospital:	85%	3%
b) Returned to Center:	15%	5%
New active patients with TB found	50 pts.	0
Subdural hematoma found	11 pts.	0
Wernicke's encephalopathy	decreased by factor of 5	0
Number of arrests for drunkenness	markedly decreased	unknown
Emergency department visits	decreased in both series	
Rehabilitation of alcoholic patients	increased in both	

detectable, and use of community facilities more efficient. Most important of all, a larger number of alcoholic patients are started into recovery and rehabilitation.[1,20]

THE HOSPITALIZED ALCOHOLIC

If a trained staff is not available to provide the abundant reassurance, reality orientation and respect needed during the first 3 days of alcohol withdrawal, or if medical complications minimize such attention, then a sedative-hypnotic drug might need to be given to the patient to help both patient and staff through the stress of withdrawal. Also requiring a sedative drug may be the "hidden" alcoholic who develops symptoms or signs of withdrawal. In such situations, chlordiazepoxide (Librium) or hydroxyzine (Vistaril) may be of help. Although other sedatives are effective, they are often potentially dangerous and/or undesirable. For example, barbiturates, diazepam (Valium) and paraldehyde are nearly as dependence-producing as alcohol. Paraldehyde may cause acidosis and, given IM, sterile abscesses. Phenothiazines decrease the seizure threshold.[19] However, the *specific depressant drug given for withdrawal is probably less important than the supportive care given by the staff, including effective treatment of serious medical consequences of alcoholism.*

As much as is possible, the patient should have an effort made to help maintain his link with reality.[1,7,9] The same techniques described above for ambulatory patients and elsewhere for delirium apply here. These would especially include:

1. Stopping the use of all restraints, IVs, and other tubes.

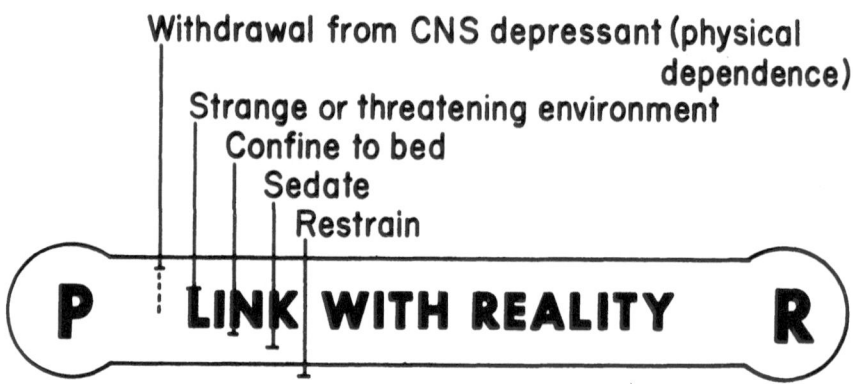

Figure 1.   Cutting the Patient's Link with Reality: A Possible Factor in the Cause of DTs
(P=Patient/R=Reality)

2. Keeping a light on in the room.
3. Keeping a radio or T.V. on.
4. Having a relative or friend sit with the patient, especially to reassure and provide reality orientation.
5. Having the patient out of bed and as active as possible, even if only sitting up in a chair or able to look out the window.

Heavy doses of sedatives and tranquilizers are probably contraindicated. This is because, as with restraints, IVs and other tubes, dark rooms, etc., they tend to cut off the patient's already precarious last touches with reality[1,7,9] (Figure 1).

Soloman[10] stresses the important aspects of sensory deprivation in medical patients, "Patients with so-called cardiac psychosis may be suffering from the effects of sensory deprivation. Elderly decompensated patients may be found wandering in the corridors of the hospital at night, when the wards have become quiet. Too much rest, silence, solitude, and darkness loosen the patients' hold on reality and make them prey to fantasy." Black patch psychosis which occurs post operatively in patients following cataract or other eye operations is often characterized by a frenzied confusion and disorientation. Bandaging only one eye or allowing a central peep hole is usually corrective or preventive. Regarding orthopedic patients, "Patients in total body casts or immobilized by head tongs or other severely restricting apparatus may develop disturbing psychotic behavior. The provision of frequent visitors, radio, and television is effective in relief." Soloman also emphasized that "the element of sensory deprivation is surely important in delirium tremens, where the best sedative is a sympathetic, attentive nurse."[10]

In short, one should do everything possible to supply clues and to maintain a receptive sensorium that will *increase the patient's link with reality*.

DURATION OF DETOXIFICATION

Depending on the severity and duration of the patient's alcoholism, and the type of treatment, detoxification usually takes from 2 to 5 days. Most patients are doing fairly well by the end of the second day and can be considered to be completed with the *acute* phase of detoxification.

Using 3 different methods of detoxification, the following durations of the alcohol withdrawal syndrome are commonly seen: non-drug = 2 days, using ethyl alcohol = 3.1 days, using benzodiazepines, low dose = 2 to 3 days, high dose = 3 to 5 days.[1,8,12,40,41]

Perhaps not formerly recognized, there appears to be a *chronic* phase of "detoxification" or recovery in which the body, and especially the central nervous system, slowly repairs itself. Based on my own and others' clinical experience, this chronic recovery phase seems to last a matter of *months*. Most of my own patients who have maintained sobriety for a year or more say that it took them from 6 to 12 months or more of abstinence to feel like their minds were functioning normally again. There is some correlative evidence for these statements, as sleep disturbance and EEG changes may persist for several months after stopping alcohol. Mood swings and emotional lability are common. Although thinking is superficially intact, judgment and memory are often unreliable. Thus, patients should be given special attention, support and monitoring for these first few months after stopping drinking.[22,39]

Decision Making in Nondrug versus Drug Detoxification

I have summarized possible decision-making in the management of the alcoholic patient undergoing withdrawal (Figure 2).

Propranolol for Withdrawal

Propranolol has been used experimentally as a treatment aid in alcohol withdrawal. However, most of the reports of such experiments have been

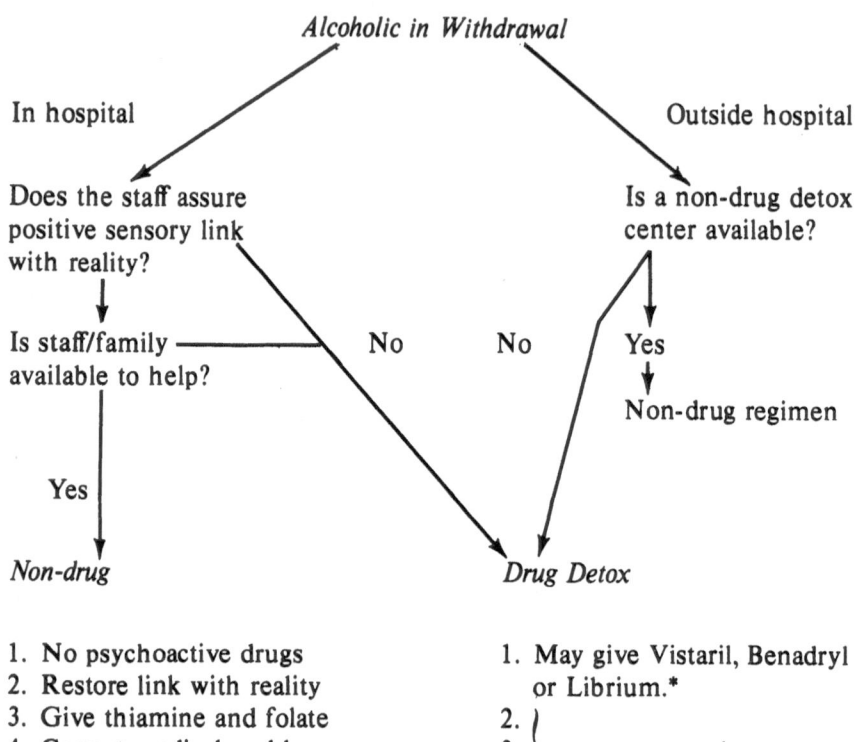

Figure 2.   Decision Tree in Alcohol Withdrawal Management.

anecedotal, uncontrolled or have used too small a patient population.[21] We know that it can worsen heart failure and asthma and is a known cardiac depressant. Becker et al.[22] write, "It should also be evident that a patient on propranolol will have a persistently slow pulse. Thus, although the slow pulse would be a good therapeutic end point to monitor compliance, the blockade of the normal adrenergic responses makes the patient vulnerable to emergencies such as gastrointestinal hemorrhage." Finally, propranolol has been tried in mice and men to decrease the CNS effects of alcohol withdrawal. It was claimed to work in mice,[23] but not in men.[24] In a double-blind controlled study, propranolol was found not to be effective in reducing anxiety among alcoholics just after detoxification, and it had no effect on sobriety maintenance or in increasing continuance in clinical therapy.[25]

Thus, until controlled trials provide positive hard data on the use of this drug in alcohol withdrawal, I believe that it should not be used for this purpose.

THE USE OF OTHER DRUGS BY ALCOHOLICS: THEIR IMPORTANCE IN WITHDRAWAL

The cross addiction and cross tolerance between alcohol and other sedative-hypnotics is well known. Alcoholics appear to be quite susceptible to becoming dependent upon other sedative-hypnotic drugs. Likewise, patients dependent upon other sedative drugs are susceptible to alcoholism. For example, heroin dependent patients are often also alcoholic, whether their treatment be with or without methadone. It is likely that such mixed drug dependencies occur in many of our own patients, often without our knowledge.

Although hard data is not available as to just how many patients are dependent upon more than one drug at one time or another, informal reports from detoxification centers throughout the country indicated that alcoholics have "misused" other sedatives in from 40 to 70% of admissions.[26,27] Often this misuse of other sedatives has been iatrogenically induced. I use the word "misuse" because I have no hard data as to how

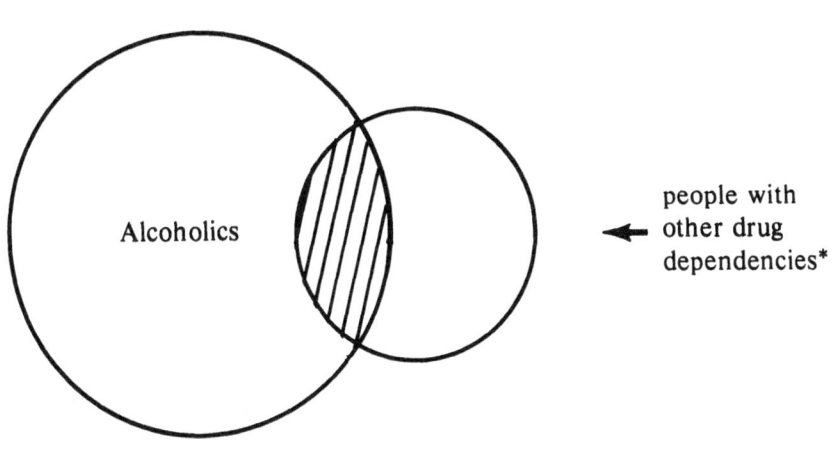

*excluding tobacco and coffee

Figure 3.   Venn Diagram Showing a Rough Estimation of People Dependent upon Alcohol and/or Other Sedative-Hypnotic Drugs

many patients are actually dependent upon both alcohol and another mind-altering drug. I would offer a rough guess of between 10–40% of alcoholics as being dependent upon another psychoactive drug (excluding coffee and/or cigarettes). A Venn diagram showing a rough estimation of these mixed problems is shown in Figure 3.

Although people may be primarily dependent upon other sedatives or mind-altering drugs, they are often at one time or another involved with alcohol in more than the usual social context. One obvious reason for this is that alcohol is readily available. Indeed, many of these people begin their drug use on alcohol and "graduate" to the other drug. Thus, this concept may be of importance in the detoxification of any of these patients.

Clues to Mixed Drug Dependence

Clues to mixed-drug dependencies can come from:

1. The history—from both the patient and his relatives;
2. The physical examination;
3. Blood or urine levels of the suspected depressant or other drug, ordered as indicated near the time of admission and
4. An abstinence syndrome lasting longer than five days, which suggests benzodiazepine dependence, due to these drugs' long half life.[42,43]

These patients may be treated as described above for their alcoholism and as described elsewhere for their other drug problem.

PROGNOSIS AND FOLLOW-UP

Results of a comprehensive, multiple-therapy program, with the detoxification and rehabilitation center as an initiating and partially sustaining factor, and with one or more of the other therapies—counseling, AA, medical, ± Antabuse, and family and job counseling—have produced from 40–90% success in reaching longer periods of abstinence.

Many physicians and even some counselors of alcoholics forget to *follow up* their patients' detoxification with a compulsive multiple-therapy program, often including *monitoring.* Such may be an *important factor in the often high failure rate* at helping a person with alcoholism. The physician and counselor can easily keep a check list as to whether the patient is receiving help from each of: AA, group or individual counseling, medical ± Antabuse, a job, and family counseling. One can do an excellent job with detoxification and with managing the medical complications. But if abstinence and recovery are not given attention and followed as carefully as we do, for example with our diabetic and hypertensive patients, then we are less likely to reach success.[44]

REFERENCES

1. Whitfield, C.L. et al. Detoxification of 1,024 alcoholics without psychoactive drugs. *J. Am. Med. Assoc.* 239:14, 1409–1410.
2. Victor, M., and Adams, R.D. The effects of alcohol on the nervous system. *Proc. Assoc. Res. Nerv. and Ment. Dis.* 32:525–573, 1953.
3. Victor, M., and Brausch, C. The role of abstinence in the genesis of alcoholic epilepsy. *Epilepsia* 8:1–20, 1967.
4. Victor, M. Treatment of alcoholic intoxication and the withdrawal syndrome. *Psychosomatic Med.* 25:636–650, 1966.
5. Victor, M., and Hope, J.M. The phenomenon of auditory hallucinations in chronic alcoholism. *J. Nerv. and Ment. Dis.* 126:451–481, 1958.
6. Adams, R.D., and Victor, M. Alcohol and alcoholism, in *Principles of Neurology,* Chap. 37. New York: McGraw Hill, 1977.
7. Simpson, R.K., et al. *Delirium tremens, JAOA* 68:123, 1968.
8. Simpson, R.K. Data on over 5,000 admissions for detoxification. Harrison Treatment and Rehabilitation Center, Des Moines, 1972.
9. Edwards, G., and Gross, M. Alcohol dependence: provisional description of a clinical syndrome. *Brit. Med. J.* 1:1058–1061, 1976.
10. Soloman, P. Sensory deprivation, in Freedman, A.M., and Kaplan, A.I. (eds.), *Comprehensive Textbook of Psychiatry.* Baltimore: Williams and Wilkins, 1976.
11. O'Briant, R.G. Social setting detox. *Alcohol Health & Res. World,* Winter 1974–75, pp. 12–18.
12. Gross, M.M., et al. Quantitative changes of signs and symptoms associated with acute alcohol withdrawal incidence, severity and circadian effects in experimental studies of alcoholics, in Gross, M.M. (ed.) *Alcohol Intoxication and Withdrawal,* New York: Plenum Press, 1975.
13. *Manual on Alcoholism.* Chicago, American Medical Association, 1967.
14. O'Briant, R.G. A new look in non-medical care for the public inebriate. *Proc. 4th Annual Alcoholism Conf. NIAAA,* DHEW Pub. No. (ADM) 76-284, pp. 236–246, 2975.
15. Kendis, J.B., referred to in LEAA project report: The St. Louis Detoxification and Diagnostic Evaluation Center. Washington, D.C. US Government Printing Office.
16. Thomas, D.W. Treatment of the alcohol withdrawal syndrome. *J. Am. Med. Assoc.* 188:316, 1964.
17. Tavel, M.E., et al. A critical analysis of mortality associated with delirium tremens. *Am. J. Med. Sci.* 242:58–69, 1961.
18. Sampliner, R., and Iber, F. Diphenylhydantoin control of alcohol withdrawal seizures. *J. Am. Med. Assoc.* 230:1430–1432, 1974.
19. Klett, C.J., et al. Evaluating changes in symptoms during acute alcohol withdrawal. *Arch. Gen. Psychiat.* 24:174–178, 1971.

20. Iber, F.L. Draft of a description of a model for community detoxification of alcoholics utilizing hospital and physician back-up. Presented at 5th Annual Meeting of the American Medical Society on Alcoholism, San Francisco, December 11, 1974.
21. Carlsson, C., and Johansson, T. The psychological effects of propranolol in the abstinence phase of chronic alcoholics. *Brit. J. Psych.*, 119:605–606, 1971.
22. Becker, C.E., et al. *Alcohol as a Drug.* New York: Medcom Press, 1974.
23. Smith, A., et al. Inhibition by propranolol of ethanol-induced narcosis. *J. Pharm. Pharmac.* 22:644–645, 1970.
24. Mendelson, J.H., et al. Propranolol and behavior of alcohol addicts after acute alcohol ingestion. *Clin. Pharm. Therap.* 15:571–578, 1974.
25. Davis, J.E., et al. A study of the anti-anxiety effects of propranolol in alcoholics during three months following detoxification. *Johns Hopkins Med. J.* (In Press).
26. Bissell, L. The treatment of alcoholism: what do we do about long term sedatives? *Ann. N.Y. Acad. Sci.* 252:396–399, 1975.
27. Williams, K. Discussion about other drugs in alcoholics. (Unpublished), Pittsburgh, 1975.
28. Martin, Drills *Pharmacology in Medicine* New York: McGraw Hill, 1971.
29. Ewing, J.A., and Blakewell, W.E., Jr. Diagnosis and management of depressant drug dependence. *Am. J. Psych.* 123:909, 1967.
30. Wikler, A. Diagnosis and treatment of drug dependence of the barbiturate type. *Am. J. Psych.* 125:6, 1968.
31. Smith, D.E., and Wesson, D.R. Phenobarbital technique for treatment of barbiturate dependence. *Arch. Gen. Psych.* 24:56, 1971.
32. Wesson, D.R., and Smith, D.E. A conceptual approach to detoxification. *J. Psych. Drugs.* 6:161–168, 1974.
33. Sapira, R.K., and McDonald, R.H. Drug Abuse 1970. Disease-a-month, November 1970.
34. Wikler, A. Opioid addiction, in Freedman, A.M., and Kaplan, H.I. (eds), *Comprehensive Textbook of Psychiatry.* Baltimore: Williams and Wilkins, 1967, pp. 89–1003.
35. Weil, A.T. *The Natural Mind.* Boston: Houghton Mifflin, 1972.
36. Frosch, W.A. Narcotic addiction. *Current Therapy* Philadelphia: W.B. Saunders, 1973, pp. 828–830.
37. Scher, J., et al. Massive vitamin C as an adjunct in methadone maintenance and detoxification. Paper presented at N. Am. Cong. Alc. & Drug Prob., San Francisco, 1974.
38. Pawlak, V. Megavitamin therapy and the drug wipeout syndrome, an introduction to the orthomolecular approach as a treatment for after-effects of drug use/abuse. Phoenix: Do It Now Foundation, 1972.
39. Bissell, L., and Mooney, A.J. The special problem of the alcoholic physician. *Medical Times.* June 1975.
40. Cohen, S. Alcohol withdrawal syndromes. *Drug Abuse and Alcoholism Newsletter,* Vista Hill Foundation, Vol. 5, No. 5, June 1976.
41. Sellers, E.M., and Kalant, H. Alcohol intoxication & withdrawal. *N. Eng. J. Med.* 294:757, 1976.
42. Smith, D.E. Valium and low dose withdrawal syndrome. *U.S. J. Drug and Alc. Depend.* 3(1):7, 1979.
43. Meletzky, B.M., and Klotter, J. Addiction to diazepam. *Int. J. Addict.* 11(1): 95–115, 1976.
44. Whitfield, C.L. Detoxification of alcoholics (letter response) *JAMA* (in press for May 1979).

Index

antidotes, 14
antihypertensive drugs, 312
antisocial adults, 273
antisocial behavior, 105, 135, 273, 277, 285
antisocial personality, 272
antisocial symptoms, 276
ANT scale, 274, 275, 277
antituberculosis drugs, 312
anxiety, 23, 26, 67, 87, 101, 106, 122, 131,
    135, 152, 153, 224, 225, 234, 237, 260,
    283, 316
anxiety neurosis, 276
apathy, 74
apomorphine, 207
arousal, 81
ascites, 74
ascorbic acid, 231
"As-If Personality", 99, 105
astringent effect, 27
ataxia, 73, 74, 75
atrophy, 70
auscultation, 231
autonomic nervous system, 308
aversive-conditioning, 88, 176, 199
avoidance, 154, 160, 161, 222, 284, 285
axon, 73
axon membrane, 77
"axonal reaction", 73

bacteria, 22
badness, 97, 107, 223
barbiturates, 128, 134, 281, 282, 283, 305,
    313
Beck Inventory, 212
behavior, 9, 12, 13, 45, 47, 49, 53, 57, 63, 67,
    81, 84, 87, 88, 105, 115, 121, 122, 123,
    131, 160, 163, 183, 187, 188, 219, 224,
    226, 247, 249, 251, 270, 271, 272, 273,
    277, 279
Behavior Rating Scale, 152
behavioral marital therapy, 121
beneficient/maleficent consequences, 153
benzodiazepines, 30, 175, 207, 208, 211, 305,
    315
Beri-Beri Heart Disease, 175
binge-drinking patterns, 252
binges, 183, 252
bipolar affective disorder, 208, 209, 211, 212,
    213, 214
blackout, 26, 47, 50, 51, 57, 60, 61, 63, 64, 65,
    66, 131, 183

blood alcohol levels, 11, 15, 24, 38, 41, 42, 66,
    130, 147, 169, 210, 262
blood aldehyde levels, 230
blood pressure, 28, 29, 169, 176, 230, 231,
    234, 235, 236, 237
blood sugar level, 270
blurring of vision, 72
borderline personality, 94-100, 102, 104-108
"borderline schizophrenia", 95
Bowen's Family Systems Therapy, 121
brain, 13, 23, 25, 26, 77, 147, 235, 248, 260
brain stem, 235
brain tumors, 25
burning dysaesthesias, 72

caffeine, 23, 81
Cage questionnaire, 38
calcium, 143
California Psychological Inventory (CPI),
    274
carbohydrates, 147
carbon dioxide, 21, 22
cardiac depressant, 316
cardiac failure, 28
cardiac functioning, 169, 175
cardiovascular system, 147, 169, 236
cataract, 314
catecholamine metabolism, 236
catecholamines, 210, 230
cell growth, 147
cell membrane, 71, 147
cellular disruption, 70
central and peripheral nervous system, 77
central nervous system, 9, 77, 140, 147, 148,
    168, 169, 243, 244, 315
centrocecal scotomas, 72
cerebellar cortex, 73
cerebellar degeneration, 23, 73
cerebellar dysfunction, 73
cerebellar function, 77
cerebellum, 73, 76
cerebral cortex, 261
cerebrospinal fluid (CSF), 230
character disorders, 105
character pathology, 98, 205, 218
child-mother relationship, 103
child neglect, 113, 120
children, 9, 80, 112, 113, 114, 115, 117, 119,
    120, 123
chlordiazepoxide, 175, 309, 312, 313
chlorpromazine, 280